Digital Removable Partial Denture Technology

Haiyang Yu

Digital Removable Partial Denture Technology

From Design Analysis to Practical Skills

PMPH PEOPLE'S MEDICAL PUBLISHING HOUSE

Springer

Haiyang Yu
Department of Prosthodontics
West China Hospital of Stomatology
Chengdu
China

ISBN 978-981-19-7922-4 ISBN 978-981-19-7923-1 (eBook)
https://doi.org/10.1007/978-981-19-7923-1

This Springer imprint is published by the registered company Springer Nature Singapore Pte Ltd.
The registered company address is: 152 Beach Road, #21-01/04 Gateway East, Singapore 189721, Singapore

Introduction

Dentures have been used to restore the beauty and function of missing teeth as early as 2500 BC. From ancient times to the present, the materials for replacing missing teeth have continued to evolve, from wood, bone, animal teeth, dead human teeth to metals, ceramics, and high-performance polymers. Each alternative material may correspond to a type of repair method, from simple simulation replacement to the pursuit of simulation bionics, and its technical connotation is often synchronized with the highest technological level of its contemporaries. Among various forms, the modern Removable Partial Denture (RPD) was once an advanced form of denture restoration. However, in the past 50 years, with the rapid development of fixed restoration and implant restoration, as well as the increasing demand for functional recovery of edentulous patients, RPD seems to be a little powerless, and professional and social attention is also declining. Whether RPD is still promising is the subject of this book.

It is not very early for RPD in the modern form to appear. In 1930 and 1937, cobalt-chromium alloys and dental acrylic resins were successively introduced into the dental field, and the modern standardized RPD appeared for the first time in dental clinics. Compared with earlier methods of restoration, the RPD at that time was extremely advanced. With decades of development, especially the empowerment of digital technology in the past decade, RPD has regained its youth. However, its overall market share has been declining.

In fact, RPD is minimally invasive and reversible, and the price is relatively low, especially when there are many missing teeth, it is the preferred repair method for patients who are sensitive to disease burden and iatrogenic damage. This is the reason why it is ordinary but lasting. How to retain its inherent advantages and reduce its disadvantages is precisely the core of this book.

However, the "removable" feature, which is favored by some patients and doctors, limits the functional reconstruction and recovery effect of RPD to a certain extent and also determines the complexity and diversity of RPD structural design. Removable and wearable increases the requirement for patients' daily cleaning and also reduces the chewing function and comfort of dentures. Also, in order to ensure sufficient retention, stability, and support under the premise of repairing defects, the iterative RPD often needs to be composed of elastic clasps, rigid framework, tooth-colored artificial teeth and gingiva-colored denture bases. Therefore, at present, patients have mainly two dissatisfaction and problems after long-term use of RPD. One problem is the lack of esthetics caused by the exposure of metal clasps. The other problem is the inadequate accuracy of framework resulting in the ill fit and poor retention of the framework. Therefore, after breaking through these two problems, the RPD can have better functional recovery and comfort, and of course, there will be more indications and a better wearing experience.

Therefore, the first chapter of this book "How to Improve the Esthetics of Removable Partial Dentures" and the second chapter "Classification and Design of Esthetic Clasp" focus on the first problem. These two problems have been driving the continuous exploration of repair materials and processing techniques by professionals. Materials and techniques complement each other and interact. The development of materials drives the progress of manufacturing techniques, and at the same time, the maturity of technology also introduces new materials. In addition, the introduction of new materials and new techniques also corresponds to the upgrading and changes of RPD design. Different denture upgrade designs have also improved the function of dentures and have continuously produced better RPD repair effects.

In Chap. 1, "How to Improve the Esthetics of Removable Partial Dentures," the authors reviewed the first esthetic problem with exposed metal clasps. As early as 1981, McCartney proposed a new design of the MGR clasp to improve the esthetics of metal clasp. Subsequently, a variety of clasp concealment designs such as lingual retention clasp, Twin-Flex clasp, and improved balance clasp were also proposed successively. In 1990, Budkiewicz proposed the design concept of minimizing the retentive arm of the clasp, which is also the source of the design of the short buccally retained clasp, the C clasp, the short-arm embrasure clasp, and other clasps shared in Chap. 2 of the book. On the other hand, scholars have also tried to replace metal clasps with thermoplastic resin materials with better esthetics. Early thermoplastic resin materials are mainly acetal resin and polyamide and other materials. These materials simulate the color of the gingiva well but are significantly less strong enough to be used as final dentures. Polyaryletherketone (PAEK) family has good biosafety and stable physical and chemical properties. With its development and wide application in the medical field, it has also been introduced into the field of oral restoration, such as its family representative materials Polyetheretherketone (PEEK), Polyetherketoneketone (PEKK) et al. On the basis of ensuring the normal performance of the RPD function, the above methods of improving the overall esthetic performance of the RPD by adopting a new clasp design or an esthetic repair material are collectively referred to as esthetic clasp technology. At the beginning of 2021, the Chinese Stomatological Association released the *Esthetic Clasp Technology* written by the author, indicating that this set of ideas and methods has been recognized and supported by Chinese counterparts.

The correct clinical pathway is also very important. This part of the content is described in detail in Chap. 3 of this book, "Clinical Pathway of Digital Removable Partial Denture Technology," Chap. 6, "Case Analysis of Digital Removable Partial Denture Technology", will show the diagnosis and treatment process and the repair and reconstruction effect through 33 typical cases.

Digital technologies effectively solve the second difficulty. In the traditional RPD manufacturing process, the steps of the cast analysis, undercut block out, refractory cast reproduction, wax-up making, and embedding casting are complicated and technically dependent, and errors are easily accumulated layer by layer. The CNC milling technology of fixed repair is difficult to realize the processing of the complex structure of RPD. Therefore, the continuous maturity and development of three-dimensional printing technology have promoted the development process of digital RPD restoration. In 2004, the method of indirect 3D printing resin wax combined with the casting method to make metal frameworks appeared. In 2006, selective laser melting (SLM) technology enabled direct 3D printing of metal frameworks. Optical scanning technology and CAD/CAM technology transform manual operation into standardized device operation, reduce human error and labor cost, shorten operation time, and at the same time, data can be stored, and the restoration has better repeatability and accuracy. The research and development of RPD expert systems such as RD-designer aim to provide standardized, diversified, and personalized framework design solutions to solve the difficult, messy, and complicated problems of RPD design. That using the convenience and flexibility of digital technology to improve the design and esthetics of dentures, and to solve difficult problems that cannot be solved by traditional technology, is so-called digital removable partial denture technology. In this book, Chap. 4 "Virtual Design and Numerical Control Manufacture of Digital Removable Partial Denture Technology" and Chap. 5 "Special Designs and Production Skills of Digital Removable Partial Denture Technology" expound the new capabilities and breakthroughs of digital technology in RPD manufacturing. In Chap. 6, "Case Analysis of Digital Removable Partial Denture Technology," from routine cases, complex cases to rare cases, with 32 cases in a step-by-step manner, a variety of RPD digital new manufacturing and new solutions are shown. Solving professional problems by combining various latest technologies empowered by the technology of the times is the only way for the development of the discipline, and it is also the driving force for the rejuvenation of RPD. This feature also supports the author's proposition that integrated restoration is the realistic development path of prosthodontics.

The chapter arrangement of this book aims to explain the current application of various digital technologies in RPD repair methods from the simple to the deep, from the part to the whole, from clinical design, processing, and manufacturing to case analysis. By adopting innovative clasps design and the application of digital new materials, the digital RPD technology displayed will help to show the new connotation of integrated prosthetics in the future.

Then, in view of the current situation that clinician-patient-technician communication and cooperation are often neglected during RPD restoration, the author also conducts detailed patient discussions in Chap. 7 "Communication and Cooperation Between Clinicians and Technicians in Digital Removable Partial Denture Technology." I hope readers can do the daily work that should be done well.

Lastly is the Conclusion. Different from traditional cognition, the author proposes that the advantages of RPD are minimally invasive, reversible, and affordable, while the disadvantages are low functional recovery, insufficient esthetics and comfort. It is emphasized that the popular implantation, esthetic restoration, and high-tech restoration techniques such as templates are inseparable from the clinical design principles and principles contained in the classical restoration methods such as traditional RPD and complete dentures, as well as the accumulation of long-term clinical practical experience, which is the basic skill that should not be overlooked. From the perspective of integrated restoration, it further emphasizes the academic value of classic RPD and digital RPD, and the thinking and suggestions that the inheritance quality of traditional restoration technology urgently needs to be improved.

The main content arrangement of this book is introduced here, please turn to the next page and start a discussion and exchange with the author.

Preface

Successful prosthetic is to let us challenge with "Nature."

Even though there are a variety of classic prosthetics for us to select, we have not overcome "Nature" overall. The final result always gives priority to short-term satisfaction and mid-long-term replacement. There are both advantages and disadvantages in each classic prosthetic technology. There's no best way but the difference of the needs of patients, profession of prosthodontist, and medical market operation, which is one of the bases that I proposed comprehensive prosthetic is one of the leading directions in the future.

The removable denture, which has been snubbed for years and might continue to be left out in the future, is actually a good option as noninvasive and reversible.

Removable prosthetic is mainly for "disabled people." This kind of patients choose removable prosthetic for four reasons. First, these patients in general have a large number of legacies like periodontal and dentin problem that have not been solved. There's no perfect case as porcelain prosthetic from the clinical intraoral photos. Only if the function can be impaired, the denture will be accepted. That means the requests of patients are not high. Second, the scheme is minimally invasive and reversible. There's room for compromise for both doctor and patient. Third, the daily maintenance is easy. Fourth, removable denture is the cheapest. But the disadvantage is more obvious: uncomfortable and unesthetic.

It is difficult to increase comfort level. Denture can only be thinner and smaller, but it is impossible to remove the saddle and big connector unless choosing other prosthetic method. The exposure of clasp is the main reason to cause unesthetic. Is there invisible "esthetic" clasp that can improve efficiency without an increase in cost?

The answer is yes. This is the original intention and goal of the book.

Since 2005, Fang Xiaoqin, Huang Wenjing, and Wang Man had been doing research about the concept, retention principle, classification, and clinical application of esthetic clasp. We have obtained two patents in this field. I also have many lectures in China. There's an episode: Before I present this topic on a meeting in 2009, a senior asked me after seeing the topic "Why do you speak on this topic?" The implication is it is too simple. Actually, I agree with him. But we have to admit that prosthodontist in China really needs it.

In the removable prosthetics dental technology published this year, I wrote an article called "the fault by simplify," listing the simplified and despised history of dental technology in China. I have discussed the influence on the design and clinical application of removable partial dentures and the main reason that causes difficulty in wearing whole casting denture and suboptimal effect. It can be said that there's no success and popularity of new prosthetic way like implant if there's no accurate acquaintance and application of classical removable prosthetic technology. Combined with the fact that more than 60% with licenses in our country do not have a bachelor's degree, the content of this book is more realistic.

Based on these understanding and preliminary work, combined with the content of general doctors, I edited this book hoping to push popularity of invisible clasp in our country. This book discusses the concept and principles, classification and design, clinical application and examples of esthetic clasp in detail. There's even work authorization (design card) with all kinds of esthetic clasp (logos). It is very practical. The learning curve is short. This book is suitable for all kinds of dental doctors, medical students, dental technicians, etc.

This book gets support from BBD, Shenzhen Jia Hong Lab, KTJ Dental Lab, Dentsply China, and many friends. Xin Chen and Na Zhang, secretary of this book, did a lot of work including text editing, image screening, and logo designing. I express my thanks to her here.

Many thanks for the editing works from the Springer and People's Medical Publishing House.

Given the limited length and my limited acknowledge, I hope your advice for the inappropriate parts!

Chengdu, China Haiyang Yu

Acknowledgment

Special thanks to Xin Chen, Yuqing Lu, Na Zhang, Bixin Wen, Chenyang Xie, Junjing Zhang, Yuxin Lou, Ziyu Mei, Jiayi Yu, and Tinglu Fang for assistance in each chapter.

Contents

About the Editor

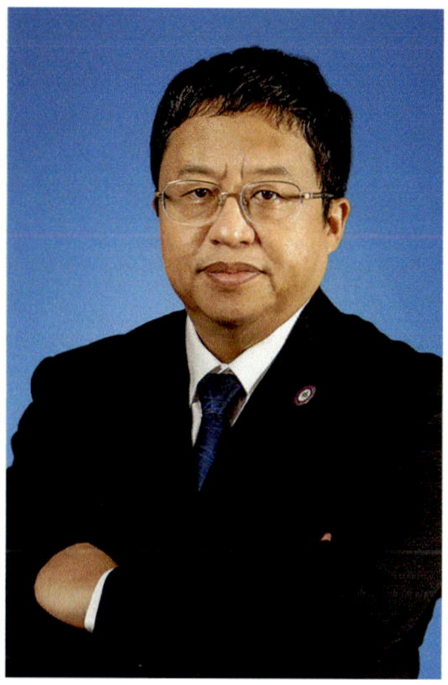

Haiyang Yu associate dean of West China School of Stomatology in Sichuan University, chair professor, Principal Investigator, and deputy director of State Key Laboratory of Oral Diseases Research, General Secretary of the guiding committee of higher dental education Chinese ministry education, Coming President of Prosthodontics Committee of Chinese Stomatological Association, well-known expert in Chinese prosthodontics and dental technology and specializes in guided esthetic restoration and digital dental implantology.Prof. Yu put forward several clinical protocols such as "the depth hole guided tooth preparation," "real-time measuring and checking protocol for correct implant site," and "RPD designer". He has given lectures around the country, published a number of papers and received widespread peer recognition as well as praises from patients. He has been teaching for 20 years and hosted online course of "Prosthodontics" of national essential resources, first enrolled undergraduates and graduate students of dental technology nationwide and obtained 2 National Teaching Achievement Prize. He is mainly engaged in research of biomechanics of implant as well as dental digital technology and has hosted more than 30 national and provincial programs. He has been rewarded the Natural Science Award of scientific and technological achievements in Colleges and Universities by the Ministry of Education. He possesses 34 national invention patents and 12 of which have been in the market. He drafted 6 national standards, edited and published 22 treatises, academic papers over 200. He created several technical protocols, such as HX-6 minimal invasive depth cutting and calibrating tungsten steel bur, e clasp esthetic framework, and measuring set of implanting site, which have made important contributions to the development of digital guided protocols in the field of Prosthodontics.

How to Improve the Esthetics of Clasps

1

From a wide view of the history of removable partial dentures (RPDs), clasp is a kind of retainer with long history. Clasp-retained RPDs were always recognized as one of the important solutions for dentition defect because of its advantages, such as noninvasive, safe and reversible, cheap, wide indications, and so on.

However, the poor esthetics is one of the most significant disadvantages of traditional clasp-retained RPDs. Do we have any protocol or solution to overcome the "metal smiling" with low cost while keeping those advantages? Make the RPDs a new life as a noninvasive and reversible cheap choice with compromised esthetic outcome for more edentulous patients. Then the first logistic question is how to improve the esthetics of clasps.

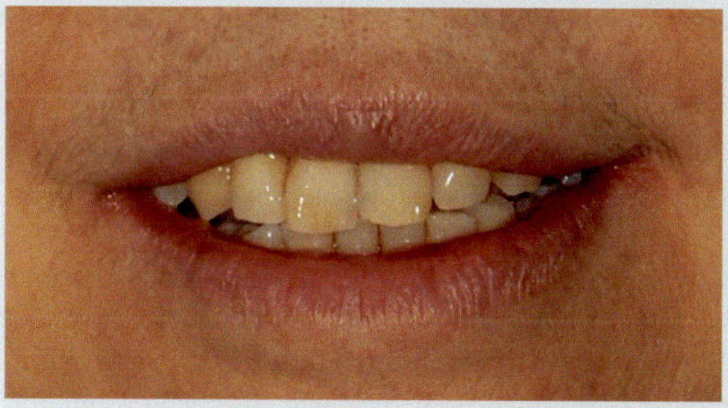

RPDs have lots of advantages, such as noninvasive, safe and reversible, wide indications, cheap, mature workmanship, and simple but reliable technological process. Though fixed denture has better esthetic effect, its indications are strictly limited and cannot totally replace conventional RPDs [1]. In developing country like China, according to the fourth practical situation and the trend of population epidemic investigation and oral epidemic investigation, for quite some time in the future, RPDs will still play an important part among quinquagenarian and low income groups in most areas [2].

But the display of metal clasps in the buccal and labial or facial surface of abutments (especially the anterior teeth and premolar teeth) has badly influenced the esthetic effect—people still looks old though with denture, and it cannot satisfy patients with their esthetic requirements. With life standard and requirement of esthetic improved, more and more patients are unwilling to choose clasp-retained RPDs. It has been the common goal of both professionals and patients to improve the esthetics of RPDs while keeping advantages of noninvasive, safe and reversible, cheap, and wide indications. Make the RPDs a new life as a noninvasive and reversible cheap choice with compromised esthetic outcome for more edentulous patients.

To remedy clasp's esthetic disadvantage [3], in recent decades, some kinds of new retainers have been used to replace regular clasps [precision attachment, dental implants with RPDs, etc. (Fig. 1.1)] for stable esthetic effect. However, resulting from its difficult technological process, higher cost, and limited indications and other factors, the popularization of these new retainers is still restricted.

At present, the main direct retainers of RPDs are still clasps, which still play an important part in prosthetics [4, 5]. So, is there a method that doesn't need to increase the cost, and is suitable for most patients and can easily improve the esthetic effect?

Synthesizing former literature and the study of our West China team, we think it can be realized from two aspects: One is to make the clasp invisible by using teeth color, gingiva color, or transparent materials. The other one is to change the design of conventional clasps to make them difficult to display during function. Based on remaining the advantages of RPDs, we try our best to make patients smile without display of metal (Fig. 1.2).

H. Yu, *Digital Removable Partial Denture Technology*, https://doi.org/10.1007/978-981-19-7923-1_1

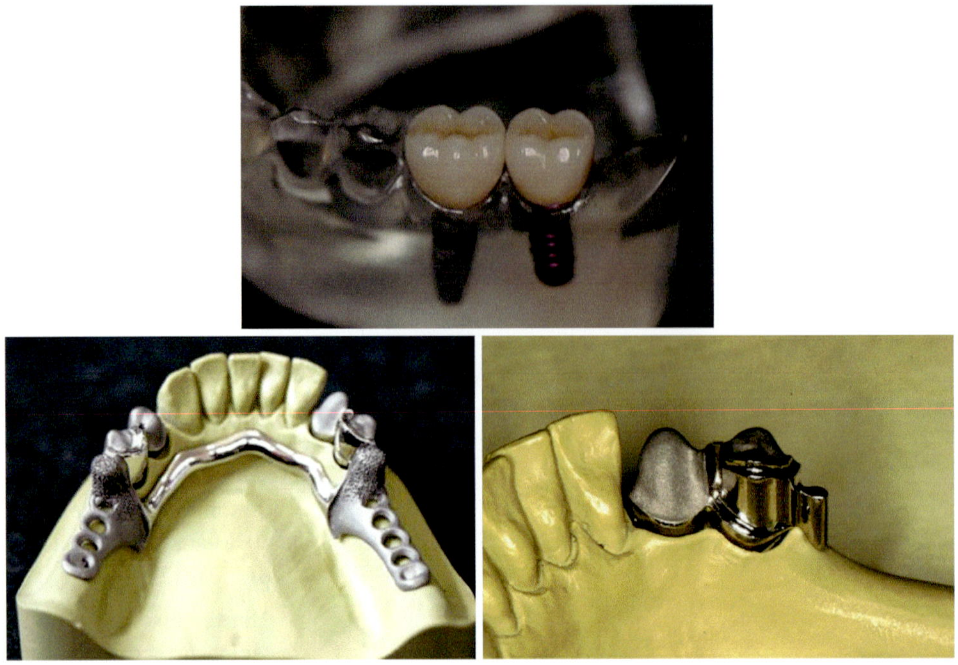

Fig. 1.1 New retention pattern: implant, precision attachment

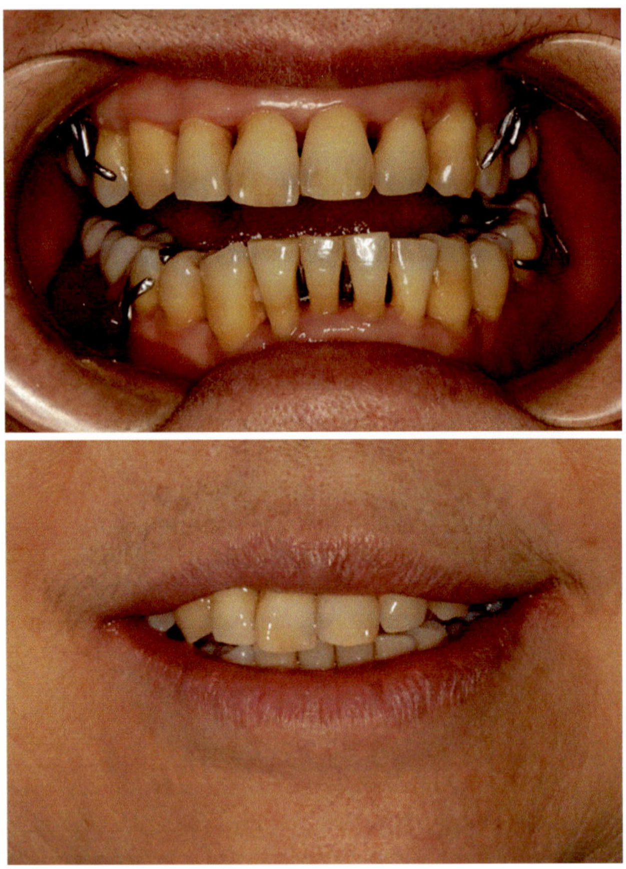

Fig. 1.2 To make patients smile with less or without display of metal

1.1 Invisibility of Clasps Characterized by Modified Material

There are two methods to make clasps invisible by modifying materials or novel stealthy design of the clasp. First, by choosing teeth color, gingiva color, or transparent resin to replace metal, we can just change the color to fit with oral tissue, but don't change the shape and retention area. Second for novel stealthy design of the clasp, we can use high elastic casting alloy to make the clasp smaller and more invisible, and we can utilize esthetic retention area to further improve the invisibility of clasp and decline or even eliminate the display of metal.

1.1.1 Elastic Resin

Elastic resin is an essential material to produce invisible denture; representative products are American Valplast elastic resin. In 1953, American dentists began to use such polymers to replace traditional metal clasp and base plate. Until now, it has been used in clinic for nearly 70 years.

Except for artificial teeth, other parts of invisible denture are all with high elasticity. Without regular clasps, the resinous base plate extends to be a clasp bracing the cervix of the abutment, and the retention is entirely provided by the elasticity of the base plate, so we also call this part base

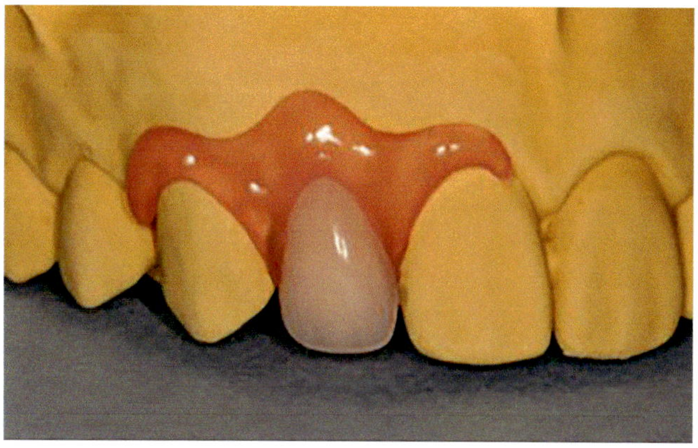

Fig. 1.3 Stealth elastic resin denture of teeth 12

plate clasp. The color and luster of invisible denture are similar to natural gingiva tissue, which has blood capillary with primary simulate effect and favorable transparency (Fig. 1.3).

However, with the resin's unavoidable aging, many problems could come, such as discoloring and the decline of elasticity [6]. The long-term effect of elastic resin denture is not good as the hot-setting traditional resin. So, it is always used to short-span temporary restoration and usually not suitable for complete denture or long cross arch denture.

1.1.2 Tooth Color Resin

Tooth color resin is a kind of polymers synthesized mainly by polyformaldehyde. To form clasp by hot setting, it is harder than common base resin. The current market has developed a variety of color options, and these can also be used with dyeing resin to fit with several colors of remaining teeth. It is suitable for RPDs, temporary restoration, periodontal splint, etc.

However, because of the limitation of resin's physical properties, it cannot replace metal to form the whole denture holder. It is fussy to get mechanical bond between metal holder and resin clasp in production. In addition, there is a problem of aging and deformation of the resin; the long-term use will lead to poor retention of clasp.

1.1.3 Transparent Resin

The texture and working principles are the same with tooth color resin. It also cannot be used to form the whole framework by itself and must be used with metal. Due to transparency, it can be used in esthetic area to replace the metal clasp on labial and buccal side. However, it also has the common disadvantage of resin and could not be used in free-end edentulous cases. Therefore, the clinical application is limited.

1.1.4 High-Elasticity Casting Alloy

Because the long-time stability of resin's mechanical property is not good, casting metal framework is still the good choice for the clasp of RPDs. But it has no transparency itself, and it is difficult to change the color, so we can but reasonably take advantage of the esthetic retention area to hide the metal and improve the design of clasps to make the metal exposed less, such as shortening or narrowing the clasp arm, hiding the clasp, etc.

However, the decline of length or width means the decline of clasp's retention. To compensate for the retention, we can put the clasp arm deeper into the undercut. But it requests enough elasticity and strength of the materials to make such clasps. In the metal used to make framework currently, the satisfactory materials are only gold alloy and vitallium.

The elasticity of gold alloy is the best, but the hardness is low, the strength is insufficient, and it is expensive. By contrast, the high elastic casting alloy, which is mainly made of Co, Cr, and Mo [7], follows proprietary proportion of ingredients and purification process in the production. So, comparing to common cobalt chromium, it possesses higher elasticity, ideal malleability, and Vickers hardness (Fig. 1.4).

The framework made of vitallium is less possible to transform or break off, so the design is more flexible. The clasp arm can be slender, and the holder can be more delicate. Vitallium not only has great retention but also improves the esthetic of clasp. It is the most suitable material for designing and producing kinds of metal esthetic clasps (Fig. 1.5). It also can be applied to traditional RPD frameworks.

There are some common vitallium brands, such as Vitallium of American Dentsply and Wironit of Germany BEGO.

Casting clasp has some advantages that clasps made of other materials can never surpass. The design of casting esthetic clasp is more flexible and various. The development of RPDs is mainly supported by the technology of casting framework. The development of materials and technology has already been rather mature, so it is worthy to popularize casting esthetic clasps for clinical use.

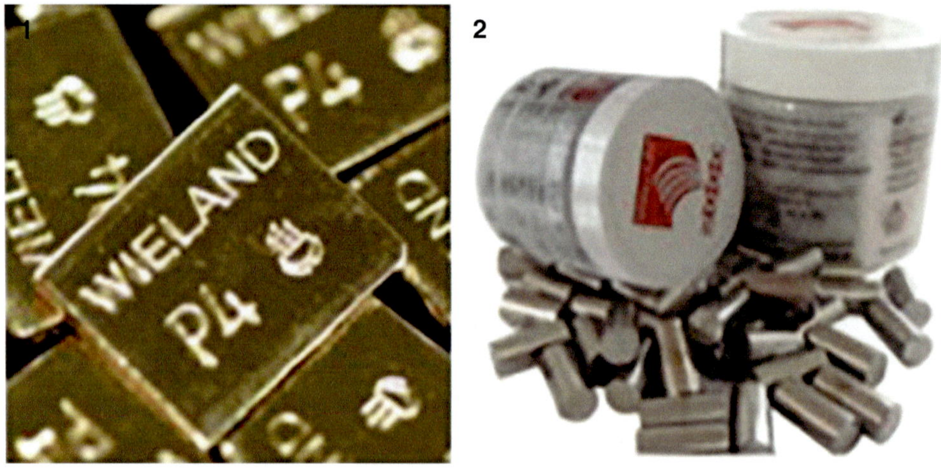

Fig. 1.4 Gold alloy and vitallium

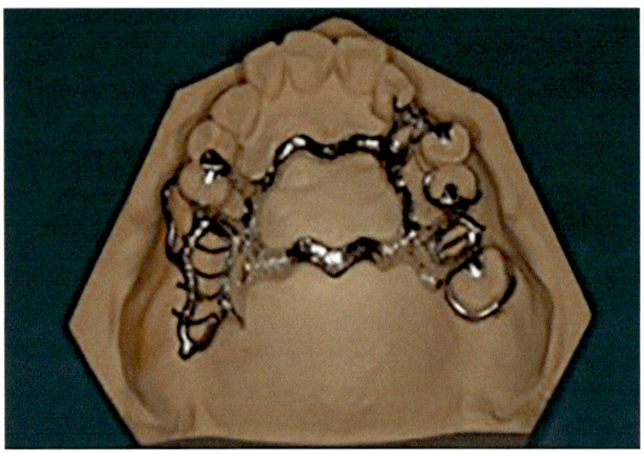

Fig. 1.5 Framework made of vitallium

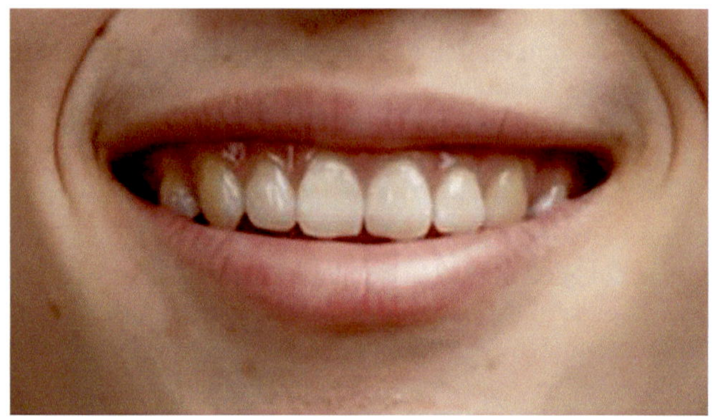

Fig. 1.6 Smiling exposed zone

1.2 Using Esthetic Retention Area to Change Clasp Design and Reduce Exposure

1.2.1 Esthetic Abutment

1. *Smiling exposed zone*: The area our soft and hard tissue exposed when grinning, which mainly includes exposed teeth and gingiva, and varies with different people (Fig. 1.6).

   Smile can make people closer without language despite of race, gender, and age. Besides, it is the window of our mind, an important factor to improve appearance charm and capital of social contact.

   The teeth crown exposure plays a critical role in our smile, which is mainly decided by the location of smile line, the width of rima oris, etc. Smile line is the fictitious line where the upper lip margin stretches when smiling (Fig. 1.7). It is usually related to age, gender, and other individual factors.

   High smile line: 75% proximal space gingiva, all the marginal gingiva, and over 3 mm gingiva above dental cervix can be seen. And what exceed the preceding scale is gummy smile.

   Middle smile line: Middle smile line is considered as the most ideal smile line, and its marginal gingiva is parallel to the under margin of the upper lip, and the incisal margin of maxillary teeth touches the inner side of the lower lip. Researches indicate that young ladies' smile line is higher than men universally.

   Low smile line: Only limited teeth are exposed.

   When young and middle-aged smile as usual, the dental cervix of the mandibular anterior teeth is hardly exposed. So, we can put low clasps on the cervix of the mandibular anterior teeth to hide claps when needed.

   Related researches show that the muscle tone of facial muscle drops and gingiva tissue shrinks back with people

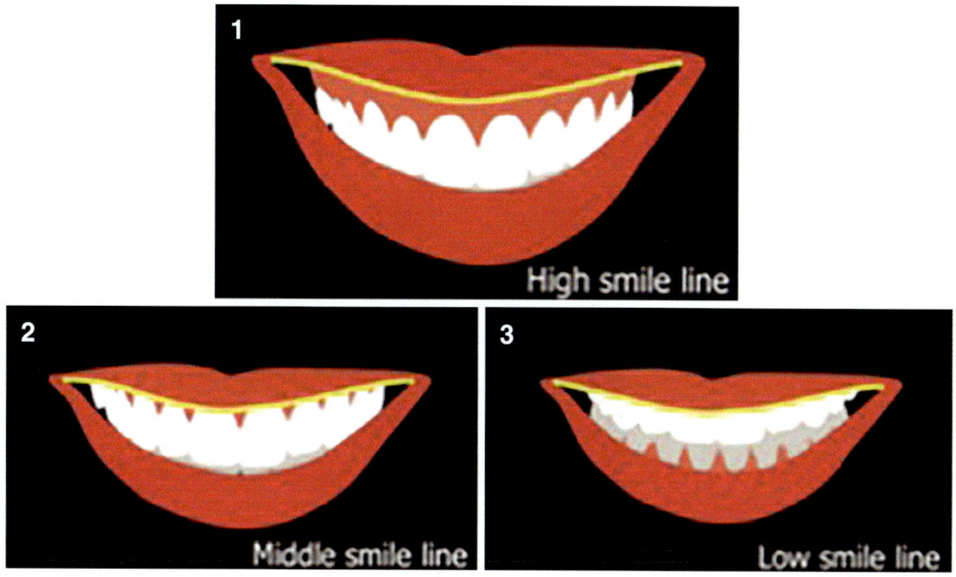

Fig. 1.7 The classification of smile line

getting older. The elderly's lip and facial muscle sag with the decline of resilience, then the smile line of the lower lip lowers (Fig. 1.8), and the exposure of anterior teeth and gingiva of mandibular increases in the meantime. Conversely, the exposure of mandibular anterior teeth and gingiva of maxillary gets less.

2. *Esthetic teeth*: The teeth which are easy to expose when smiling or talking (Fig. 1.9).

   A great number of people expose their anterior teeth and premolar, and a few of people can expose first molar even the second molar.

3. *Esthetic abutment*: A nature tooth in the esthetic zone chosen to be abutment

   The choice of abutment plays a critical part in RPDs. When it is distal extension or some anterior teeth get lost, the nature tooth in the esthetic zone is always chosen to be abutment (Fig. 1.10).

   On condition that we need to set retainers on canine or premolar, we had better put it on the premolar. When it is necessary to use mandibular anterior teeth as abutment, we can set clasp on the cervix of abutment to get esthetic effects. On the premise that the design is reasonable, we should choose the most esthetic teeth as possible as we can. How to choose esthetic abutments will be stated in the third chapter in detail.

   Traditional clasps should brace the abutment as far as possible to get retention, but the labial (or buccal) part of mental clasp is easy to be exposed. The metal color that doesn't match with the oral tissue would severely influence the entire esthetics. The esthetic teeth lie in the front of dental arch, so the negative influence of mental clasps on the appearance is more apparent, and traditional clasps cannot meet the esthetic requirement of esthetic teeth.

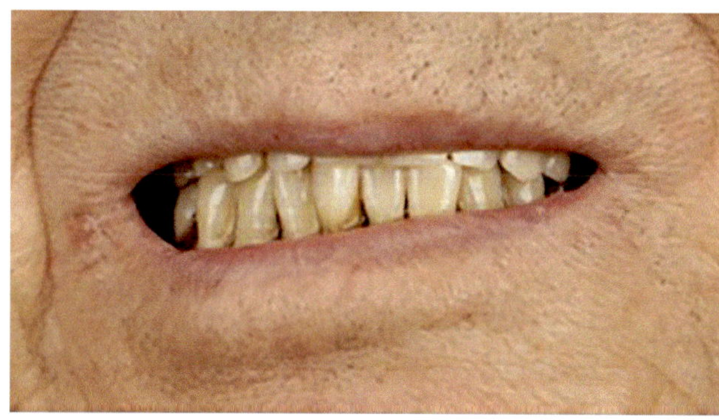

Fig. 1.8 The elderly's smile line of the lower lip

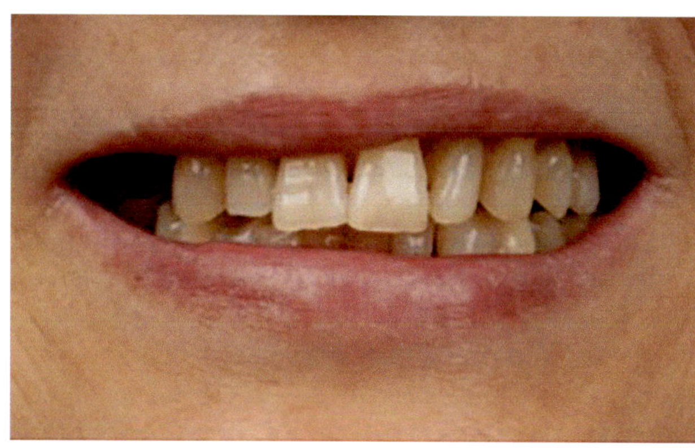

Fig. 1.9 Esthetic teeth (A3–B5 in this figure)

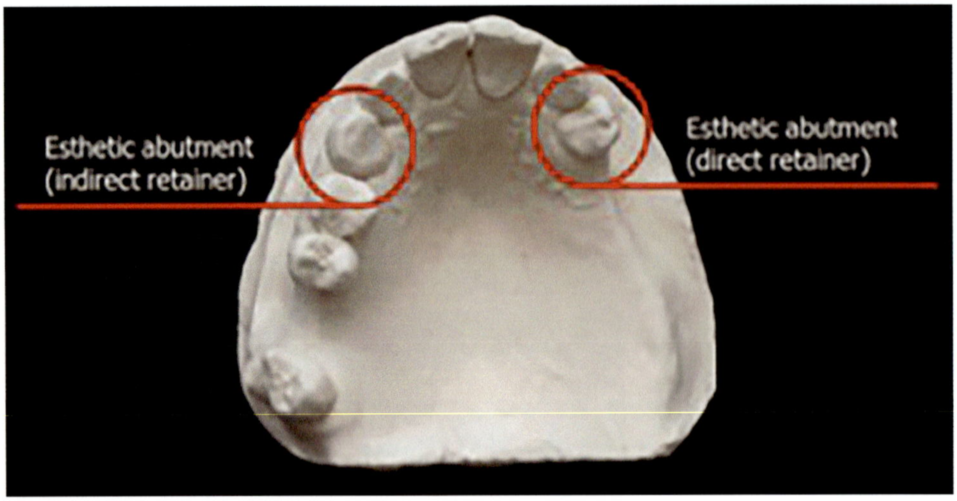

Fig. 1.10 Esthetic abutment. A3 and B3 are both esthetic abutments. We designed an indirect retainer on A3 and an direct retainer on B3

1.2.2 Esthetic Path of Insertion

1. *Esthetic path of insertion*: One of the path insertions which can eliminate or reduce the metal exposure on the esthetic abutment and improve the esthetics of denture.

   Usually, when surveying a model, determine the direction of path of insertion first and then draw the survey line. The model can be tilted to the angle that the clasp on the esthetic abutment is not easy to be exposed, and then the path of insertion can be determined according to the oral condition.

2. *Rotary path of insertion*: Denture revolves on lateral axis to get retainers seated in turn, which can effectively reduce the exposure of anterior teeth clasp. Rotary path of insertion is one type of esthetic path of insertion [8].

   When applied, the front end of framework should be designed to be rigid retainer, combined with one or several traditional clasps on the backend. Rigid retainer is composed of occlusal rest and minor connector, and the part of minor connector extending to the gingiva plays a main part in retention.

   When you try denture on, rigid retainer gets seated at first, and then the back clasps get seated in turn. Rotary paths of insertions are divided into two categories according to the different rotation center:

   First-class rotary path of insertion: The center of rotation is at the tail end of occlusal rest's extension part, and rigid retainer lies on the gingival extension part of minor connector. When tying the denture on, the center of rotation, O point, gets seated first, then the gingival extension of minor connector gets into undercut to get retention while denture rotating, and finally the rest part of denture is seated (Fig. 1.11).

   Second-class path of rotary insertion: The center of rotation lies on the gingival extension part of minor connector, which works as rigid retainer. It has double path of insertions. The first step is to let the center of rotary get seated along the vertical path of insertion. The second step is to make occlusal rest and other parts of framework get seated along the rotary path of insertion (Fig. 1.12).

   Although the advantages of the rotary path of insertion outstand, disadvantages still exist:

   (a) The clinical operation is difficult, and it is not convenient to take on or off, and it really takes time for initial placement.
   (b) The cancel of the clasp on anterior teeth makes some influence on stability, so we have to take some measures, such as increasing the thickness and length of occlusal rest.

   Some clinicians may not fully grasped the theory of rotary path of insertion, or it is hard to get support from technicians, or there is no evidence to prove the long-term success of rotary insertion so as to lack indispensable confidence; the application of rotary insertion denture is few.

3. *Esthetic survey line*

   When surveying a model, by adjusting the tilt angle of model, to get a survey line below which the undercut should all be in esthetic retention area, this survey line is called esthetic survey line (Fig. 1.13). We can predict the

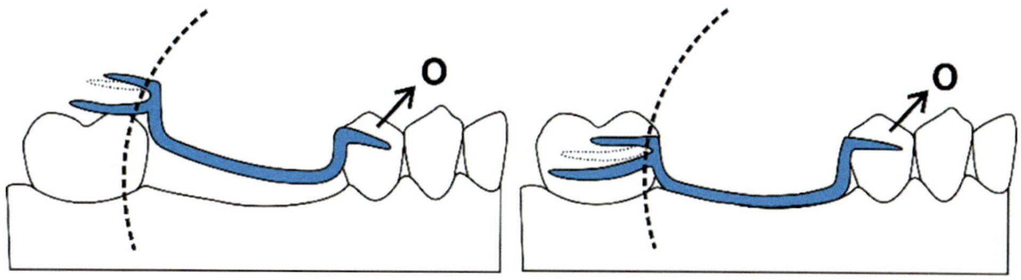

Fig. 1.11 The first-class rotary path of insertion to eliminate anterior clasps

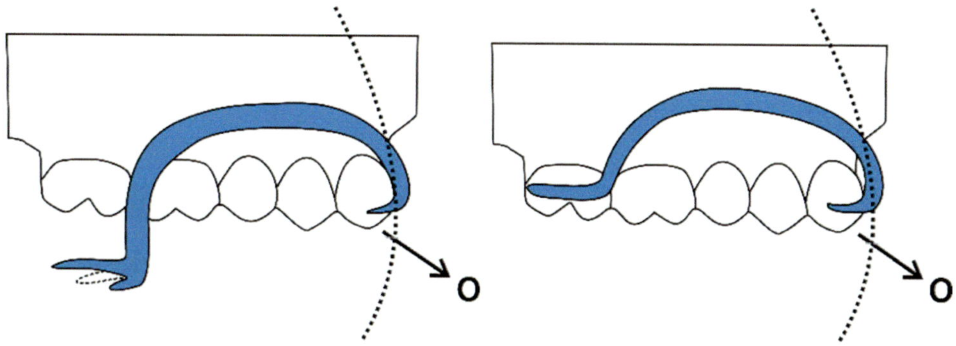

Fig. 1.12 The second-class vertical-rotary path of insertion to eliminate anterior clasps

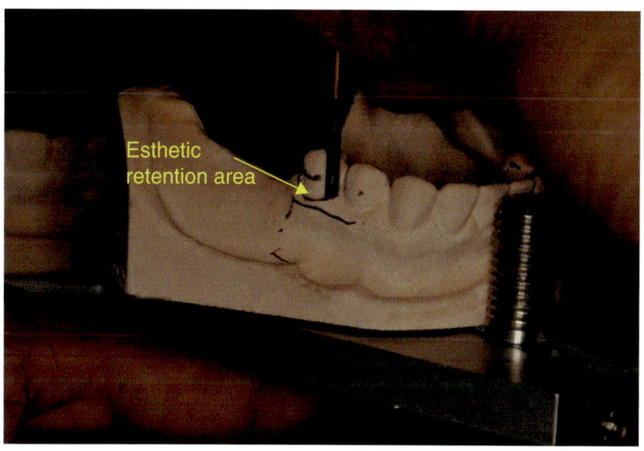

Fig. 1.13 Esthetic survey line

location of esthetic survey line in terms of esthetic retention area and then decide the angle of esthetic path of insertion.

1.2.3 Esthetic Retention Area

1. *Clasp exposed area*: The area that displays metal part of clasps on abutment when opening mouth.

   On account of anatomical features of abutment and oral tissues or the different angles of observing, the mental part of clasp would not be seen totally, only part of it can be seen, and the other parts are hidden by abutment, adjacent teeth, or labial-buccal muscle.

No matter what kind of the clasp is, the metal on abutment's lingual side is definitely hidden by abutment. But the buccal part of clasp is relatively complicated to be hidden. The main factors influencing labial-buccal cover are the height of smile line and the width of rima oris. For example, in the case, we have to set clasp on central incisor, if patient's smile line is high, the gingiva of anterior teeth will all lie on exposed area in smile. So the mental clasp on the labial side of abutment is hard to be hidden, and clasp arm even can be seen totally. On the contrary, if the smile line is low, clasp can be hidden by the lip, and the area where is not hidden is exposed area of clasp (Fig. 1.14).

The main factor that influences the clasp's cover from adjacent teeth and abutment is the location of the abutment selected in the dental arch. If we use the clasp arm with the same length to brace the abutment in different location, the closer to the facial center line and the front of the dental arch the tooth is, the more the labial-buccal clasp arm is exposed. Taking the maxillary as example, if the clasp is set on the second incisor, it may not get any cover from adjacent teeth. If the clasp is set on the cuspid at the corner of dental arch, the distal part of axis ridge will be hidden by itself (Fig. 1.15). If it is set on the first molar whose location is backer, not only its axis ridge will be hidden by itself, but also its mesial part would be hidden by next cuspid, and the exposed area of clasp is less.

There is a special statement: Because of different observing angles such as frontal view and lateral view from 45°or 90°, the cover area formed by abutment and adjacent teeth would change. In addition, looking hori-

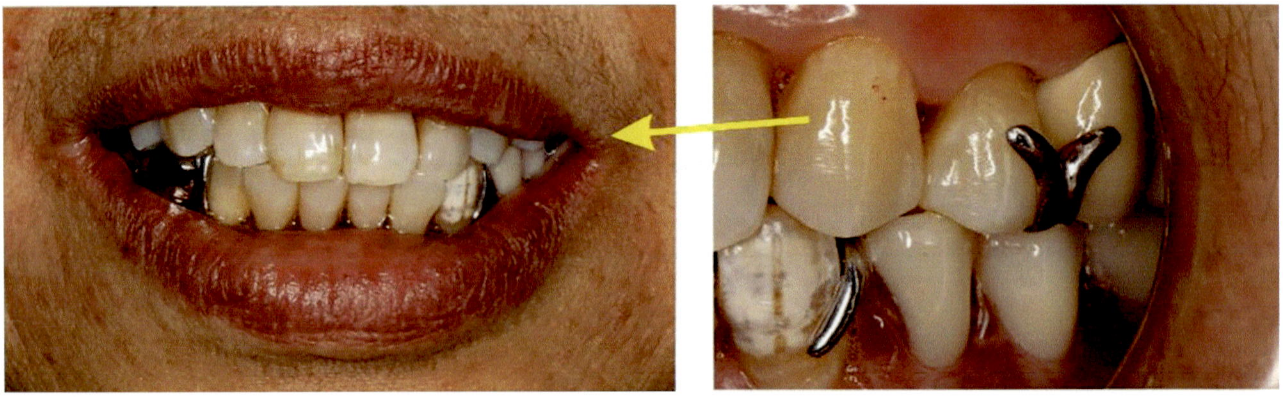

Fig. 1.14 The explosion and shelter of clasps (clasps are sheltered by the lip)

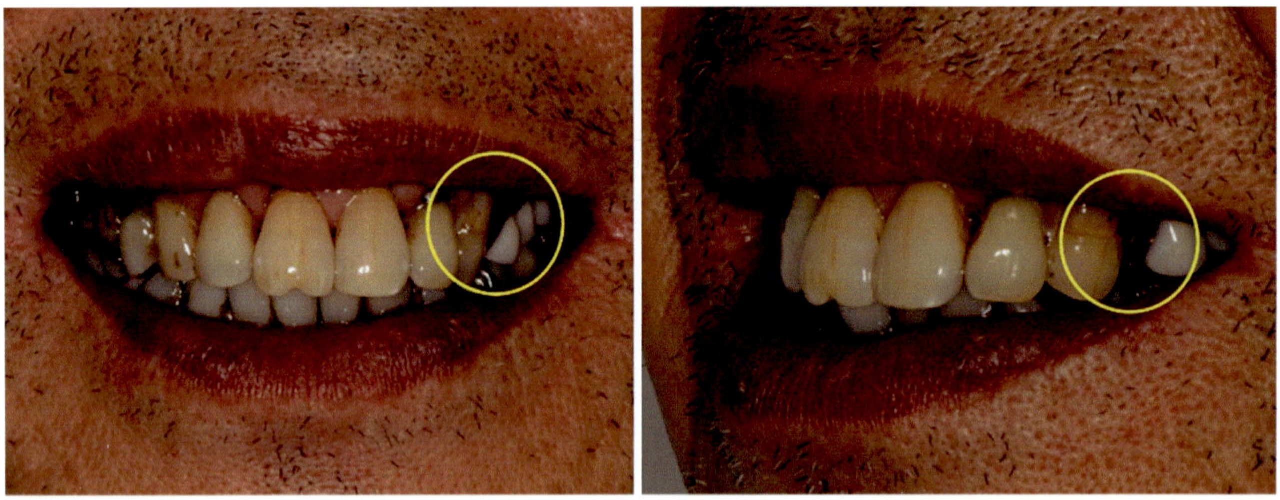

Fig. 1.15 The different shading effects from different observation angle. It was showed from the front view that the clasp on the distal area of cuspid buccal axial ridge was sheltered by itself

zontally, looking down, and looking up would lead to the visual change of the cover area, too. In daily social life, we usually talk to others face to face, so frontal view and horizontal view are more valuable in clinical application.

The esthetic clasp aims to reduce display of clasps as much as possible, hide the metal part exposed of traditional clasps on the buccal-labial side, and improve the esthetics of RPDs.

2. *Clasp retention area*: It is the undercut on the abutment that provides retention [9]. The retention generated by the clasp terminus extends into this area can ensure the normal function of denture.

   The retention of clasp mainly comes from the friction force between clasp arm and nature teeth [10]. The shape of nature teeth is convex, and the area under the most salient points is undercut. Usually, the free end of clasp arm clings to the undercut; when dislocated, the elastic deformation of the clasp arm will happen to pass through the salient point. And there is a pressure on abutment at the same time, and then the friction force is occurred to prevent clasp from dislocating. The retention must be strong enough to ensure that denture can function normally.

   There is nonquantitative proper undercut on all nature teeth that is available for selection, and we can change the range and the location of undercut by adjusting the direction of path of insertion. If there is no appropriate undercut, we can get necessary undercut by tooth preparation.

3. *Esthetic undercut area*: All the undercuts on the esthetic abutment that have no effect on esthetics, including distofacial undercut, distal proximal undercut, lingual undercut, and so on.
4. *Esthetic retention area*: The part of tooth which is included both in the area below esthetic survey line and esthetic undercut area.

According to the statement above, balancing the esthetics and the function, the scope of exposed area of clasp in exposed area of smile should be reduced as much as possible to improve esthetics in social life and oral function. In the meantime, the size of clasp retentive area selected should ensure that the retention produced by the clasp reaches the minimum that the clinical application requires. This is the principle of esthetic clasp design, which leads to a brand-new concept: esthetic retention area (Fig. 1.16). This kind of undercut area is not exposed

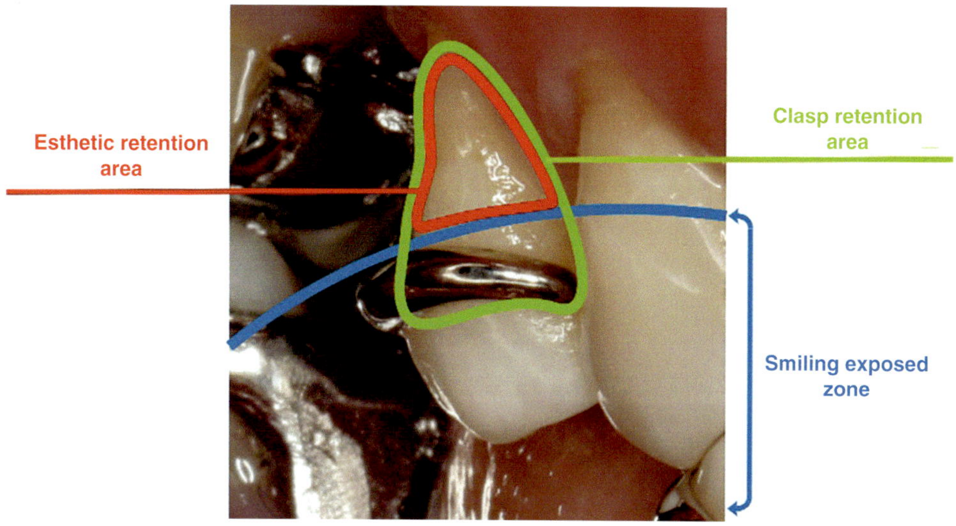

Fig. 1.16 Esthetic retention area

due to the shelter from lips, cheeks, and adjacent teeth during normal functional activity.

As for framework removable dentures, retention is the premise of function, and it mainly relies on the clasps, so it is impossible to completely eliminate clasps. Among all the undercuts of abutments, there are at least some cryptic undercuts we can use. The clasp tip can get into the esthetic retention area to get necessary retention and esthetics as well.

The existence of esthetic retention area can be said to be the important premise of designing and producing esthetic clasps.

1.3 Mechanics Principles and Comparison of the Retention of Esthetic Clasps

1.3.1 Mechanics Principles

1. *Retention*

Retention refers to the RPDs would not dislodge during oral function activities with RPDs in mouth. The force resisting the dislocation on the occlusal direction or the direction opposite to the path of insertion is called retention. Retention mainly includes the friction force between the retainers and abutments, the adsorption force between the base plates and mucous membranes, and the atmospheric pressure. In terms of the supporting type of RPDs, the proportion of these three kinds of retention is different.

The retention of retainers is mainly influenced by three factors: undercuts, materials, and the shape of clasps [11, 12].

Undercuts can be described by three elements: location, depth, and slopes.

First of all, we decide the location of undercuts according to the tooth contour, for example, the buccal axial ridge on the buccal surface of B4 and the lingual surface of C5.

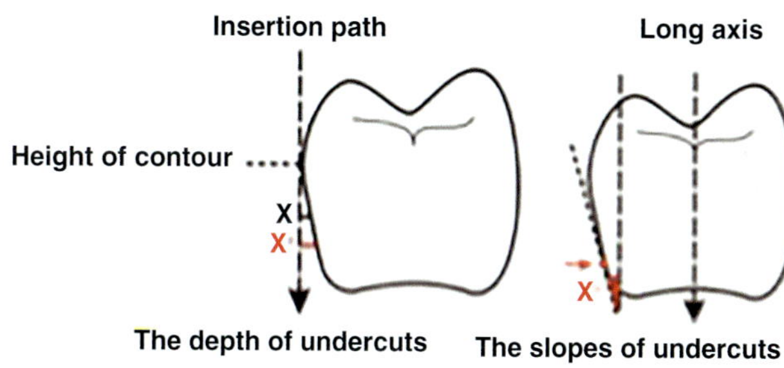

Fig. 1.17 The depth and slopes of the undercut

The depth of undercuts is the horizon distance from the analyzing rod of the surveyor to certain point on the undercut area. The deeper the undercut, the larger the retention. The slopes of undercuts are the angles formed by the tangent of certain point on the undercut area and the major axis of the abutment (Fig. 1.17). The retention increases with the slopes increasing.

Commonly, the rulers measuring the undercut of clasp have three different specifications: 0.25, 0.5, and 0.75 mm. The depth that the clasp enters the undercut varies with the materials. The larger the elasticity of the materials, the smaller the force needed to make the clasp deformed or moved. So to improve the retention, we should put the clasp into the undercuts deeper. The wrought wire gets into undercuts by 0.5~0.75 mm. The gold alloy is 0.5 mm, and the cobalt-chromium alloy is 0.25~0.5 mm.

Clasp tips should be elastic, and clasp arms should get into the undercut by half to one third. This principle is essential. If the clasp is not elastic, patients cannot put the RPDs on. RPDs have the function of retention, only if the force that the retention arm of the clasp generates is larger than the force needed when removing RPDs from the abutment, when crossing abutment's height of contour.

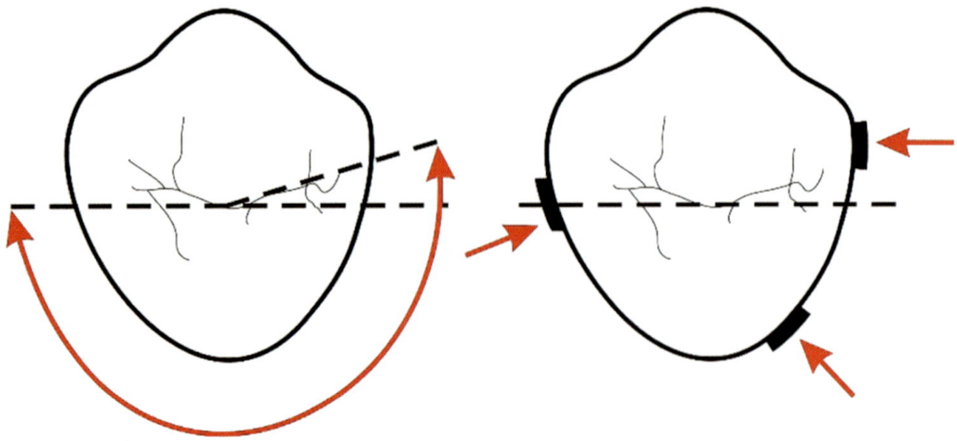

Fig. 1.18 Bracing at least 180° (the left is three-point discontinuous contact)

But the retention should not be too strong to make wearing and removing difficult and even damage the abutment. We should try to decline the retention if only it can resist the dislocation force.

2. *Bracing*

   Clasps must brace the maximal circumference of the abutment at least 180° from the undercut area to non-undercut area of the axial surface. It can be a continuous contact or discontinuous contact (point contact) and at least in contact with three areas of tooth surface (Fig. 1.18). On the one hand, that can prevent clasp from separating from teeth when pressed. On the other hand, that can prevent abutment from moving under eternal force.

3. *Stability*

   The abutment should try to avoid bearing gradient force, and the clasp is able to decline the movement of abutment. Especially for the abutment near the free-end gap, we had better make it equip stress interruption effect by adjusting the design and structure of frameworks. We can achieve that through using the mesial occlusal rest to change the balance point (Fig. 1.19).

4. *Supporting*

   Occlusal rests should be designed to prevent the RPDs from sinking.

5. *Resisting*

   The resisting arm is the rigid part on the opposite tooth surface to the retention arm. Its function is to balance the lateral force caused by the retention arm when it crosses the maximal circumference in the process of dislocation. Then it compels the retention arm to be deformed to protect the abutment (Fig. 1.20). In general, every retention arm needs a resisting arm to interact with each other. Furthermore, the resisting arm also can be replaced by lingual plate or high base plate, which has the same resistance effect.

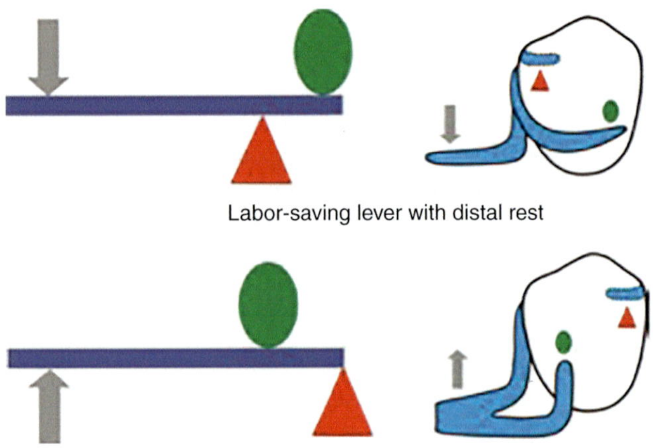

Fig. 1.19 The different leverage effects occurred on different clasp locations

6. *Passivity*

   Except for when functioning with RPDs and seating and removing the RPDs, there should not be any compressive stress between the retention arm and the abutment. All in all, when the clasp is put on the abutment, it should be passive, still and with no compressive stress.

7. *Balance*

   Clasps should be dispersed on two sides of dental arch, so they can restrict each other. The retention of two sides of dental arch should be even to get balance.

   If there is no guiding plane to control the direction of path of insertion, the retention arm should be symmetrically designed. In other words, the retention arm on both sides of dental arch should all be put on the buccal side or the lingual side. As for the bilateral abutment of Kennedy III type, the retention arm can be designed heterochiral.

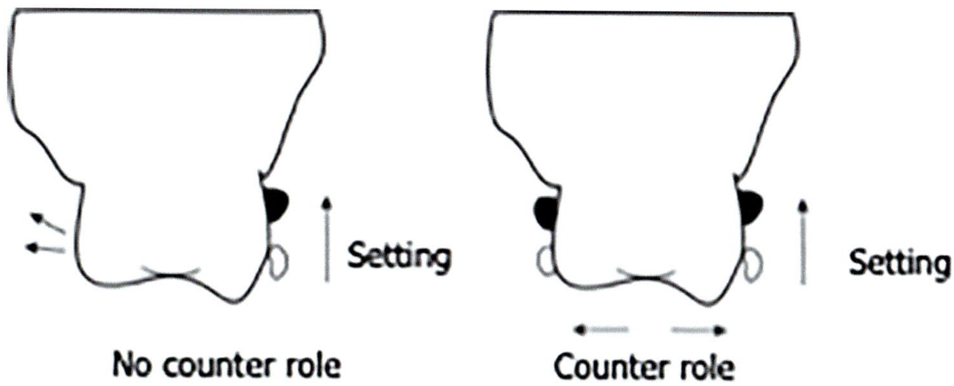

Fig. 1.20 Resisting

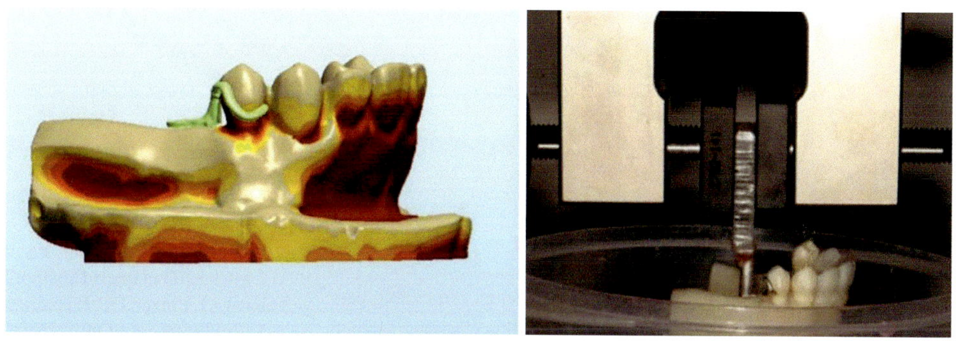

Fig. 1.21 We designed clasps using CAD/CAM and then use Instron tensile elongation measuring device to test the retention force

1.3.2 Comparison of Retention

Until now, reports about esthetic clasp design are almost descriptive and lack of scientific evidence. The fundamental function of clasps is retention, but clasp arms of most esthetic clasps are shorter than regular design ones. The cut of length would cause the decline of contact area and the increase of metal deformation resilience force, but what influence it has on the retention of esthetic clasps on Earth? Would it satisfy the retention requirement in clinical use? These questions decide the application value of clasps, so it is necessary to carry out the retention test to esthetic clasps.

The material, used to produce samples of carrying out the retention test of esthetic clasps, is the most suitable material for esthetic clasps—high-elasticity vitallium. We took natural premolars with standard size as abutments and then designed and produced ten kinds of esthetic clasps, such as buccal short retention arm clasp, lingual retention short buccal shoulder clasp, modified RPI clasp, RLS clasp, saddle-lock clasp, plate-rod clasp, lingual retention L clasp, C clasp, L clasp, and Terec hidden clasp. And the control group was traditional three-arm clasps. The undercut depth was 0.25 mm, and we carried out tensile dislocation force test on Instron tensile elongation measuring device (Fig. 1.21).

According to the results (Fig. 1.22), it could be considered that the retention force of all ten kinds of esthetic clasps was smaller than traditional three-arm clasps, but all can meet the demand of clinical use. The retention of modified RPI clasps, C clasps, lingual retention L clasps, and saddle-lock clasps was almost the same, and the retention effects were better than other esthetic clasps. The RSL clasp showed the lowest retention. Terec hidden clasp and saddle-lock clasp were the most invisible ones, and the retention also satisfied the clinical requirement, so both are worthy to be popularized.

The detailed design of various esthetic clasps will be introduced in the next chapter.

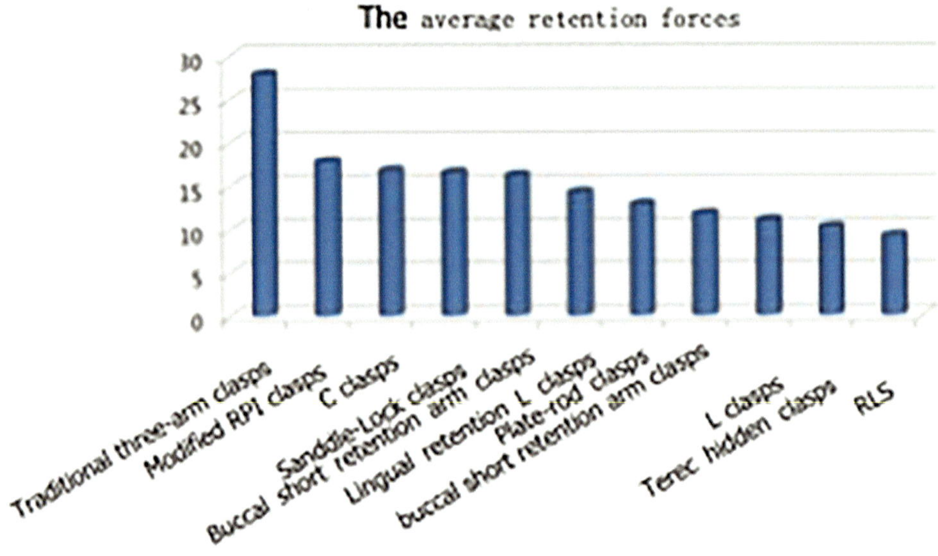

Fig. 1.22 The comparisons of average retention forces between ten kinds of esthetic clasps and traditional three-arm clasps

References

1. Alan BC, Glen PM, David TB, et al. McCracken removable partial prosthodontics. Zhang FQ, translated, 11 ed. Beijing: People's Military Medical Publishing House; 2007.
2. Chao Y. Stomatology. Beijing: People's Health Publishing House; 2006.
3. Beaumont AJ. An overview of esthetics with RPDs. J Quintessence Int. 2002;33(10):747–55.
4. Rodney D. Stewart's clinical removable partial prosthodontics. Batavia: Quintessence; 2008.
5. Alan B. McCracken's removable partial prosthodontics. St. Louis: Elsevier Science Health Science div; 2004.
6. Fitton JS. The physical properties of a polyacetal denture resin. J Clin Mater. 1994;17(3):125.
7. Bridgeman JT, Marker VA, Hummel SK. Comparison of Ti and Co-Cr RPD claps. J Prosthet Dent. 1997;78(2):187–93.
8. Krol AJ, Finzen FC. Rotational path removable partial dentures: part 1. Replacement of posterior teeth. Int J Prosthodont. 1988;1:17–27.
9. Hebel KS, Graser GN, Featherstone JD. Abrasion of enamel and composite resin by removable partial denture clasps. J Prosthet Dent. 1984;52(3):389–97.
10. Sato Y, Abe Y, Yuasa Y, et al. Effect of friction coefficient on Akers clasp retention. J Prosthet Dent. 1997;78(1):22–7.
11. Prothero JH. Prosthetic dentistry. 2nd ed. Chicago: Medico-Dental; 1916. p. 332.
12. Jepson NJA. Removable partial dentures. Wang J, translated. Beijing: People's Military Medical Publishing House;2006.

2 Classification and Design of Esthetic Clasp

Esthetic clasp (e-clasp) is the generic terms of new classified design clasps which improve the overall esthetic appearance of removable partial denture on the basis of balancing both esthetics and normal function of the denture. It could be one of the traditional clasps or brand-new designed one. According to the teeth where the clasp is set, it can be classified into anterior e-clasp and posterior e-clasp, while it also can be classified into buccally retained clasp, proximally retained clasp, and lingually retained clasp according to the retention site on the abutment teeth.

Taking the abutment teeth as classification standard, this chapter will state the designs, characteristics, and indications of e-clasp in detail.

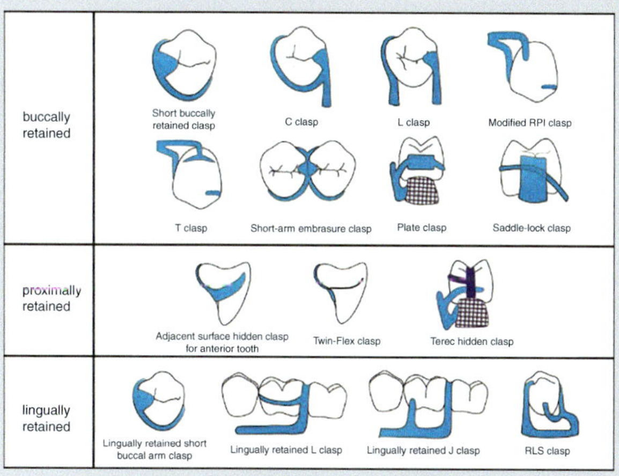

2.1 Concept of Esthetic Clasp

Esthetic clasp, the generic term of new classified design clasps which use esthetic retention area of the abutment teeth to retain or are made of esthetic restoration materials [1–3], can improve the overall esthetics of denture on the basis of ensuring the normal function performance of RPDs.

E-clasp is a new classification of clasps in terms of overall esthetics of denture, including some traditional clasps and newly designed clasps [2, 4]. At present, it is mainly made of highly elastic Co-Cr-Mo metal [5] or tooth color, gingival color, or colorless nonmetallic composite materials. The metal esthetic clasps are usually placed on the teeth on the esthetic teeth, and the retention comes from the hidden esthetic retention area of abutments. Metal esthetic clasp can make patients smile with less or without display of metal during function, which is more common in clinic. On the other hand, nonmetallic composite materials have a stealth effect because their colors are similar to that of teeth and gingiva but possess lower mechanical and antifatigue properties, and so they are often used in temporary or transitional restoration of RPDs [6].

2.2 Esthetic Clasp for Anterior Teeth

For anterior teeth in esthetic zone, including incisors and canines, it is difficult to determine the esthetic retentive area and design e-clasp due to their special features like no occlusal surface, small lingual retention area, and the exposure of buccal retention area, which has a great impact on esthetics [7].

H. Yu, *Digital Removable Partial Denture Technology*, https://doi.org/10.1007/978-981-19-7923-1_2

Therefore, the following seven kinds of anterior e-clasps mainly take advantage of distofacial undercut and distal proximal undercut to obtain retention and decrease or even eliminate the display of metal, which can be applied for posterior teeth as well.

2.2.1 Short Buccally Retained Clasp

Modified from the traditional circumferential clasp that consists of occlusal rest, retentive arm, and reciprocal arm, the short buccally retained clasp shortens the length of the retentive arm and lies on the distal side of the buccal axial ridge rather than across it, to minimize the display of metal clasp.

1. *Structure*

   Short buccally retained clasp consists of short buccally retained clasp arm, lingual reciprocation, distal guiding plate, and distal rest (Fig. 2.1).
2. *Characteristic*

   The short buccally retained clasp arm is placed on the distal side of the buccal axial ridge rather than across it. In this way, reduced encirclement makes facial and buccal clasp arm hidden in the mouth. The distal guiding plate can also provide supplementary retention for the denture (Figs. 2.2 and 2.3).

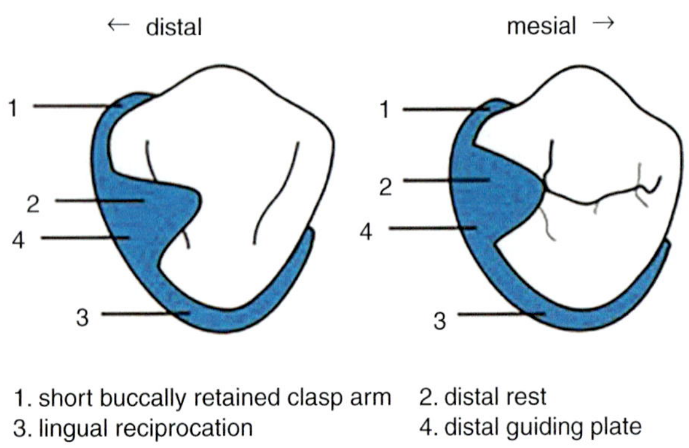

Fig. 2.1 Short buccally retained clasp (lingual view of the anterior type, occlusal view of the posterior type)

3. *Indication*

   This kind of e-clasp is applied to both anterior and posterior teeth with appropriate undercuts. It is also required that there must be distal and mesial abutments on both sides of edentulous space meanwhile. However, it is not suitable for distal extension abutment.

2.2.2 C Clasp

C clasp is modified from the traditional ring clasp, whose clasp arm encircles the lingual, buccal, and proximal surface of abutment. Due to the excessive contact with abutment, the self-cleaning of traditional ring clasp is poor. So, the modification of C clasp improves both esthetics and self-cleaning [2].

1. *Structure*

   C clasp consists of shortened retentive arm, minor connector, and mesial occlusal rest (Figs. 2.4, 2.5, and 2.6). The retentive arm originates from the mesial rest and encircles the lingual surface of abutment and then terminates at the proximo-facial line angle. If there is no contact between the adjacent tooth and the abutment to reciprocate, a reciprocal plate can be set connecting with the mesial rest.
2. *Characteristic*

   Because the clasp terminus is closed to the denture artificial teeth and the rest is positioned on the mesial side of the abutment, the lock structure can effectively prevent the saddle from tilting when dislodging force is applied. And when masticatory loading is applied, both saddle and retentive arm sink, reducing the pressure on the abutment and decreasing or removing the torsion.
3. *Indication*

   Wide application scope of C clasp, especially for distal extension cases. However, for abutment whose non-undercut area is too closed to the occlusal surface or anterior teeth with insufficient lingual encirclement area, its arm is likely to affect occlusion. Thus, another modification clasp, L clasp, is derived.

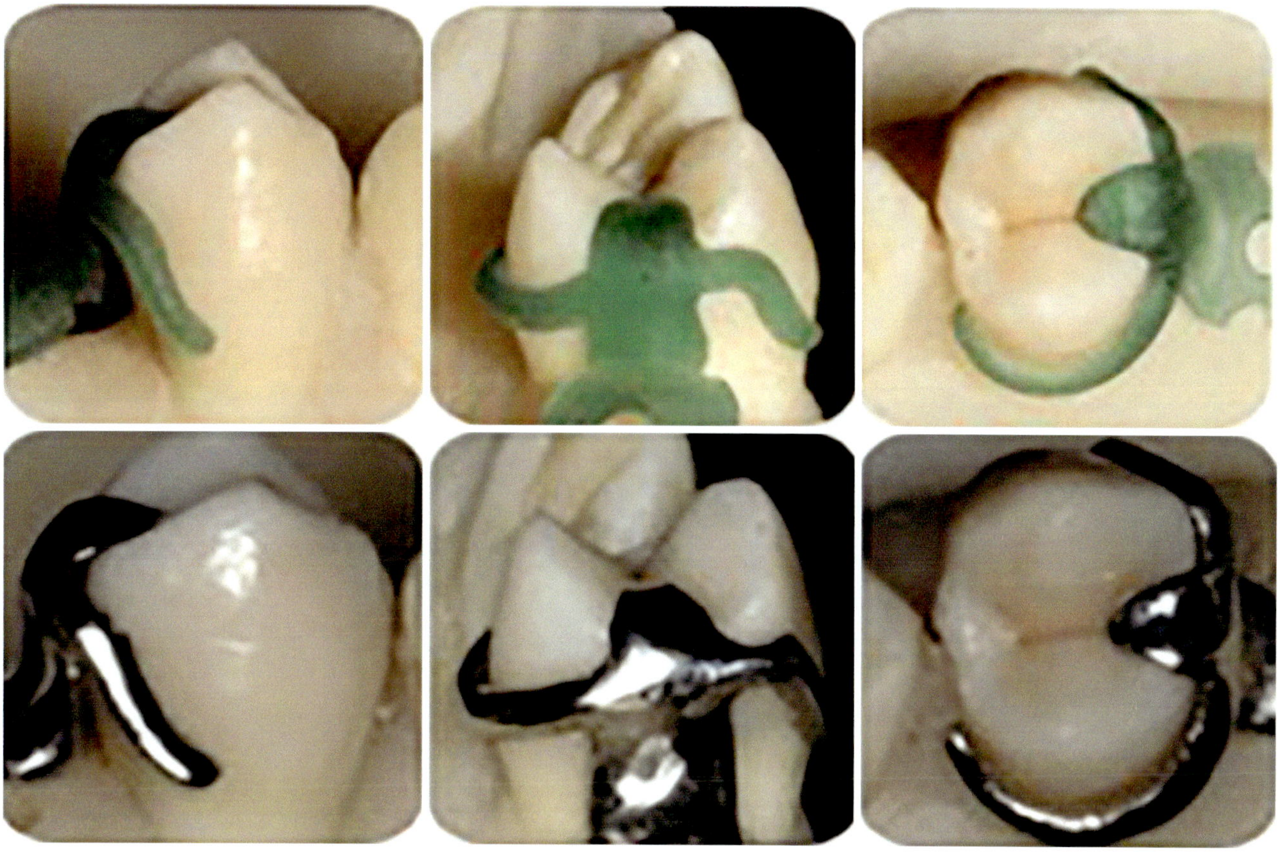

Fig. 2.2 Short buccally retained clasp (wax pattern type, cast metal type)

Fig. 2.3 Short buccally retained clasp (intraoral effect)

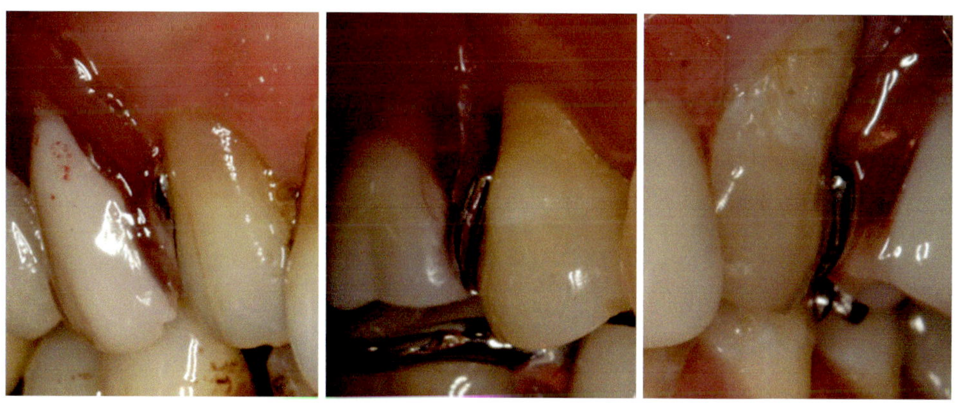

Fig. 2.4 C clasp (lingual view of the anterior type, occlusal view of the posterior type)

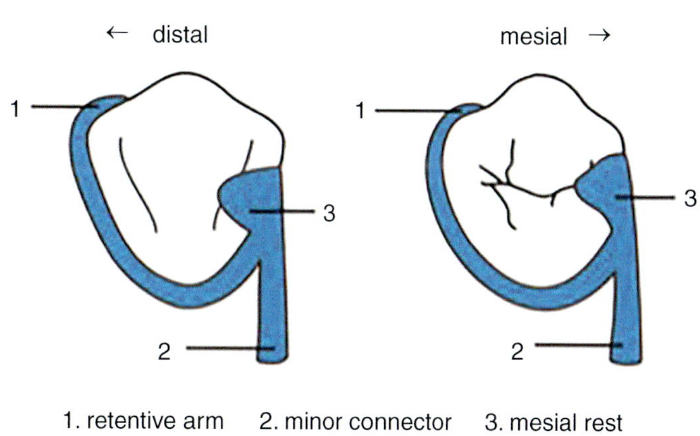

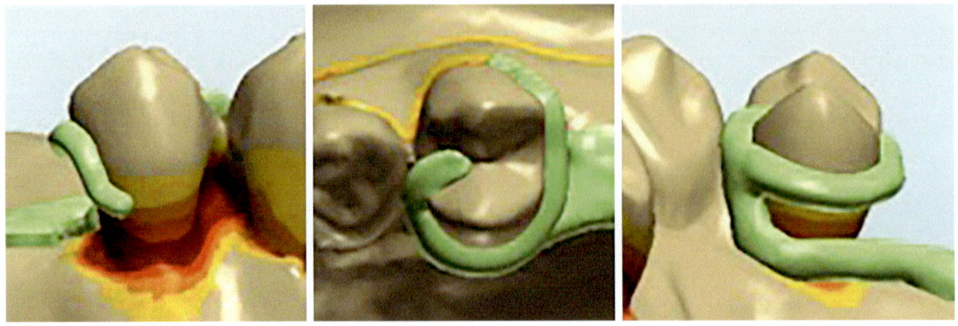

Fig. 2.5 C clasp (CAD drawing: buccal, occlusal, lingual view)

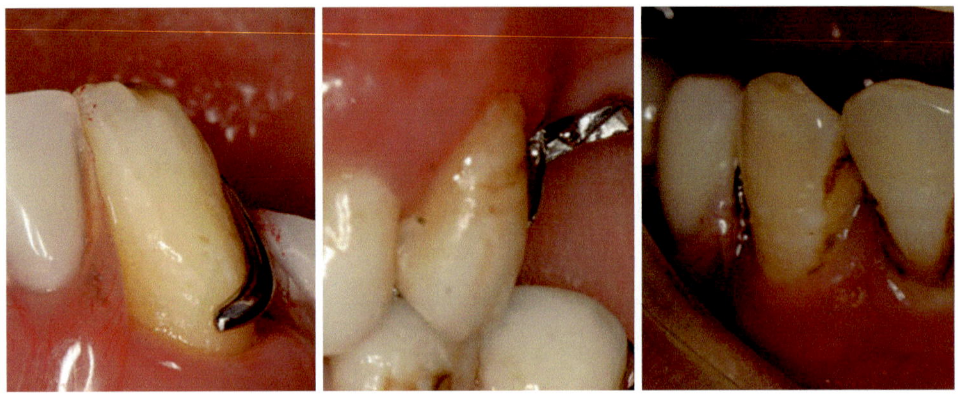

Fig. 2.6 C clasp (intraoral effect)

2.2.3 L Clasp

L clasp is a further modification of C clasp [2]. Its retentive arm is separated from the occlusal rest and is connected with the minor connector so as to improve self-cleaning of the abutment by reducing metal covering on the lingual surface and prevent the forming of abnormally high occlusal points. It is also applicable for distal extension cases. For the separated retentive arm that looks like "L" when viewed from the proximal direction, it is called L clasp.

L-type clasp is applicable for both anterior and posterior teeth, but it should be in accordance with the actual conditions to avoid metal exposure.

1. *Structure*

   L clasp consists of retentive arm, minor connector, and occlusal rest (Fig. 2.7).

2. *Characteristic*

   The main structure is formed by independent L-shaped retentive arm and mesial rest (Figs. 2.8 and 2.9).

   When there are edentulous spaces at the mesial and distal sides of the abutment with no adjacent teeth for reciprocation, a mesial reciprocal plate, which the mesial rest could connect with, should be added to separate the rest from the retentive arm.

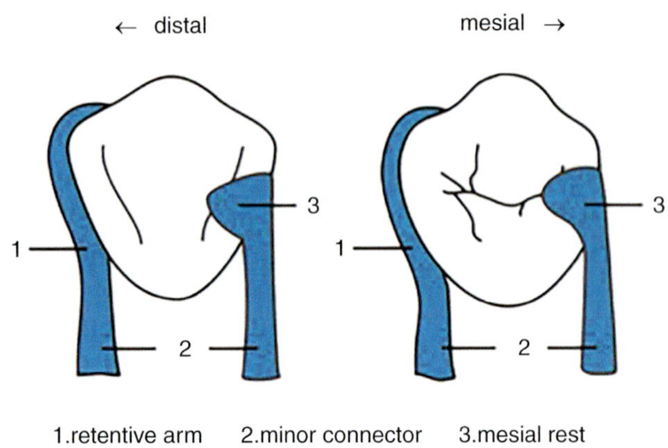

Fig. 2.7 L clasp (lingual view of the anterior type, occlusal surface of the posterior type)

3. *Indication*

   Similar extensive application scope as C clasp, especially for distal extension removable partial dentures. On the condition that lingual non-undercut of abutment gets too close to occlusal side and influences occlusion or abutment is low and flat, C clasp isn't applicable, and then we can choose L clasp.

   When L clasp is applied to incisor or canine, clasp arm does not look like L-shaped because abutment arm is lim-

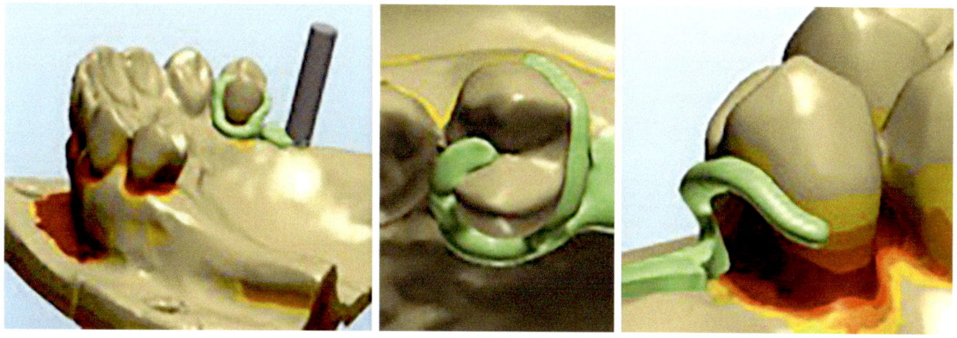

Fig. 2.8 L clasp (CAD drawing: lingual, occlusal, distal side of the buccal surface)

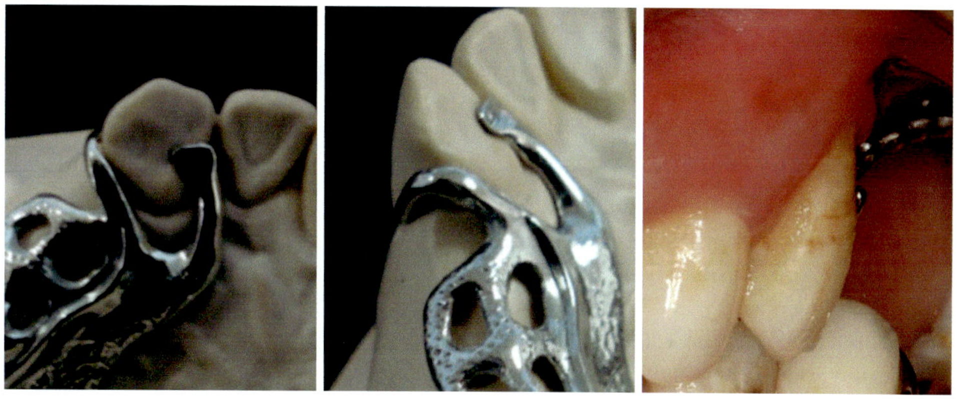

Fig. 2.9 L clasp (lingual view, proximal view and intraoral effect of cast metal)

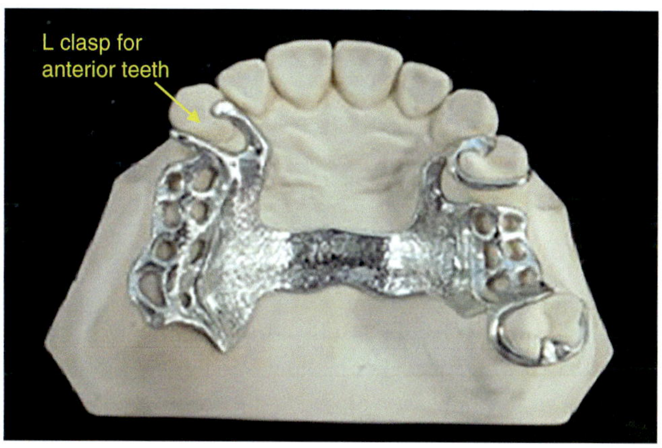

Fig. 2.10 L clasp is applicable for distal extension edentulism

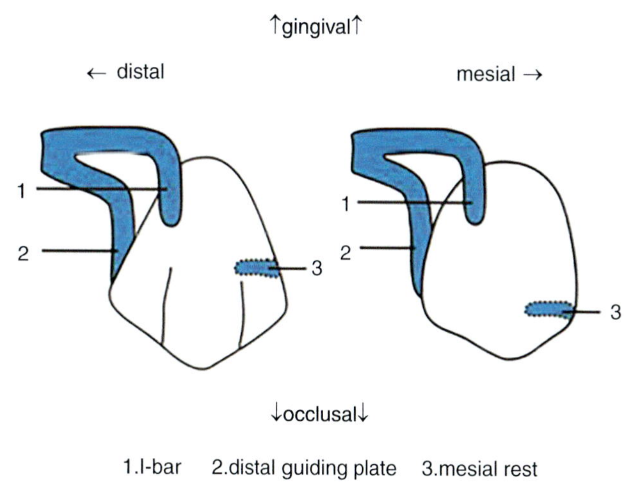

Fig. 2.11 Modified RPI clasp (buccal view of the anterior type, buccal view of the posterior type)

ited and its retention and stability are slightly decreased additionally. Hence, using both L clasp and other clasps of distal abutment is advised (Fig. 2.10).

2.2.4 Modified RPI Clasp

Traditional RPI clasp is a classic infrabulge clasp and also considered as e-clasp [1, 3]. The I-bar of RPI clasp is positioned on the gingival third undercut area of the buccal or labial surface of the abutment, and only a small surface area is contacted, so just a little esthetic impact is caused. However, the I-bar is also likely to display if the patient gets a high smile line.

The modified RPI clasp is designed to apply to a variety of situations. It is still composed of I-bar, distal guiding plate, and mesial rest, but the I-bar is positioned on the distal side of the buccal axial ridge instead of the mesial side to be less visible and can prevent the distal extension saddle from tilting to occlusal side.

1. *Structure*

   The modified RPI clasp consists of I-bar, distal guiding plate, and mesial rest (Fig. 2.11).

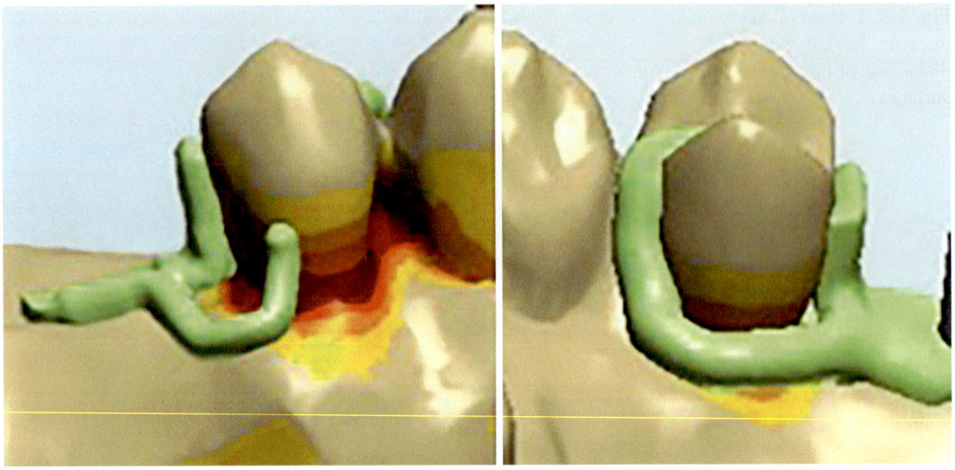

Fig. 2.12 Modified RPI clasp CAD drawings (buccal and lingual view)

2. *Characteristic*

   The I-bar is positioned on the distal side of the buccal axial ridge and engages the distofacial undercut, which makes it more invisible (Fig. 2.12).

3. *Indication*

   It is suitable for the last distal abutment whose survey line is close to the gingival third. It is contraindicated when severe buccal or lingual tilts of abutment teeth, severe tissue undercuts, or shallow buccal or labial vestibules exist.

   The I-bar of this modified RPI clasp is positioned on the distal side of the buccal axial ridge to help prevent the distal extension saddle from tilting to occlusion side. When denture is under masticatory process, the distal extension saddle sinks and rotates around the mesial rest, and the direction that distal I-clasp moves is perpendicular to gingival side. Then the I-bar gets out of touch with abutment, reducing or avoiding the torsion applied to abutment and protecting abutment ultimately.

2.2.5 T Clasp

T clasp is also infrabulge clasp [1, 2] similar to I-clasp with almost the same structure and indication. But its retentive arm changes to T-shaped extending from approach arm, causing a better retention by covering more tooth surface.

1. *Structure*

   T clasp consists of T-bar, distal guiding plate, and mesial rest (Figs. 2.13, 2.14, and 2.15).

2. *Characteristic*

   Its concealment is favorable, and two clasp terminus of the T-bar can be adjusted according to the actual situations.

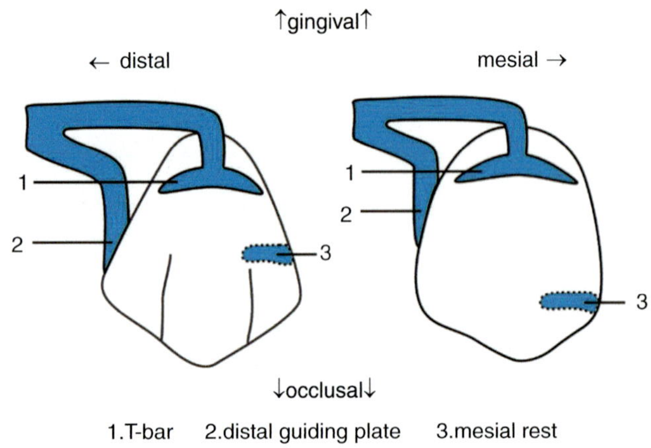

Fig. 2.13 T clasp (buccal view of the anterior type, buccal view of the posterior type)

3. *Indication*

   It is suitable for the last distal abutment and is contraindicated when buccal or labial vestibules are too shallow or the survey line is too closed to the occlusion surface for there would be a large interspace between T-bar and oral tissue that may cause food impaction and a higher risk of display of metal.

   The five kinds of clasp described above are all modified from traditional clasps. Their esthetics are improved by reducing the contact area of metal on the labial or buccal surface. However, if the patient gets a high smile line and the clasps cannot be hidden by either lips or adjacent teeth, esthetic effect would be unacceptable. Thus, it is also essential to make the full use of proximal undercuts in e-clasp design. The following section is going to describe two types of proximally retained e-clasp: adjacent surface hidden clasp for anterior tooth and Twin-Flex clasp.

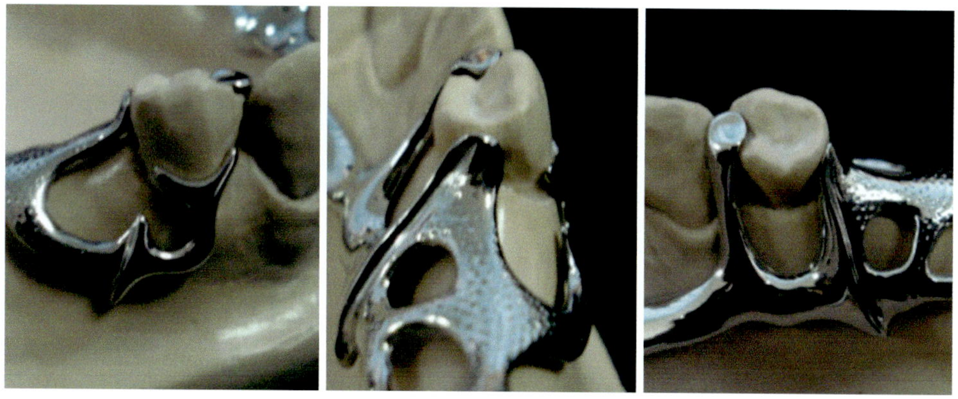

Fig. 2.14 T clasp (buccal, distal, and lingual view)

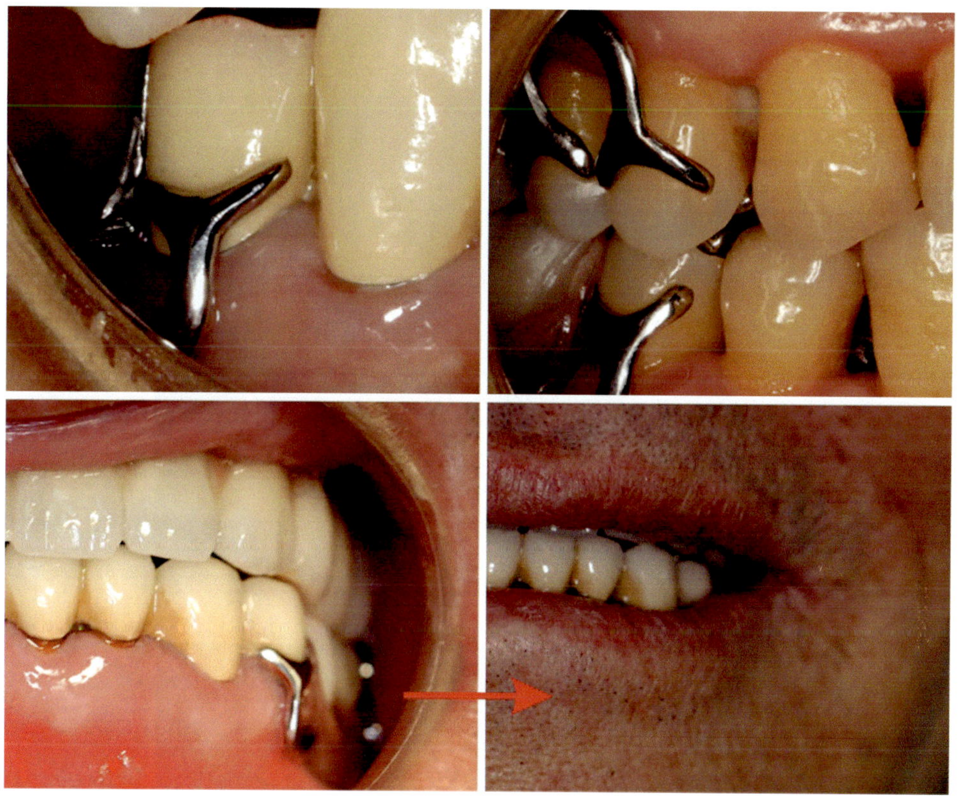

Fig. 2.15 Intraoral effect of T clasp

2.2.6 Adjacent Surface Hidden Clasp

Adjacent surface hidden clasp for the anterior tooth accomplishes retention by engaging the proximal undercut. Its crescent-shaped retentive arm originates from the distal side of palate plate, then extends into the undercut, and terminates at the proximo-buccal line angle without buccal metal exposure, so it is esthetically pleasing.

1. *Structure*

   It consists of retentive clasp and palate plate. The crescent-shaped retentive clasp is located on the proximal surface and does not extend into the buccal area (Fig. 2.16).
2. *Characteristic*

   It accomplishes retention by engaging the proximal undercut and has platelike retentive arm (Figs. 2.17 and 2.18).
3. *Indication*

   It is suitable for incisors or canines with enough proximal undercut for patients with high requirement of appearance. It has to be used in conjunction with other clasps on distal abutment due to insufficient retention. It is contraindicated in distal extension cases.

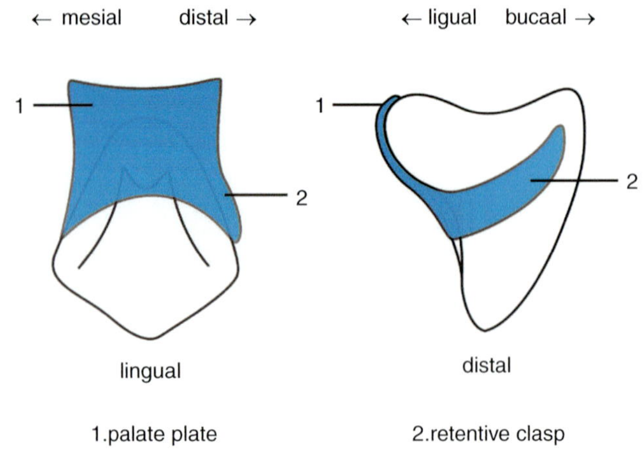

Fig. 2.16 Adjacent surface hidden clasp for anterior tooth (lingual and distal view)

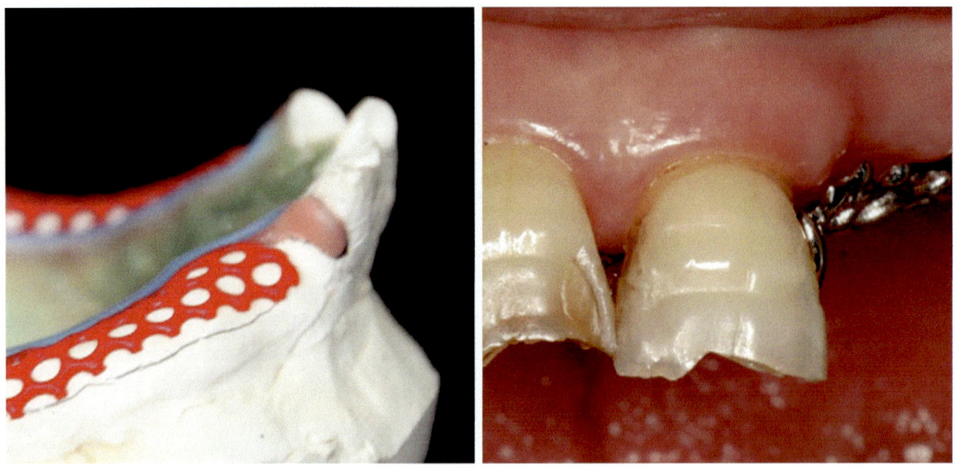

Fig. 2.17 Adjacent surface hidden clasp for anterior tooth (wax pattern and intraoral effect)

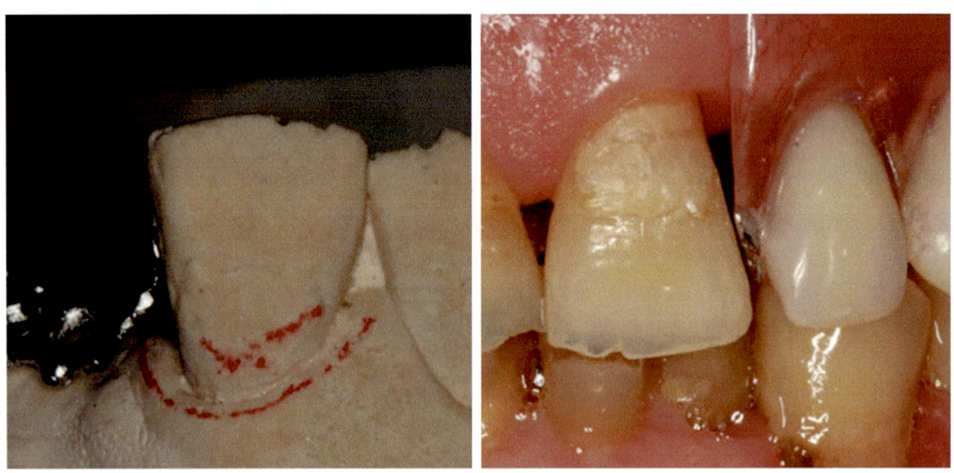

Fig. 2.18 Adjacent surface hidden clasp for the anterior tooth (effect on model and intraoral effect)

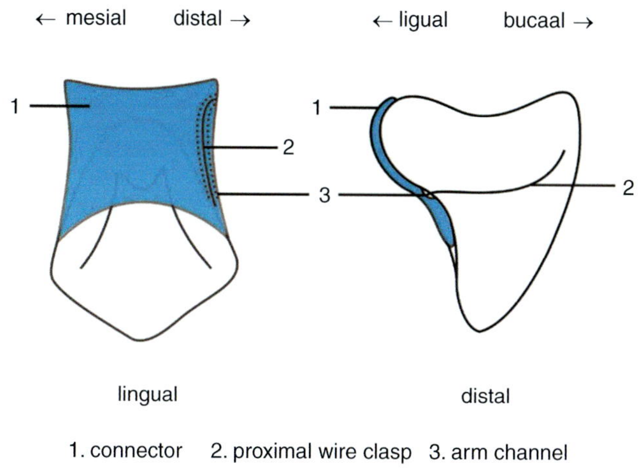

Fig. 2.19 Twin-Flex clasp (lingual and distal view)

2.2.7 Twin-Flex Clasp

Twin-Flex clasp, designed by Ticonium (USA), is a kind of e-clasp with special structure [8, 9]. There is a precast channel on the tissue surface of the metal major connector for the connector of clasp arm to pass through. It is very suitable for anterior teeth due to no buccal display of metal.

1. *Structures*

   Twin-Flex clasp consists of proximal wire clasp, minor connector, and arm channel (Fig. 2.19).
2. *Characteristics*

   The elastic retainer made of wire does not generate as much torsion to abutment, and its retention force can be adjusted. Moreover, there is little display of metal for no buccal clasp.
3. *Indication*

   Twin-Flex clasp is not suitable for deep undercut because the retentive arm is comparatively short and less elastic [10]. It can be applied only when the depth of the undercut is less than 0.25 mm. In addition, it is also suitable for the posterior teeth with insufficient buccal or lingual undercuts and has to be used in combination with other clasps. Twin-Flex clasp can be fabricated by whole-casted or the laser-welded method [9].

2.3 E-Clasp for Posterior Teeth

2.3.1 Short-Arm Embrasure Clasp

Short-arm embrasure clasp is modified from the traditional embrasure clasp. Its buccal retentive arms are shortened, and the clasp terminus lies at bucco-proximal line angle of the two adjacent abutments so as to be hidden in the embrasure. This is our design.

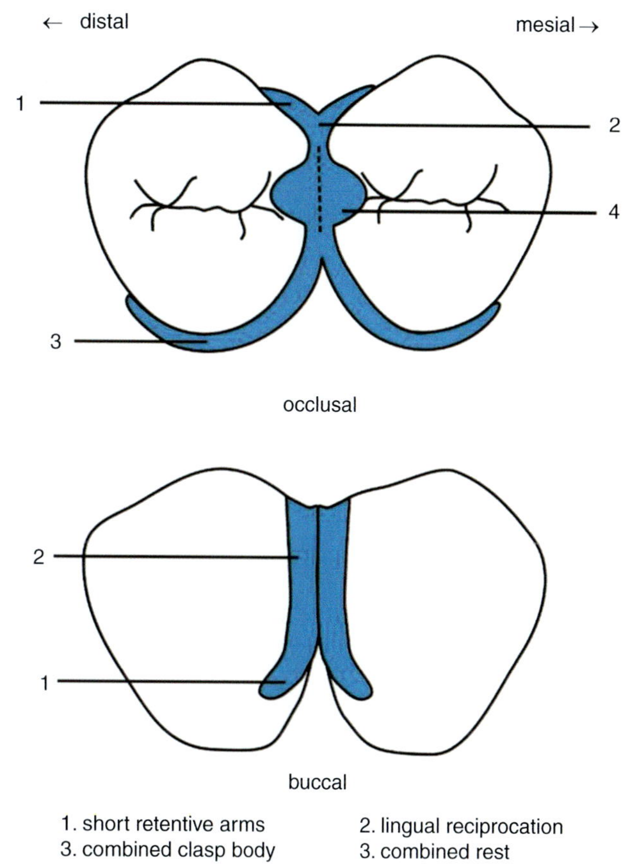

Fig. 2.20 Short-arm embrasure clasp (occlusal and buccal view)

1. *Structure*

   Short-arm embrasure clasp consists of short retentive arms, lingual reciprocation, combined clasp body, and combined rest (Fig. 2.20).
2. *Characteristics*

   The shape of the retentive arms looks similar to embrasure hook, but the difference is that there are clasp tips emerging and entering the undercuts. The two short arms which end at buccal-proximal line angle of the two adjacent abutments can provide retention while hiding in the embrasure, which enhances esthetics dramatically (Figs. 2.21 and 2.22).
3. *Indication*

   It is applied to abutments of distal extension edentulism, which are short and solid, or there is space between them.

2.3.2 Plate-bar Clasp

L clasp does harm to the abutments when applied to independent posterior abutments without adjacent teeth to reciprocation. Besides, the L retentive arm on the distal surface would be pressed down when overloaded, causing abutment rotat-

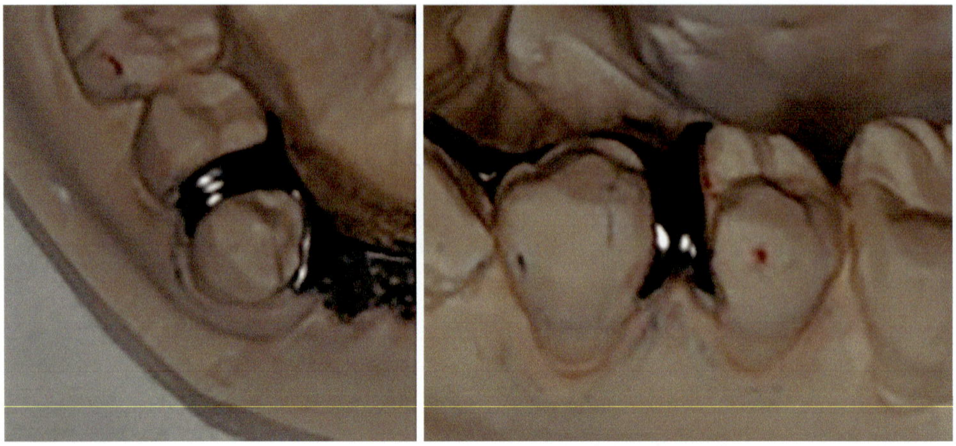

Fig. 2.21 Short retentive clasp arms (occlusal view)

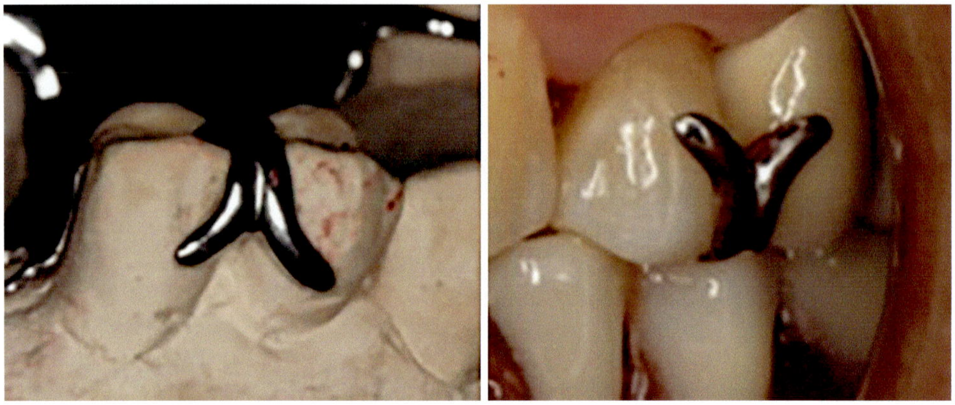

Fig. 2.22 Short-arm embrasure clasp (effect on model and intraoral effect)

ing and influencing the occlusal function. To solve this problem, plate clasp is designed to adapt to the occlusal features of posterior teeth based on the L clasp. This is also our design.

1. *Structure*

   Plate clasp consists of short retentive arm, rod-shaped connector, distal guiding plate, and mesial rest (Fig. 2.23).

2. *Characteristic*

   The rod-shaped connector projects from the major connector, connecting with the distal guiding plate, from which the short retentive arm extends. Similar to L clasp, mesial rest is separated from clasp arm (Fig. 2.24).

   The distal plate maintains plane contact with the guide surface along its path of insertion or removal, which can protect the abutment, aid retention, and prevent food impaction between abutment and denture. To ensure the elasticity of the retentive arm, the plate does not connect with the saddle.

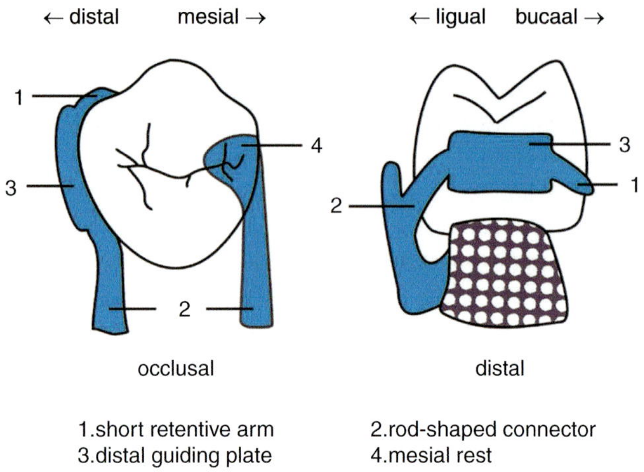

Fig. 2.23 Plate-bar clasp (occlusal and proximal view)

3. *Indication*

   It is applied to premolars and molars and is applicable for distal extension cases. A guide surface should be prepared.

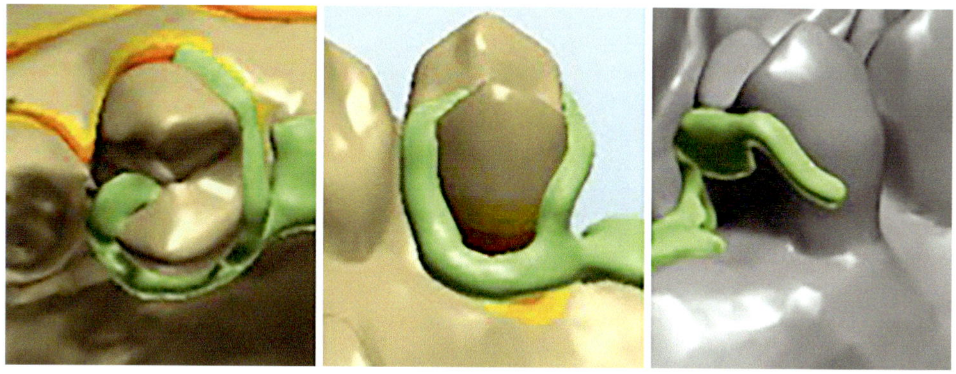

Fig. 2.24 CAD drawings of plate-bar clasp (occlusal, lingual, distal side of the buccal surface)

2.3.3 Lingually Retained Clasp

For anterior teeth, their buccal and proximal surfaces are usually taken into consideration of esthetic design due to the insufficiency of lingual retentive area. However, for posterior teeth with sufficient height, lingually retained e-clasp is an option [11]. There are three types of lingually retained clasp including lingually retained short buccal arm clasp, lingually retained L clasp, and lingually retained J clasp.

1. *Lingually retained short buccal arm clasp*

   Lingually retained short buccal arm clasp looks similar to the short buccally retained clasp. The difference is that the retentive arm of the former lays on the lingual surface, with its short reciprocation on the buccal surface, while the short retentive arm of the later is located on the buccal surface with its reciprocation on the lingual surface. Whatever, the buccal exposed clasp has to be shortened while keeping involvement of more than half of the circumference of the tooth.

   (a) *Structure*

   Lingually retained short buccal arm clasp consists of lingually retained arm, short buccal reciprocation, and distal rest (Fig. 2.25).

   (b) *Characteristic*

   The short buccal reciprocation is positioned on the distal side of the buccal axial ridge of the abutment and near the occlusal surface since it is over the contour (Figs. 2.26 and 2.27).

   (c) *Indication*

   It is often used on premolars which lie on both sides of the edentulous space and is commonly used with other types of clasps or used as indirect retainer.

2. *Lingually retained L clasp*

   There are other two kinds of lingually retained clasp, whose reciprocation is the short plate that extends to the buccal surface and connected with the occlusal connector across the occlusal surface of the two abutments instead of clasp arms. They are named lingually retained L clasp and lingually retained J clasp according their shape.

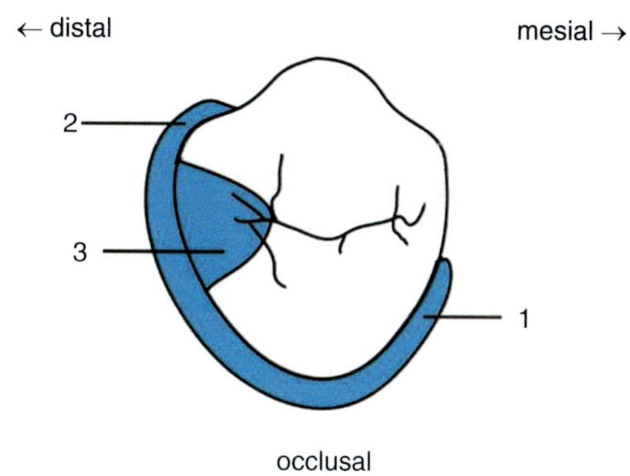

1. lingually retained arm 2. short buccal reciprocation 3. distal rest.

Fig. 2.25 Lingually retained short buccal arm clasp

   (a) *Structure*

   Lingually retained L clasp consists of occlusal rest, tiny reciprocal palate, lingual retentive arm, and occlusal connector (Fig. 2.28).

   (b) *Characteristic*

   The reciprocal arm is removed, and a tiny palate that extends to the buccal surface forms reciprocal plate instead. Its retentive arm is L-shaped from the lingual view.

   (c) *Indication*

   This clasp can be used on the abutment opposite to the space in unilateral distal extension cases. The self-cleaning of gingival papilla is weakened because of the large contact area between the lingual retentive arm and the abutment surface.

3. *Lingually retained J clasp*

   Because of the bad self-cleaning of L-type clasp, the lingual retentive arm of J-type clasp has changed from surface contact to point contact to ensure the normal self-cleaning of gingival papilla.

   (a) *Structure*

   Lingually retained J clasp consists of occlusal rest, tiny reciprocating plate, lingual retentive arm (J-type), and minor connector (Fig. 2.29).

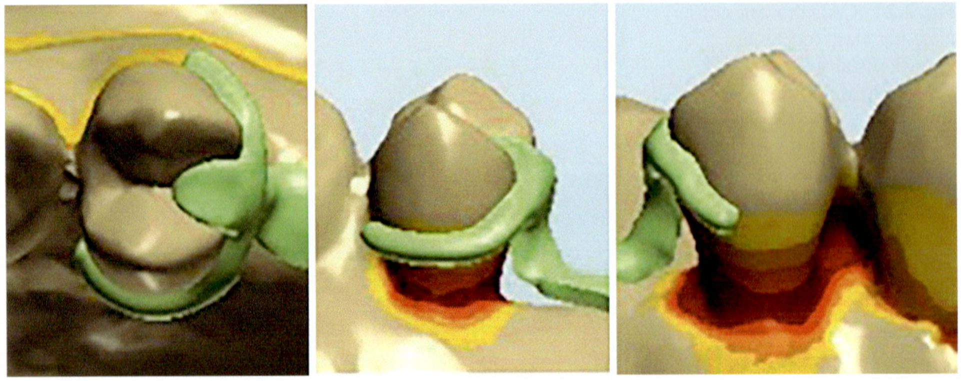

Fig. 2.26 CAD drawings of lingually retained short buccal arm clasp (occlusal, lingual, buccal)

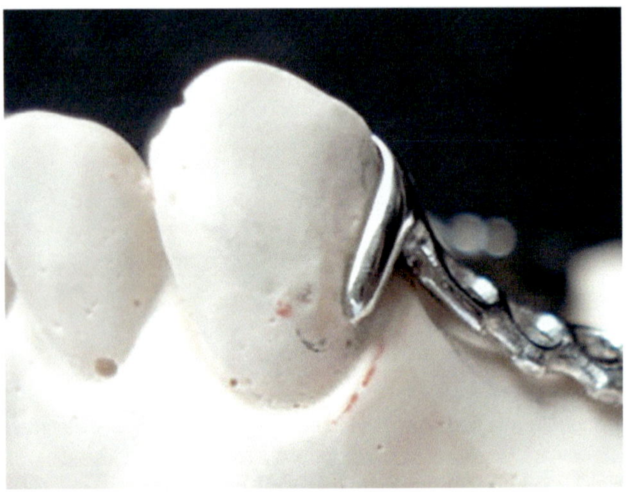

Fig. 2.27 Lingually retained short buccal arm clasp (effect on model)

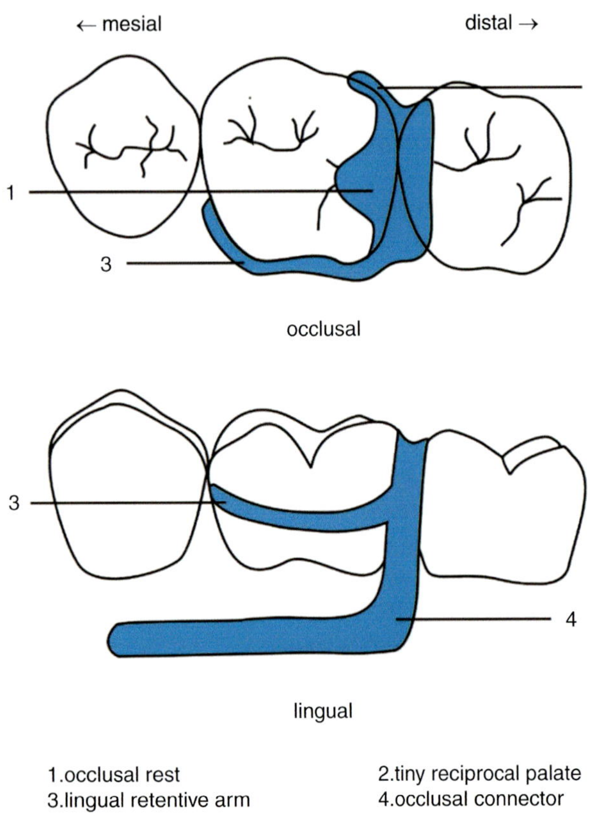

Fig. 2.28 Lingually retained L clasp (occlusal and lingual view)

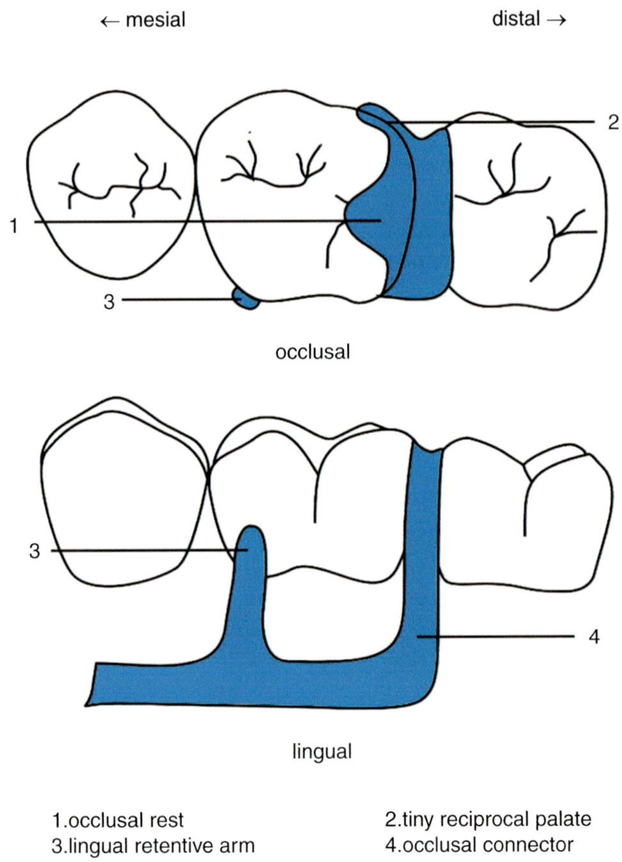

Fig. 2.29 Lingually retained J clasp (occlusal and lingual view)

(b) *Characteristic*

J-type retentive arm instead of L-type. Surface contact instead of point contact.

(c) *Indication*

Similar to L clasp, lingually retained J clasp is also applicable for abutment on the opposite arch to the space in unilateral edentulous cases. However, it requires careful consideration because of the certain loss of the retention.

2.3.4 RLS Clasp

RLS clasp (rest L-bar stabilize clasp) is another type of lingually retained e-clasp. Due to its similar structure to RPI clasp except that the I-bar is placed at the lingual undercut of the abutment, it is called "reverse RPI" and "lingual RPI" as well.

1. *Structure*
   RLS clasp consists of lingual I-bar, distal stabilizer, and mesial rest (Fig. 2.30).
2. *Characteristic*
   RLS clasp can be regarded as "reverse RPI" with mesial rest, distal stabilizer similar to guiding palate that interacts with the retainer for stability, and retentive I-bar designed on the lingual surface. It is visually satisfied without display of metal on the buccal surface (Fig. 2.31).
3. *Indication*
   It is applicable for distal extension cases on premolars or molars with appropriate lingual undercut. Alert your patient to pay special attention to oral hygiene in case of plaque deposits on the lingual surface of abutment.

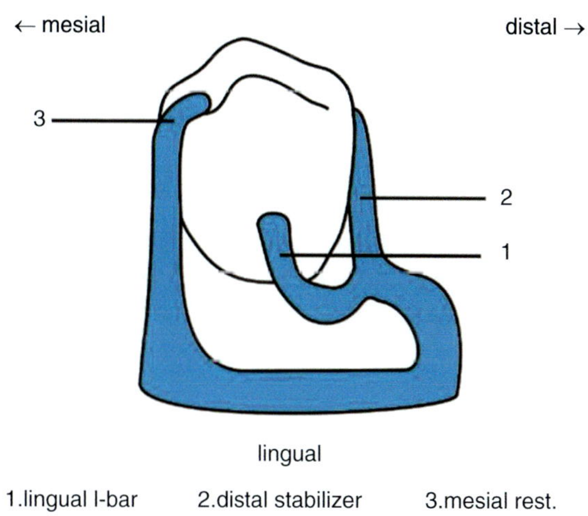

Fig. 2.30 RLS clasp (lingual view)

Fig. 2.31 CAD drawings of RLS clasp (buccal, occlusal, and lingual view)

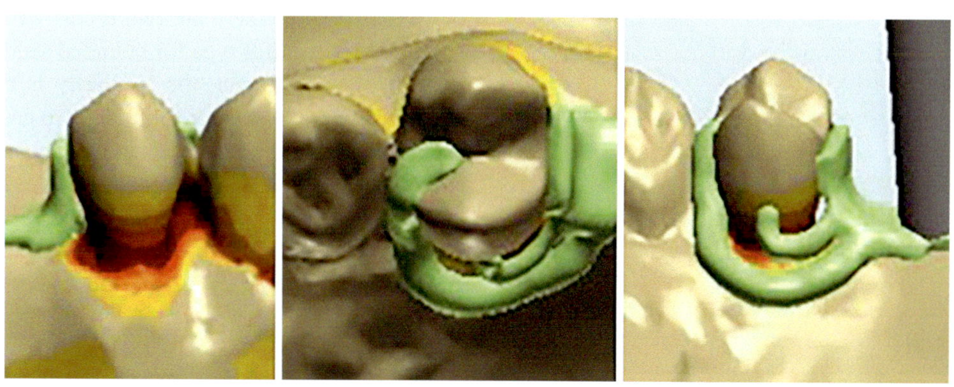

2.3.5 Terec Hidden Clasp

Terec hidden clasp, invented by TEREC dental lab, can be regarded as a separated lingually retained three-arm clasp. To obtain retention from the proximal undercut, its retentive arm has to be separated from the reciprocation and the minor connector with sufficient length to ensure elasticity as well as retention.

1. *Structure*
   Terec hidden clasp consists of proximal retentive arm, lingual reciprocation, minor connector, and occlusal rest (Fig. 2.32).
2. *Characteristic*
   The proximal retentive arm starts from the major connector, then extends beneath the lingual reciprocation, and finally hides in the proximal undercut. The minor connector is only connected with the rest and the reciprocation without contact with the proximal retentive arm.
   There is seldom buccal display of metal since only proximal undercut is used for retention, which makes it visually satisfied. There are also disadvantages including its complex structure that is difficult for fabrication, insufficient undercut, and low elasticity of cast clasp that may cause permanent deformation (Fig. 2.33).
3. *Indication*
   Appropriate undercut at proximal surface that is near the edentulous space is necessary because of the complex proximal structure. It is applicable for distal extension cases considering its stress-interrupting design that separates retainer and reciprocation (Fig. 2.34).

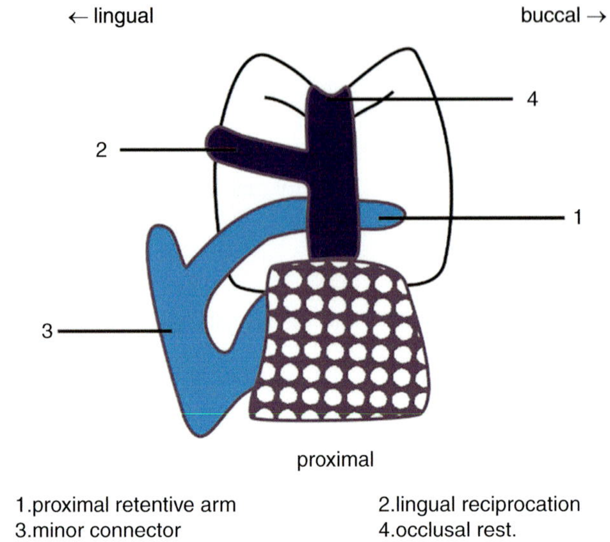

Fig. 2.32 Terec hidden clasp (proximal view)

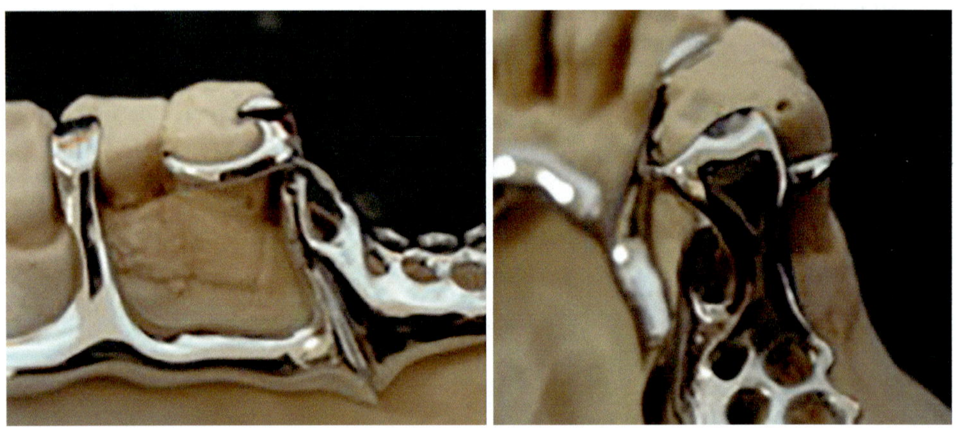

Fig. 2.33 Terec hidden clasp on model (lingual and proximal view)

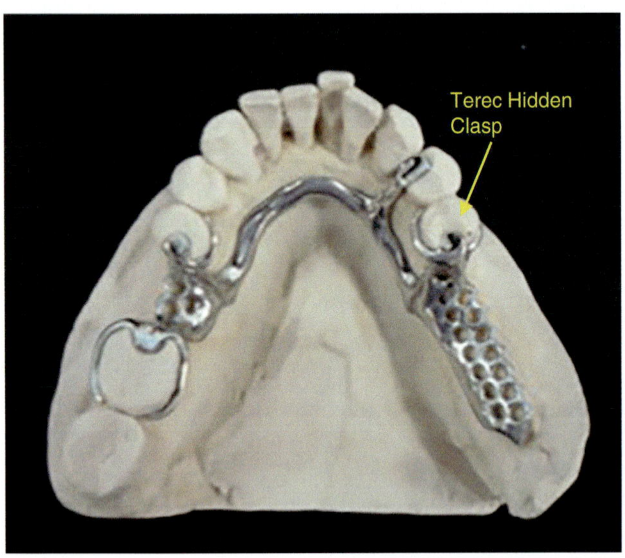

Fig. 2.34 Terec hidden clasp applied to distal extension edentulism

2.3.6 Saddle-Lock Clasp

The saddle-lock clasp is an e-clasp system designed for the elasticity of the retentive arm and named after its inventor saddle-lock dental lab [12].

There are two types—A type for distal extension saddle and B type for bounded saddle. Though their indications are different, the similarity is that both of them have an arm channel for the retainer to pass, which means that the guiding plate and the retentive arm are separated though they do contact to each other. And the main difference is if the rest is connected to the plate.

1. *Type A Saddle-Lock Clasp*
   (a) *Structure*

   Elastic retentive arm, reciprocal plate (when there are spaces on both sides of abutment and no adjacent tooth to provide reciprocation), guiding plate, mesial rest (Fig. 2.35).

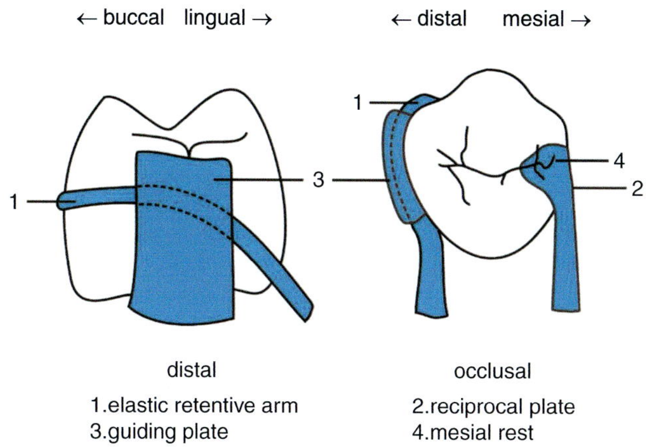

Fig. 2.35 Type A saddle-lock clasp (distal and occlusal view)

(b) *Characteristic*

The retentive arm starts from the major connector, passes through the channel in the plate, and ends at the distobuccal line angle or proximal-buccal line angle. There is no contact between the retainer and the plate, so the arm has a tensile elastic range. The mesial rest moves toward the gingival to decrease its torque to protect the abutment while masticating.

(c) *Indication*

It is applicable for last abutment of distal extension. To ensure sufficient space for the retainer and the plate, appropriate height of the abutment is needed (4–5 mm from marginal ridge to gingival papilla is desirable).

If the distal abutment of bounded saddle is diagnosed loose and is risky to be lost, A-type saddle-lock clasp is suggested.

2. *Type B Saddle-Lock Clasp*

B-type saddle-lock clasp is applicable for bounded saddle, and it has two types—type I and type II.

When there is remaining teeth on the mesial side of the abutment that provide reciprocation, the mesial rest can be removed and directly connected to the distal plate. This is type I (Fig. 2.36), and it can be placed on the mesial abutment beside the edentulous space.

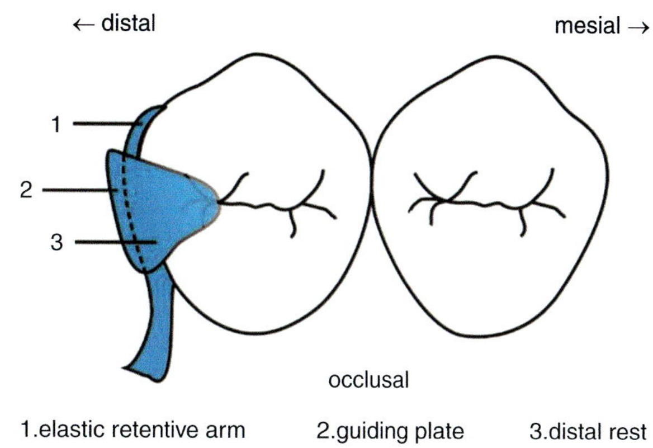

Fig. 2.36 Type B saddle-lock clasp (I) (occlusal view)

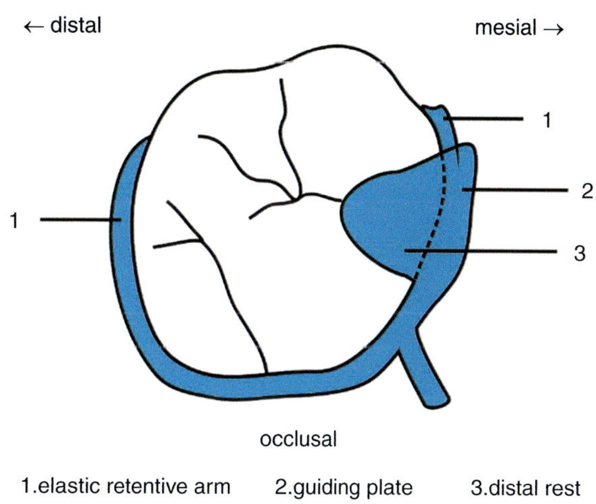

Fig. 2.37 Type B saddle-lock clasp (II) (occlusal view)

For distal abutment, type II is suggested. Its reciprocation is obtained from the lingual arm encircling around the distal surface of the abutment (Fig. 2.37).

2.4 Comparison

It is easy to be confused when the prosthodontists clinically use several kinds of e-clasp similar in shape, and for better understanding, the comparison of the characteristic is shown as take-home messages in Fig. 2.38.

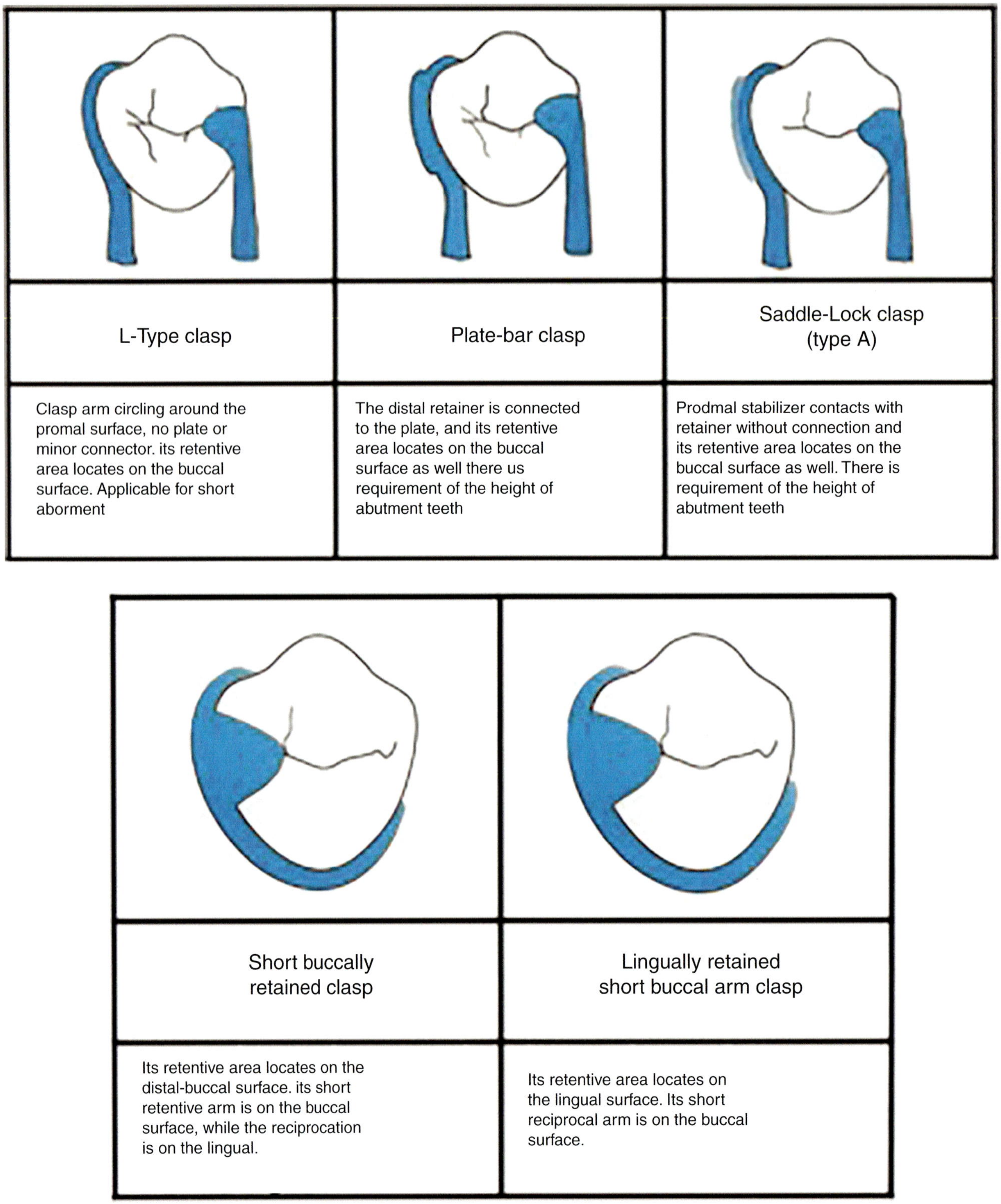

Fig. 2.38 Similar-looking e-clasps

References

1. Chu CH, Chow TW. Esthetic designs of removable partial dentures. Gen Dent. 2003;51(4):322–4.
2. Donovan TE, Cho GC. Esthetic considerations with removable partial dentures. J Calif Dent Assoc. 2003;31(7):551–7.
3. Cibirka RM, Lefebvre C, Goldstein RE. Esthetic removable partial dentures. In: Goldstein RE, editor. Esthetics in dentistry, vol. 2. 2nd ed. Hamilton: B.C. Deker; 2002. p. 669–702.
4. Beaumont AJ. An overview of esthetics with RPDs. J Quintessence Int. 2002;33(10):747–55.
5. Vallittu PK, Kokkonen M. Deflection fatigue of a cobalt-chromium, titanium and gold alloy cast denture clasp. J Prosthet Dent. 1995;74(4):412–9.
6. Tannous F, Steiner M, Shahin R. Retentive forces and fatigue resistance of thermoplastic resin clasps. J Dental Mater. 2012;28(3):273–8.
7. Oh WS, Basho S. Esthetic removable partial denture design in replacing maxillary antetior teeth. J Gen Dent. 2010;58(6):252–6.
8. Perezous LF. The twin-flex clasp: An esthetic removable partial denture approach. J Prosthod. 2003;12(4):325.
9. Mansueto MA, Phoenis RD. The Twin-flex removable partial denture: design, fabrication, and clinical usage. J Prosthod. 1998;7(4):268–72.
10. Santana-Penín U, Mora MJ. An esthetically attractive twin-flex clasp for removable partial dentures. J Prosthet Dent. 1998;80(3):367–70.
11. Brudvik JS, Palacios R. Lingual retention and the elimination of the visible clasp arm. J Esthet and Restor Dent. 2007;19(5):247–54.
12. Cherkas L, Jaslow E. Saddle lock hidden clasp partial dentures. J Compend Cotin Educ Dent. 1991;12(10):746–75.

3 Clinical Pathway of Esthetic Clasp Technology

The clinical pathway of esthetic clasp technology is very important for clinicians to design esthetic clasp on RPDs conveniently. The process can be carried out successfully as long as clinicians follow it.

The purpose of this chapter is to help clinicians to complete the clinical process of esthetic clasp technology and provide patients a perfect or compromised esthetic RPD denture

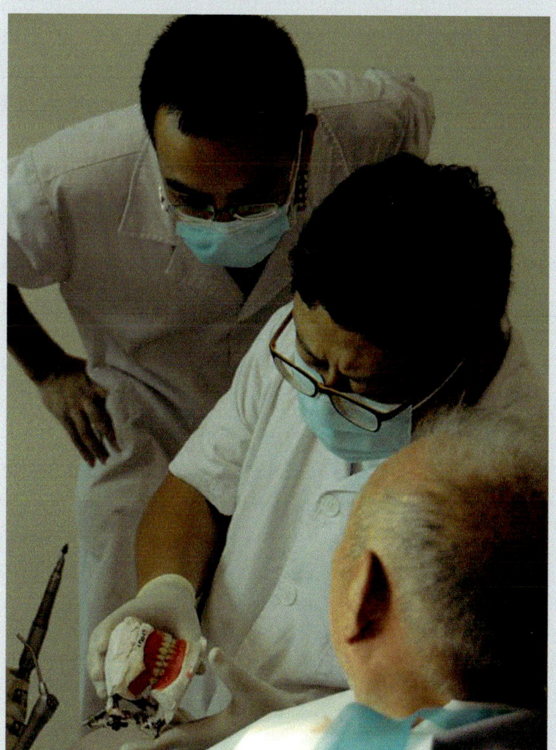

3.1 The First Visit

3.1.1 Reception

1. *Record essential information and complaints.* When edentulous patients first come to your dental office, they should be welcomed friendly and led to a dental chair. Then clinicians are supposed to ask and record the essential information of the patients, including name, gender, age, and contact way [1].

   Obtain the authentic details, for example, whether the patient has systemic or contagious disease, such as hepatitis B, AIDS, etc. Patients with heart disease, hypertension, and other systemic diseases need real-time monitoring and special clinical skills.

   Record patient's chief complaint (Fig. 3.1), and exam oral condition preliminarily.
2. *Oral examination.* The content of oral examination including:
   (a) *Missing teeth*: Record the position of the missing teeth by site recording method.
   (b) *Loose teeth*: Check and record the mobility of remaining teeth.

      I°loose: The mobility in the buccolingual direction is within 1 mm, and in other directions, there's no moving.

      II° loose: There are two types. One is the mobility in buccolingual direction between 1 and 2 mm, and the other is that the tooth in two directions (buccolingual and mesiodistal) has mobility.

      III° loose: There are also two types. One is the teeth with buccolingual direction mobility of more than 2 mm. The other is that the tooth is movable in three directions (buccal lingual, mesial, vertical)
   (c) *Teeth*: Check whether there is movement, inclination, and elongation in remaining teeth. Whether there is occlusal interference. First, make sure if orthodontic

H. Yu, *Digital Removable Partial Denture Technology*, https://doi.org/10.1007/978-981-19-7923-1_3

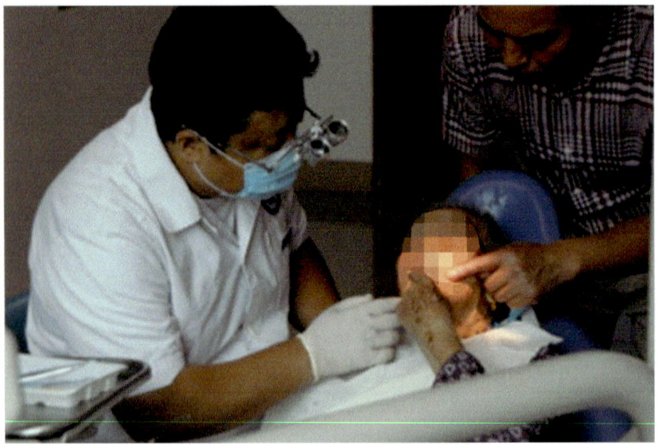

Fig. 3.1 Reception and record basic information and complaint

treatment is necessary. If there's too much grinding capacity for severely elongated and inclined teeth, clinicians can do root canal therapy first. Then regain the natural occlusal curve by a full crown prosthesis.

(d) *Dentin*: Check the defection and caries on remaining teeth—whether there's wedge-shaped defection or percussed pain. Check whether there's probing or percussion. Clinicians can estimate with the dental radiograph.

(e) *Dental periphery*: Check the condition of the periodontium, including bacterial plaque, dental calculus, periodontosis, gingiva, and gingival recession. If there's too much bacterial plaque or bad oral condition, clinicians should do periodontal scaling treatment before prosthetic treatment.

(f) *Mucous*: Check whether the color of mucous is normal. Estimate if the patient has a mucous disease.

(g) *Other oral treatments*: Ask patients if they have received other oral treatment before, and check the effect, for example, if the tooth extraction wound is healed and fixed denture is well preserved. If the patient accepted root canal therapy, clinicians should estimate the periapical condition by dental radiograph.

Before restoration, the oral condition should meet the following requirements:

(i) Necessary surgical procedure is finished (remove residual root and III°loose tooth).
(ii) No defective denture.
(iii) No pulposis; The defect tooth has been repaired.
(iv) Periodontal disease has been treated perfectly. Dental calculus and tartar have been removed completely.
(v) No mucous disease. The condition of oral mucous is good.
(vi) Optimal designed necessary orthodontic treatment is finished (correct over inclination tooth).

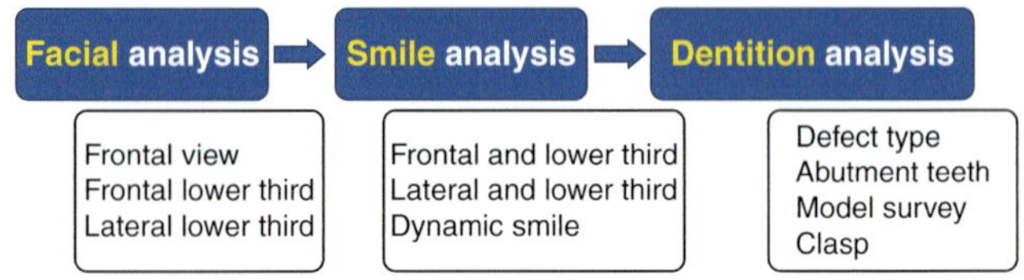

Fig. 3.2 Three major parts of analysis and design process

3.1.2 Analysis Design

After the reception, clinicians can begin the second step flow analysis design. This procedure includes analysis and design based on patients' facial features, smile, and dentition (Fig. 3.2). Analysis and design play a decisive role in the final esthetic effect of a removable denture.

1. *Facial analysis*: The first step of analysis is facial analysis, which means observing facial features at rest position, estimating, and information recording.

(a) *Frontal view*

(i) *The height of the lower third of the face*

According to the rule of thirds, make a line along with the patient's glabella and subnasal, which separates the face into three equal parts horizontally: the upper third (hair line to glabella), the medium third (glabella to subnasal), and the lower third (subnasal to gnathion) (Fig. 3.3). When the patient loses too many teeth, the height of lower third face would be short. This can be used to confirm the height of the lower third face.

(ii) *Position and form of facial reference points and lines*

Nasolabial groove: Nasolabial groove consists of a nasal groove (lateral nasal depression) and labiofacial groove (diagonal depression between the upper lip and genal region) (Fig. 3.4). Patients with deep nasolabial grooves might give others an aging impression.

Angulus oris: Observe the coordinate position of angulus oris in the face horizontally.

Rima oris: It is the horizontal fissure between upper and lower lips. Observe the feature of rima oris at rest position (concave, horizontal, convex) before prosthetic treatment.

(b) *Frontal lower third*

The vertical range of the frontal lower face is from the nasal tip to gnathion. Its significance is to help observe the proportion of the upper lip and lower lip. According to the lower third proportion, the rate of the distance between subnasal and rima oris and the distance between rima oris and gnathion should close

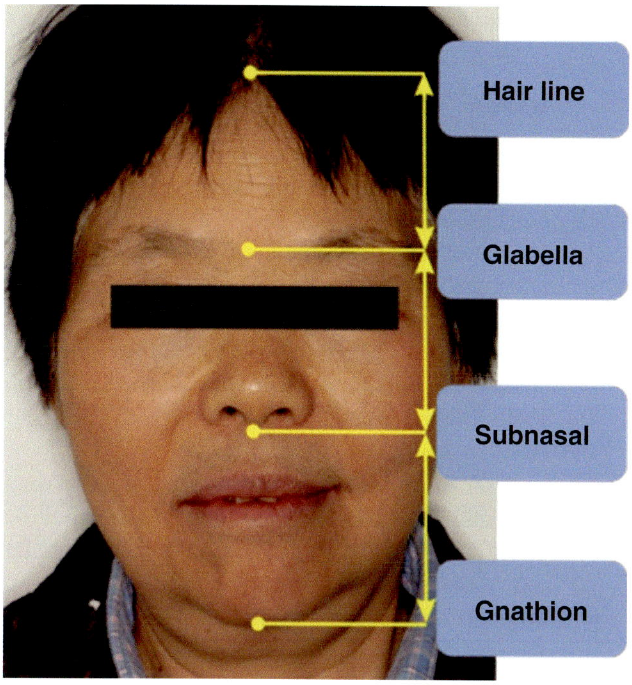

Fig. 3.3 Frontal view (long tri-stop)

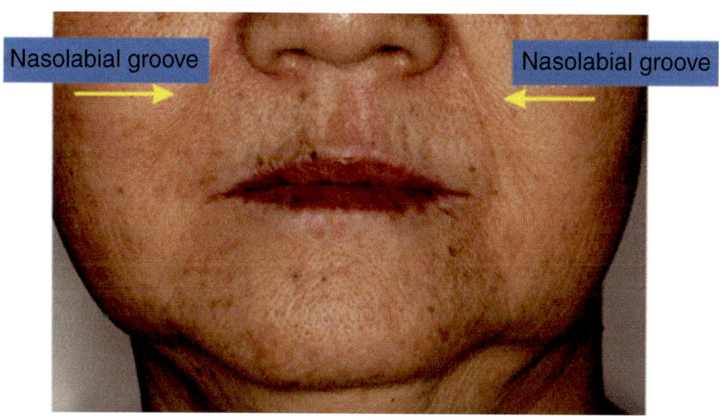

Fig. 3.4 Nasolabial groove and rima oris

1:2 (Fig. 3.5). The insufficient height of lower 1/3 face may be caused when the two parts are all too short.

(c) *Lateral lower third*

The vertical range of frontal lower face is the same with frontal lower third face, including nasal tip and gnathion. And the angle includes 45°and 90°:

(i) *Lateral lower third face in 45°*

Philtrum: Observe whether philtrum and philtrum ridge (the parallel skin ridges along with philtrum) is depression inward, droop, or asymmetry. If the fatness of philtrum is insufficient, clinicians can restore facial profile by proper thickness base plate (Fig. 3.6).

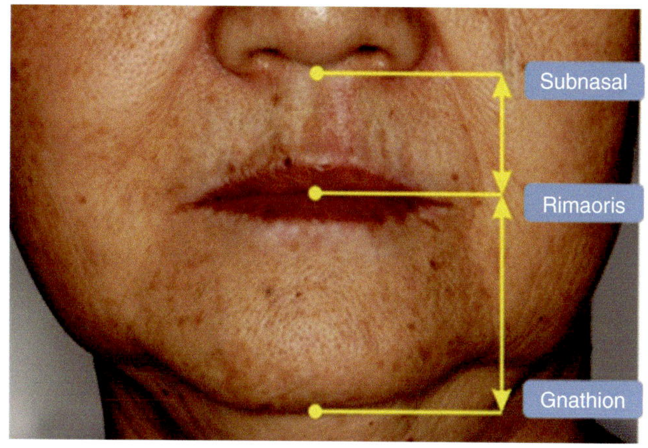

Fig. 3.5 Frontal lower third face (short tri-stop)

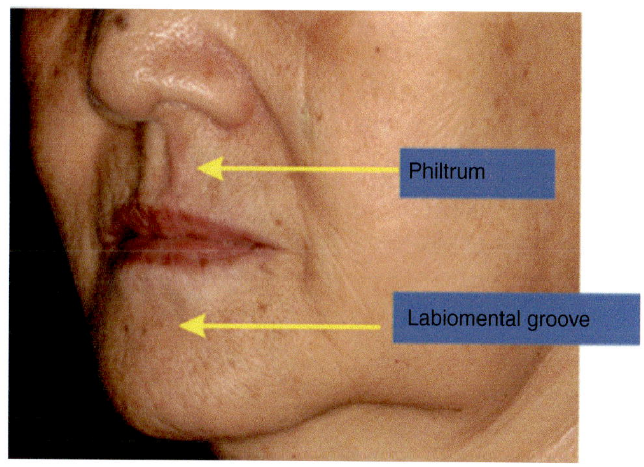

Fig. 3.6 Lateral lower third face in 45° (philtrum, labiomental groove)

Labiomental groove: Observe whether the horizontal depression between the lower lip and the mental region is sunken (Fig. 3.6).

(ii) *Lateral lower third face in 90°*

Lateral tri-stop: Draw lines from the center of tragus to the midpoint of hair line, glabella, nasal tip, and pogonion, which form three angles. It fits in with estheticism when the difference is less than 10°.

Ricketts esthetic line: The lower lip should set on the line from patient's nasal tip and pogonion (Fig. 3.7).

Nasolabial angle: The normal angle between the nasal columella and the upper lip is 90°–100°, which helps estimate fullness of the upper lip should be restored.

Nasomental: Clinicians can restore patient's vertical height of lower 1/3 face by estimating the optimum nasomental. Draw two lines from

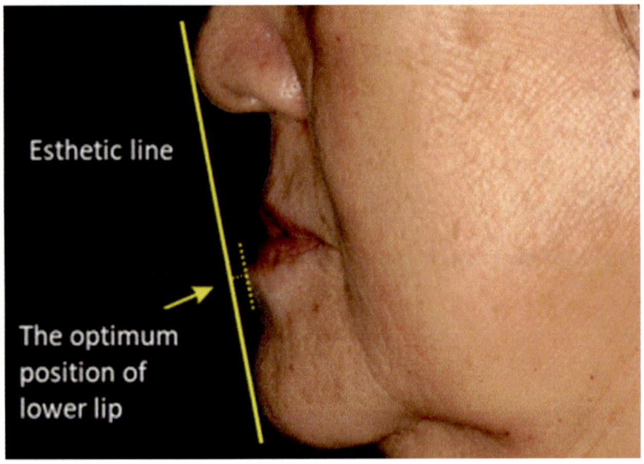

Fig. 3.7 Lateral lower third face in 90° (esthetic line)

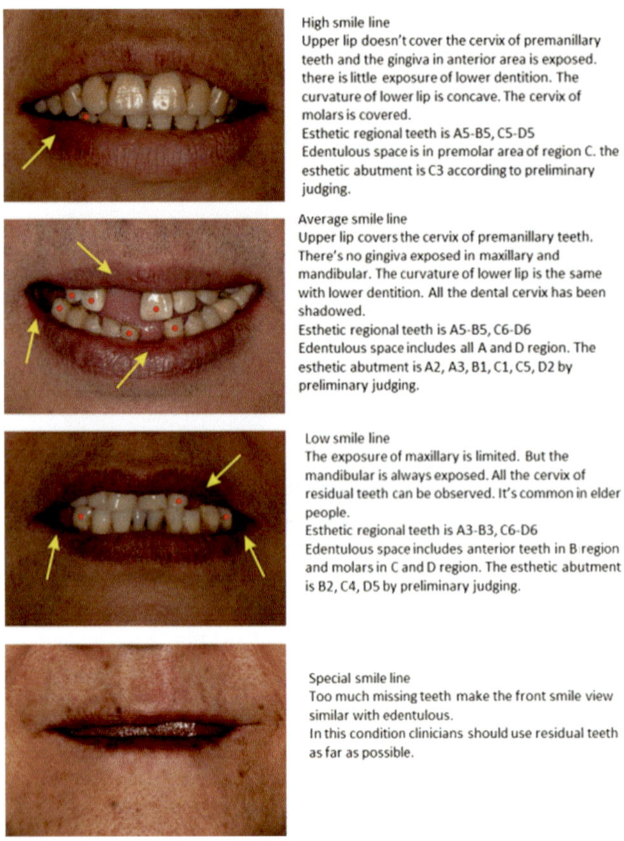

Fig. 3.8 Static smile analysis (frontal lower 1/3 face)

the nasal tip to nasion and gnathion, which intersect and form nasomental, whose normal range is 120°–132°.

2. *Smile analysis*

When the facial analysis is finished, the next step is to analyze smile [2]. Observe smile exposed area, estimate teeth in esthetic zone, and provide a reference to selecting esthetic abutment (Fig. 3.8).

(a) *Frontal lower third*

Observe the smile exposing area before prosthetic treatment. Choose the smile line type. Then analyze the explosion of tooth tissue and soft tissue. Record the esthetic teeth. At last, choose the esthetic abutment according to the gap position.

(b) *Lateral lower 1/3 face*

Lateral lower 1/3 face in 45°and 90° is auxiliary reference of front feature. Observe the exposure of esthetic abutment laterally by estimating the esthetic regional teeth when the patient smiles. Besides, observe the facial sufficient signs when the patient smiles (Figs. 3.9 and 3.10).

(c) *Dynamic smile analysis*

After finishing analyzing the static oral exposing area, clinicians can observe the exposure condition when patient opens and closes the mouth naturally and speaks and smiles by communicating with them. Through this procedure, clinicians can choose the abutment and the type of esthetic clasp.

Because of the variability of dynamic smile, we can record it dynamically by camera, to obtain abundant and accurate information. Hold the camera in the same horizontal plane with patient's lower 1/3 face. Both frontal and lateral views should be recorded. Let patient read a paragraph of words or have a conversation, to record the dynamic image of lips meanwhile. It helps clinicians and technicians to select the optimum denture, the position, the type of clasp, and the color of the base by watching the video.

Video recording is an important case data. It is also the reference for next prosthetic treatment. From now on, the second part of the analysis-smile analysis is complete. The main processes are presented in Fig. 3.11:

3. *Dentition analysis*

The third part of analysis and design is dentition analysis, which means analyzing patient's study cast, because different types of dentition defects are corresponding to different design rules. First, determine the type of dentition defect. Then confirm abutments by analyzing esthetic abutment and study cast. The esthetic retention area in abutment can be confirmed by model surveying. At last select optimum esthetic clasp according to esthetic retention.

Select a proper tray to get a model for patient. It can not only help clinicians to analyze dentition and make custom tray but also be preserved as record model. It serves multiple purposes.

(a) *Types of dentition and design rules*

Dentition defect includes missing one tooth to remaining one tooth. There are many classification methods. We can't introduce them in details one by

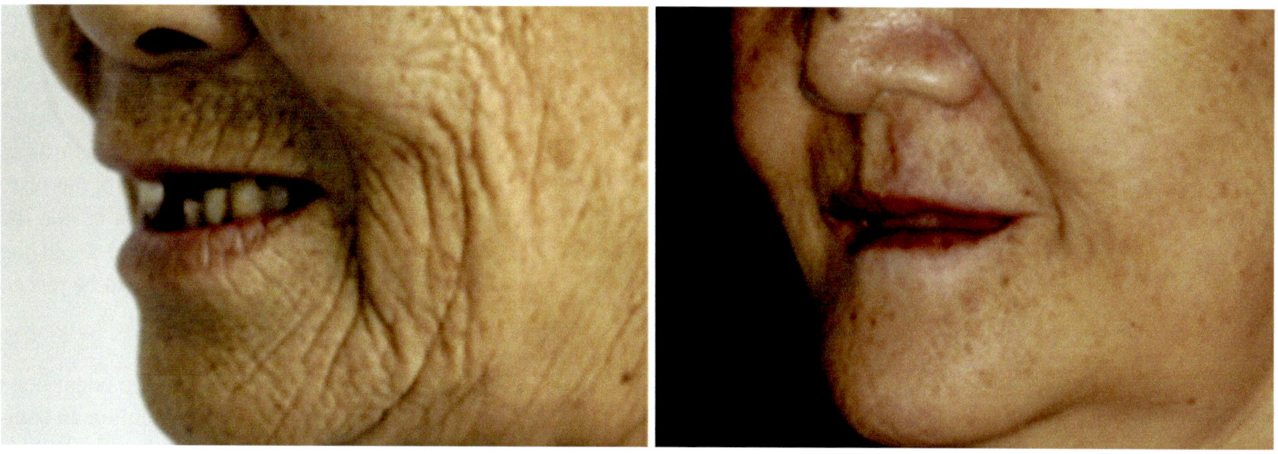

Fig. 3.9 Static smile analysis (lateral lower face in 45°)

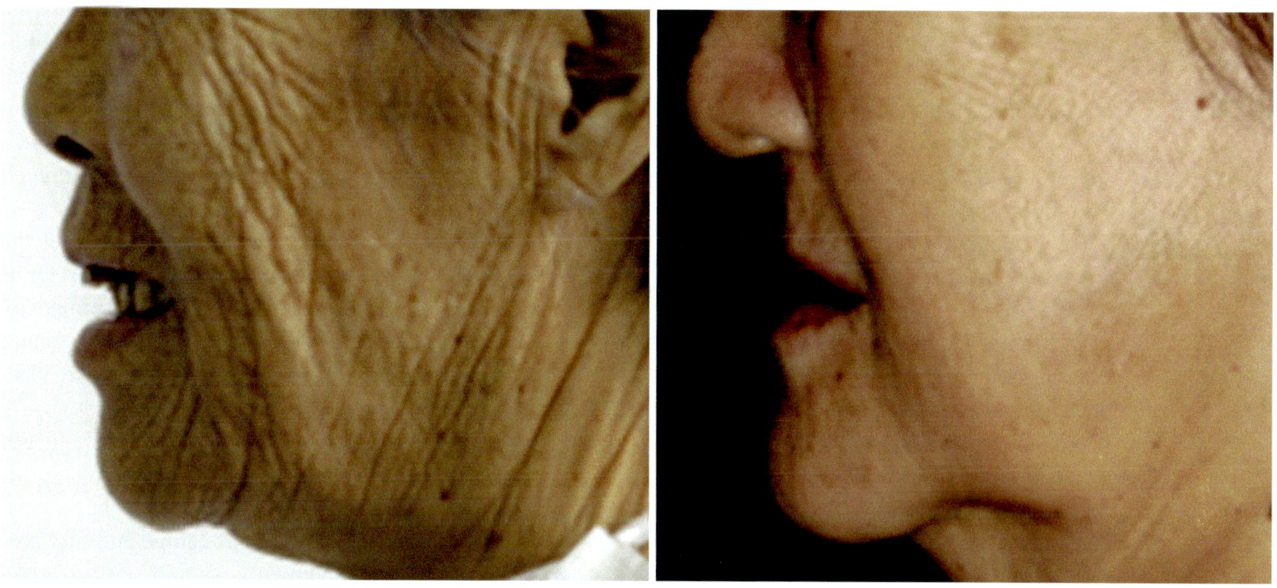

Fig. 3.10 Static smile analysis (lateral lower face in 90°)

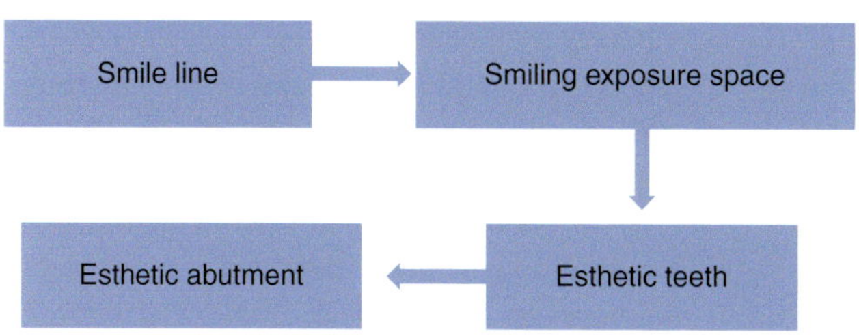

Fig. 3.11 Key point of smile analysis

one. Now, we introduce Kennedy dentition defect classification [1]. The main design points are as follows:

(i) *Kennedy classes I and II distal extension*:

Where tooth support is considered inadequate, additional mucosal support should be planned. When mucosal support is used, an attempt should be made to reduce the load acting on the tissue [3]. This may be achieved by extending the fitting surface of the denture as widely as possible and by reducing the number or the width of the teeth on the denture.

When there're many remaining teeth and the oral condition is good, combined support can be considered mucosal and teeth support. The design of teeth and mucosa-supported RPD is the most complex. Improper design can lead to abutment loose, mucous tenderness, and alveolar bone absorbing. When designing this kind of RPD, clinicians should pay attention to three "reduces":

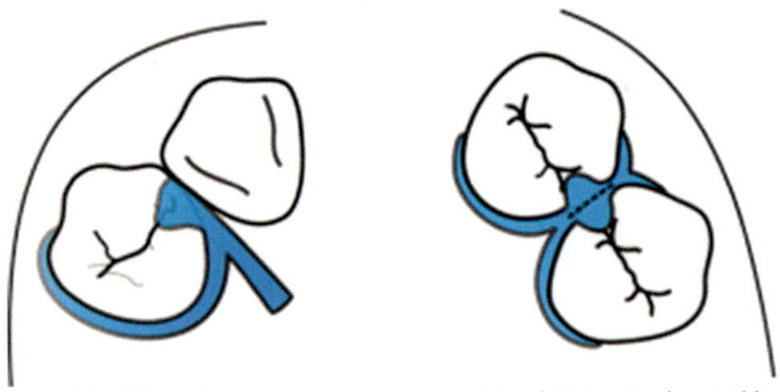

Fig. 3.12 Reduce the denture sinking

Reduce sinking: The rest at the mesial abutment of edentulous space should be designed at mesial as far as possible to confirm lever effort. Clinicians can also combine retainer in two abutments in the mesial side of edentulous space to improve retention (Fig. 3.12). The distal extension edentulous space should be impressed under pressure. The fitting surface should be relined in time when the denture is used a period of time.

Reduce revolving: Set indirect retainer in the opposite of fulcrum. It should be away from distal extension base as far as possible. Enlarge base properly to make the bases on both sides of arch restrict each other.

Reduce swing: Big connecter with rigid connection can resist swing. Reduce the width of the teeth and the height of cusps. Set proximal plate on the distal surface of abutment at the proximal edentulous space.

(ii) *Kennedy class III nondistal extension*:

There are teeth both at the head and the back of the edentulous space in Kennedy class III defect, which indicates the type of the denture is tooth support [4]. This kind of support method can provide great retention, support, and stabilization. There's one point to pay attention to: we can choose the invisible denture only when the gap is small. We should avoid designing unilateral denture—there's denture only on one side of the dental arch to avoid the coronal rotation of the denture.

(iii) *Kennedy class IV anterior defect*:

Kennedy class IV dentition means the losing of anterior teeth. An esthetic abutment is generally located in the esthetic area [5]. From an esthetic point of view, the design of the buccal clasp should be avoided in the edentulous side abutment, as well as the design of proximal retain clasp (anterior proximal plate clasp, Twin-Flex clasp). The proximal retain clasp must be used with other clasps because it can't meet the requirement of retention. The traditional clasp can be placed in the unesthetic area.

If there are not many missing teeth, the plate will be only placed on the abutment beside the edentulous space. If not, in order to avoid the subsidence of the denture, rest should be placed on the abutment.

(b) *Selecting abutment*

(i) Select the abutment adjacent to the edentulous space preferentially. Improve retention and stability and reduce denture structure.
(ii) When the patient has fewer teeth (less than four), clinicians should try to make as full use of every abutment as possible. When there's a large number of remaining teeth in good condition, the number of abutment has to be less than 4. An overcomplex framework structure is not conducive for patient to wear and clean. What's more, because of the increase of lateral force, it may cause periodontal trauma.
(iii) The distribution of abutment should meet the requirement of three-point distribution as far as possible. The center of the plane formed by direct retainers should be located in the center of the denture, which helps to achieve ideal stability.
(iv) On the basis of reasonable design, try to use wrapped clasp at nonesthetic area.
(v) Try to choose the abutments with large periodontal members, such as canine and first premolar. The abutments should be in good periodontal condition. If the patient has dental calculus or periodontal disease, it is suggested that the treatment should be done after periodontal treatment. The long axis direction of abutment should be vertical with the bite force. Increase periodontal potential. Reduce excess load on abutments.
(vi) Try to choose the abutments with complete crown, good retention form, and a certain depth of concave and concave slope. The wrap of clasp to caries tooth can influence its self-cleaning effect and accelerate the decay process. So treatment must be done first for this kind of abutment. In the case of defective abutment, the shape of the retainer should be restored by inlay or filling.
(vii) Teeth with endodontic disease must be treated with root canal therapy before loading. The hard tissue of devital teeth has low strength, and

the stress of the retainer may lead to fracture. Therefore, the application of post core and crown prosthesis is necessary to strengthen the devital teeth. Dentin hypersensitivity tooth shouldn't be selected as abutment if it is still sensitive to external stimulation after desensitization.

(c) *Model surveying*

Determinate the insertion path of removable partial denture, and control the factors affecting the selection of insertion path by surveyor called model surveying [1] (Fig. 3.13). Surveying is the key step in designing removable denture. The main purpose of model surveying in esthetic clasp technology is to determine the esthetic retention area.

The surveyor essentially comprises a vertical rod that is held perpendicular to a horizontal platform which can be adjusted on the 3D direction. The rod can be moved horizontally, up and down. It represents the path along which the denture is inserted and removed. The path of insertion can be altered by changing the tilt of the model on the horizontal plane. By positioning this vertical rob against the teeth and soft tissue area on the model, their morphology can be examined.

(i) *Positioning esthetic insertion path*

There are three main factors that affect the esthetic insertion path: retention area, interference area, and esthetics [6].

Retention area: The existence of undercut provides the retention force. The area of undercut in every abutment should be distributed equally, which means it shouldn't be very deep on some abutment and very shallow on others.

In addition, the guide plane can provide partial retention by rubbing with the tooth. The guide plane should be parallel to the insertion path and each other.

Interference: Tooth and soft tissue may be formed so as to physically obstruct the RPD along an otherwise appropriate path of insertion. The common interference area includes the dentin lingual tilted area (Fig. 3.14). The effect of positioning can be eliminated by modification in general. However, if there is much grinding, it should be restored by a full crown prosthesis, or change the location of denture units.

Esthetic: For the loss of anterior teeth, if the undercut of the tooth adjacent to edentulous space is too deep, clinicians can adjust the insertion path to reduce nonesthetic gap (Fig. 3.15).

After facial analysis and smile analysis, clinicians should know the position of esthetic retention area fairly well. For example, in order not to expose the metal, the only adjacent surface can be used in A2. Only a little bit of the distal-buccal axis ridge can be shadowed to rely

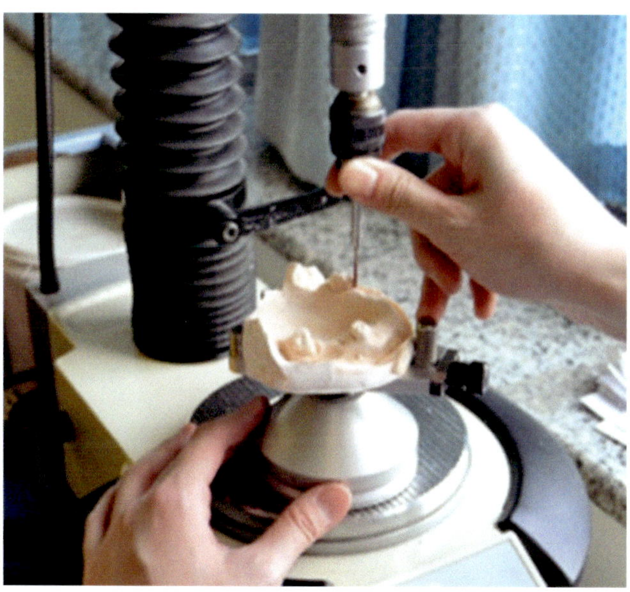

Fig. 3.13 Model surveying

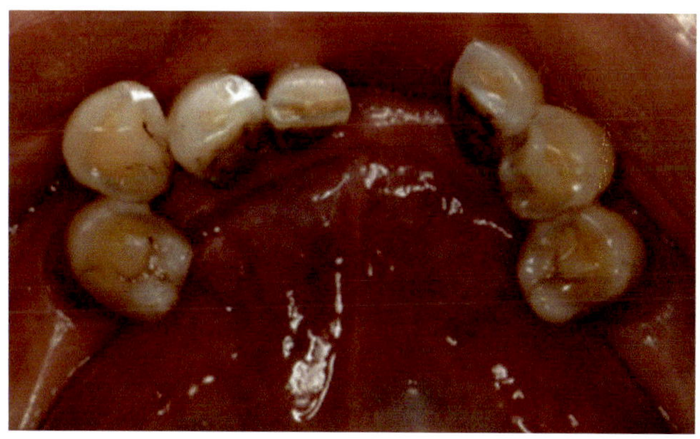

Fig. 3.14 Lingual abutment

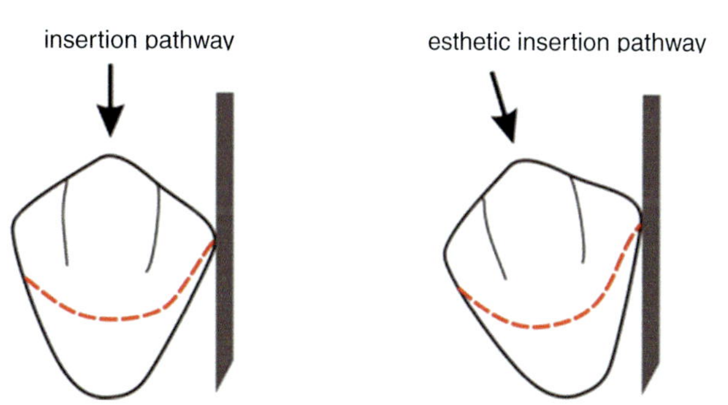

Fig. 3.15 Esthetic insertion pathway to reduce anterior gap

on dentin in A3. The dental convex can be covered by the lip completely in A4. According to these judgments, survey esthetic abutment, position esthetic insertion path, and check the depth and slope of retention area.

Esthetic insertion path focuses more on esthetic factors. Meanwhile, other factors must also meet the requirement of clinical practice.

(ii) *Drawing esthetic survey line*

Once the path of insertion has been decided upon, the final design of the prosthesis can be completed. The contour line formed by joining points of maximum bulbosity on the teeth or soft tissue is termed the "survey line." There are many kinds of survey lines on one model. The choosing of survey lines depends on physician's experience and the emphasis of denture design.

All the inelastic parts of the denture should be located above the survey line. Only the elastic parts like clasp tip can extend under the survey line. If the path of insertion and removal are not in the same direction, the terminus of the clasp should enter the common undercut area (Fig. 3.16).

(iii) *Confirming esthetic retention area*

Confirm esthetic retention area by esthetic survey line. Commonly, the clinical esthetic retention area includes distofacial undercut, cervical third, and proximal undercut [5] (Fig. 3.17).

(d) *Choosing esthetic clasp*

According to the tooth surface in esthetic retention, choose an esthetic clasp [7] (Fig. 3.18). Then on the basis of esthetic abutment (anterior, molar), confirm the type of the esthetic clasp at last.

From now on, the dentition analysis is finished completely. Let's review the main processes (Fig. 3.19).

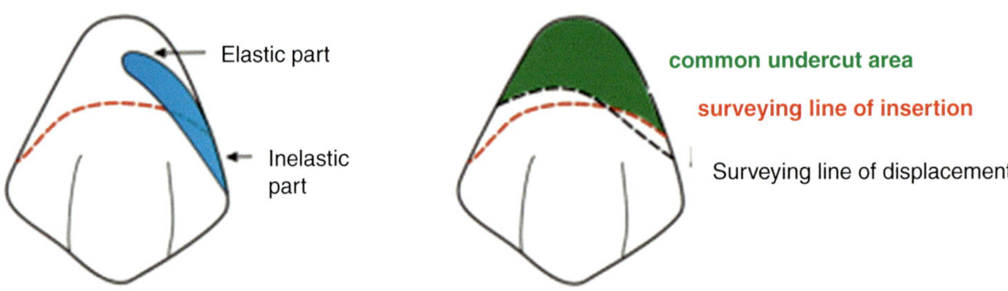

Fig. 3.16 Right figure: The only elastic tip of clasp can expend under the survey line. Left fig.: The tip of clasp enters common undercut area

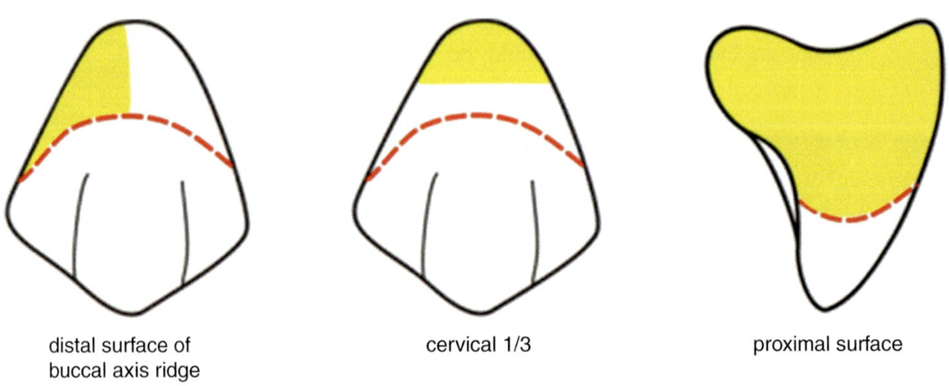

Fig. 3.17 Commonly esthetic retention area

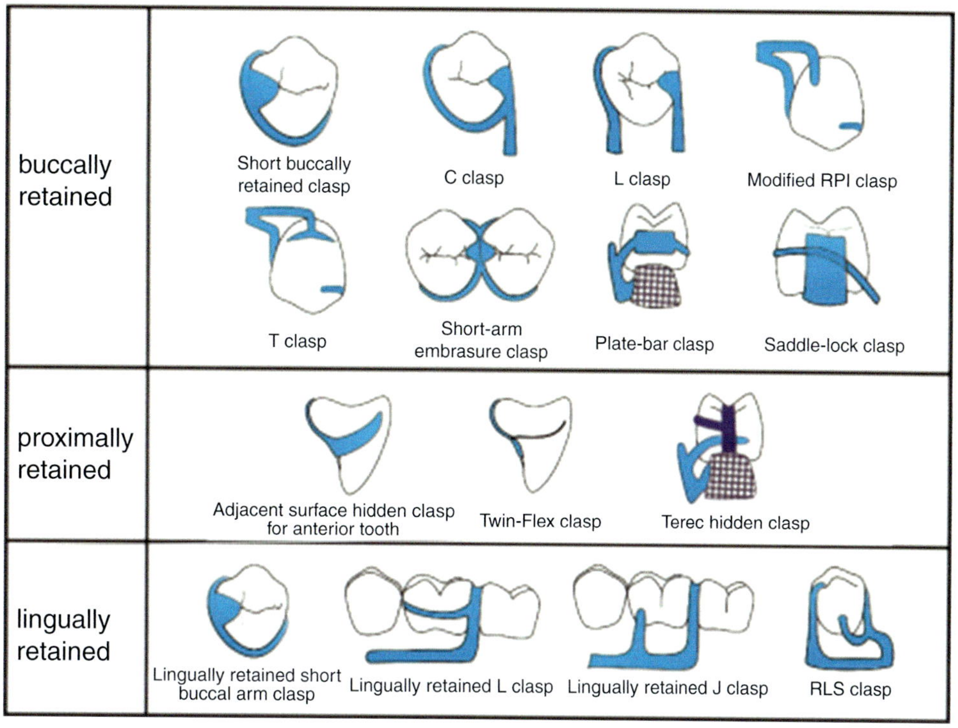

Fig. 3.18 Esthetic clasp classification according to the location of retention area

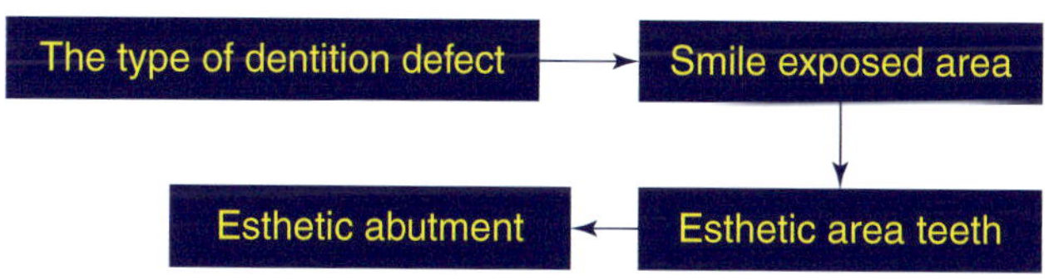

Fig. 3.19 Flow chart of dentition analysis

3.1.3 Fill Work Authorization

After selecting the esthetic clasp, the work authorization should be filled at once, which helps to check the prepared tooth. The following figure is the design of 15 kinds of esthetic clasp design diagrammatic sketch (Fig. 3.20). They are simple, legible, and unique. The main purpose is to transfer information between physicians and technicians. The detailed process of filling work authorization and <esthetic clasp prosthesis technology work authorization> provided only in this book will be introduced in the fifth chapter.

3.1.4 Make Custom Tray

Because there are differences among individuals, trays in consulting room may not be suitable for all patients [5]. The individual differences of patients include the morphology and size of the dental arch, arrangement of dentition, and condition of the frenum and other soft tissues. In order to get a complete and accurate impression, it's necessary to make custom trays for most patients. This part will introduce how to make custom tray quickly with self-curing resin.

Draw Lines Draw the boundary of tray on the study cast with a soft pencil. Be careful to leave the mucous at a distance to give out the channel for overflow of impression material.

Fill the Undercut and Buffer Soak the model in water for 1 min. Heat the wax knife to fill the undercut area at the model. The sharp ridges on the alveolar ridge can be buffered by 0.5 mm wax.

Wax Coating Heat two layers of red wax slices soft covering the model. The part with remaining teeth is thick (about 4–5 mm). Mucosal pat is thin (about 2–5 mm). The impression material is not easy to lose in this way. Be careful not to cover the pencil line.

Coat Separating Agent The separating agent is applied to the model on where self-curing resin may flow over. There must be enough separating agents on the surface of the wax layer. Otherwise, it will be difficult for the next polishing to work.

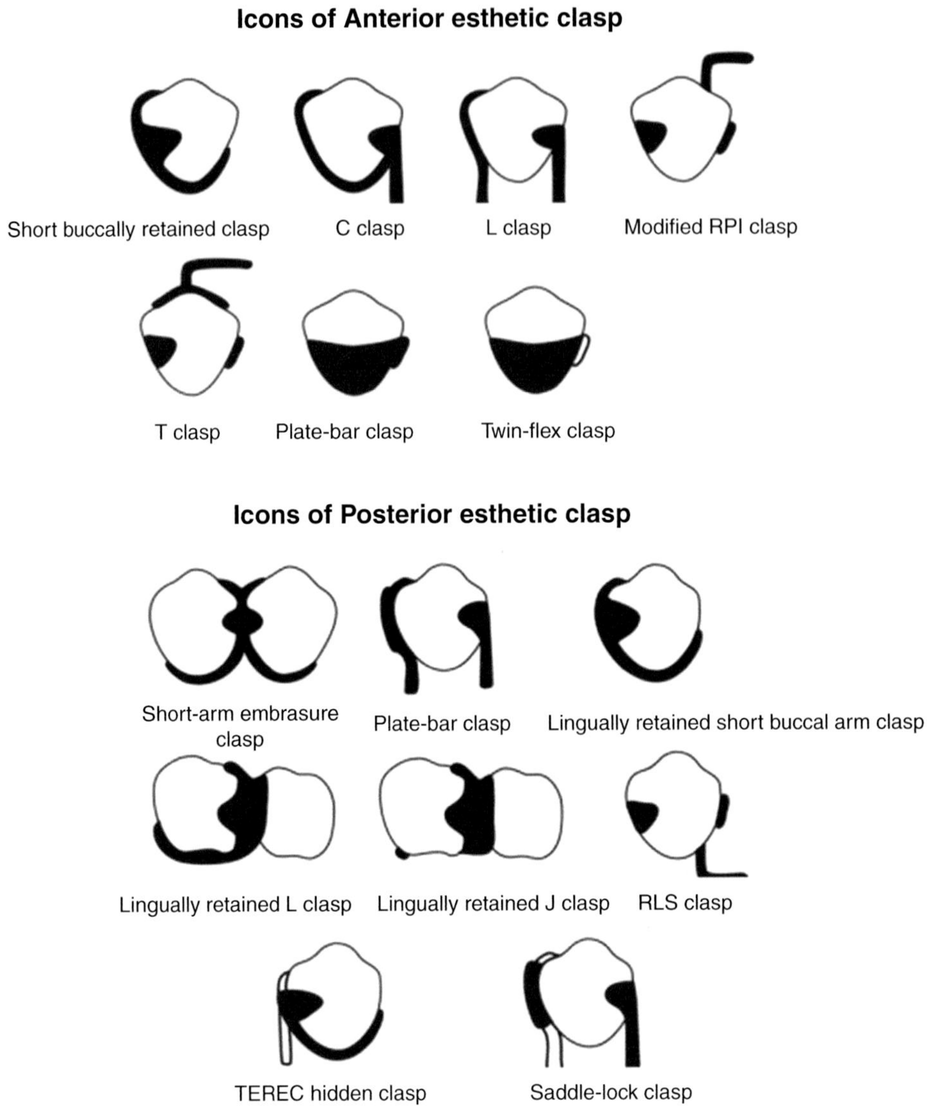

Fig. 3.20 Diagrammatic sketch of anterior esthetic clasp

Prepare Self-curing Resin Material Self-curing dental resin consists of dental base acrylic resin liquid and powder. According to the instruction of manufacturers to take the powder in a certain amount, drop the liquid into the container until the powder is completely immersed. It can be taken out to shape when it is in the dough stage.

> **Tips**
> Remove the resin with a little amount of water under the tap. Washing while rubbing can keep the dough from sticking to hands.

Press Slices Press the resin with hand or smooth stick. Thickness is preferably less than 2 mm.

Cover and Cut The resin slice is covered on the surface of the wax layer. Press the resin making it fit the wax. Trim off the excess material following the boundary.

Make Handle Form the excess material into needful shape. Dip the connection with dental resin liquid. Then place it on the tray. Be careful that the handle can't hamper the lip movement.

Burnish and Polish Wait for 20–30 min until the resin cures completely. Separate the tray and model carefully. Remove excess wax and separating agent. Grind off the small lips with emery wheel. Leave soft tissue like frenum. At last, polish the surface with cotton wheel to avoid scratching patient's mucous.

Try-In The last job is to put the tray into the patient's mouth to check if there's enough space for impression material and whether it effects the movement of soft tissue.

3.1.5 Tooth Preparation

Clinicians can start to prepare teeth after finishing a custom tray. The purpose of tooth preparation is to provide reliable support, retention, and stability [1].

Rest Seat Preparation Rest is an important part to provide support in RPD. Rest should seat at the occlusal tooth surface to transmit axial loads to abutment and avoid hurting supporting tissue.

The rest seat in the abutment provides rest space to ensure the thickness of the mental. The position of the rest seat means a lot for bite force to transfer accurately.

Occlusal Rest It looks like a rounded triangle. It's widest at the marginal ridge and tapers down into the adjacent fossa [5]. The tip points to the center. Its width is 1/3–1/2 of edge ridge. Its length is 1/3–1/4 of tooth distal diameter. The margin of rest seat should be round. It also should transit naturally to the edge ridge. Avoid a sharp line angle.

The thickness of rest seat should be deeper than 1 mm to ensure rigidity of selected material's recommendations. Clinician can make patient bite a softened wax to check the thickness. The bottom of rest seat should be inclined to the center of a tooth, which forms an angle less than 90° with the proximal surface (Fig. 3.21). The purpose of this way is to ensure positive seating. Denture wouldn't slide along the direction of abutment.

Cingulum Rest The ideal position for cingulum seating should be apical to the area of contact with opposing teeth (Fig. 3.22 left).

Start at the edge ridge of abutment, and stop at the incisal surface of cingulum with round diamond bur. Observed from lingual surface, it is like semilunar (Fig. 3.22 middle). It should be widened properly in edge ridge. The margin should be rounded.

What's more, there's also lingual rest, seating at cingulum located on the cingulum near the gingival, which along the cingulum as U shape (Fig. 3.22 right). It requires a certain height of abutment. This kind of rest not only can transfer occlusal force but also can be a resistant arm to improve the stability of the denture.

Carry out embrasure widening. The abutment teeth should be taken into account when the space is enough for a metal framework. For example, the clasp shoulder and small con-

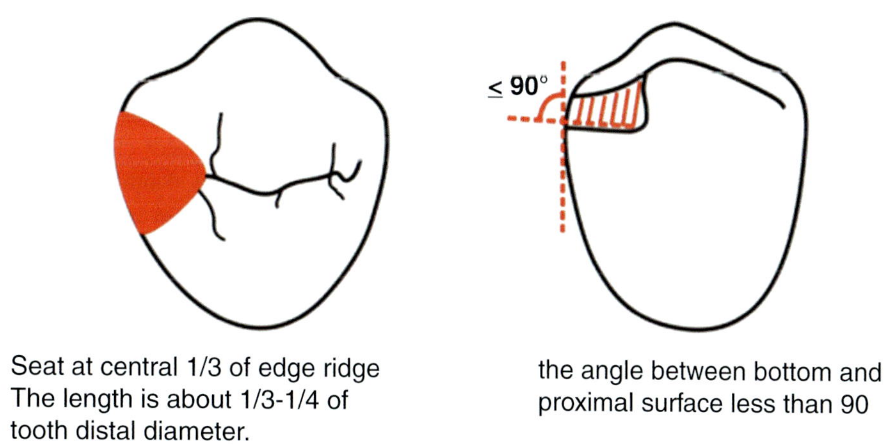

Fig. 3.21 Occlusal rest seat

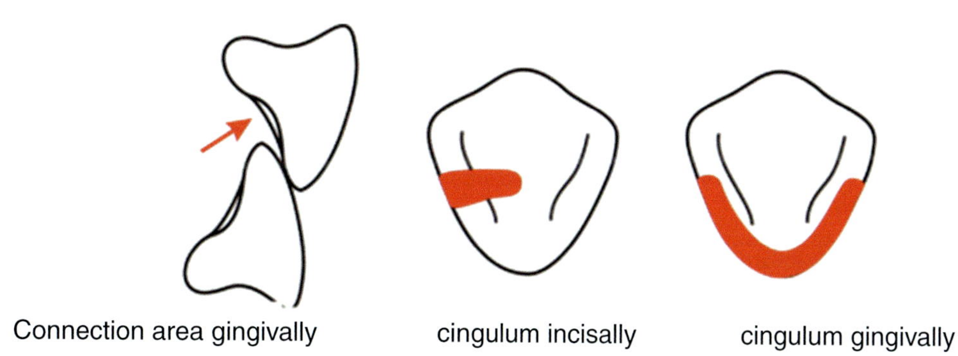

Fig. 3.22 Tongue rest

nector may affect occlusion (Fig. 3.23). Apply thin cone car to mill off a small amount of enamel. The line angle should be round.

Prepare guide space. Guide plates are most frequently prepared on the proximal surfaces of abutment teeth adjacent to the edentulous space, which guide the direction of denture wearing in and out. They also need to be parallel with the pathway of insertion and displacement. The structure contacting guide surfaces called adjacent panel in RPD. Because the guide surfaces and adjacent panels have friction when they contact, so guide surfaces can also provide some retention effect. Key points to prepare include the following:

Apply a cylindrical bur to prepare along with the abutment teeth. A guide surface should be prepared by even reduction of the surface of the tooth maintaining its contour and not as a flat surface (Fig. 3.24).

A proximal guide surface should be 2–4 mm high and about as wide as the distance between the buccal and lingual cusp.

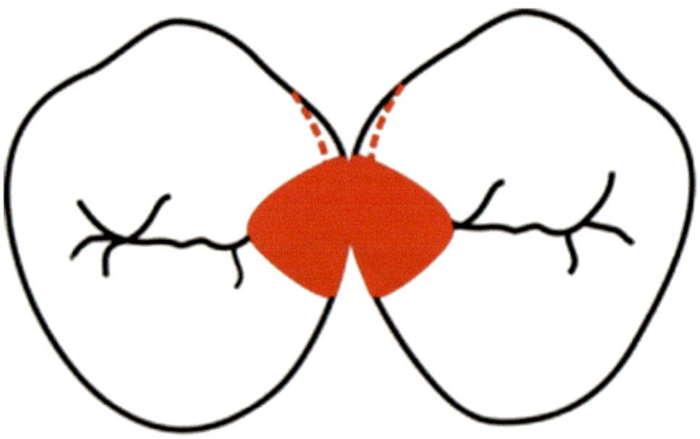

Fig. 3.23 Carry out embrasure widening to obligate enough space for metal framework

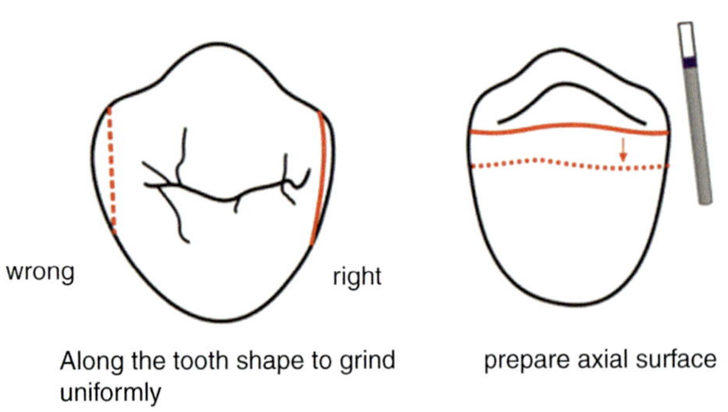

Fig. 3.24 Guide surface should fit the shape of abutment teeth

The anterior guide surface should be in proximal tongue surface, but not affect the labially axiomesiodistal surface.

Prepare teeth axial surfaces. The propose of preparing teeth axial surfaces is to lower survey line and improve clasp placement. Declining and dislocated teeth make the position of the survey line improper. If the clasp can't enclasp the ideal retention area, it would affect the denture to be in place.

Firstly, we should refer to the survey line on the study cast. Apply cylindrical diamond bur positioned alongside the enamel surface to be prepared. Tip slightly to form a new angle. Remove the enamel to form a new height. Pay attention to protect the teeth. The surface should be polished or mineralization and desensitization treatment. If the tilt angle is too large resulting in a large amount of tooth modification, the ideal solution is to make a crown for abutment teeth.

3.1.6 Impression and Working Model

1. *Impression*. We present alginate, the most commonly used in the clinic, as an example to introduce the key point. Firstly, we introduce two different impressions: anatomic impression and functional impression [5].
   (a) *Anatomic impression*: It records the soft and hard tissue in static. It is suitable for tooth support and mucosa support denture. Anatomic impression records oral anatomy in one go.
   (b) *Functional impression*: It records the surface feature when alveolar ridge bears occlusal force, which can protect soft and hard tissue better. It is suitable for tooth and mucosa support dentures. It is commonly used in Kennedy classes I and II free-end dentition. When free-end dentition bears occlusal force, denture in the mucosa and abutment is in different sinking degrees. A denture made according to anatomic impression will make abutment teeth withstand large torsional force. So, it needs to make a functional impression.

   Apply selective tissue placement impression to make a functional impression. A denture can get support in the primary bearing area (mucosa in free-end alveolar ridge) by controlling the flowability of impression material.

   Reduce buffering capacity in primary bearing area of custom tray (e.g., lay a wax slice in fitting surface or other unflow material) to increase tension.

   Buffering by wax and increasing overflow hole can control the flowability of impression material, which can help form different displacement capacity. In that way, it can record the organization functionally.

Operation steps and outcome

(a) *Check tray*: Put the custom tray into patient's mouth to check the size and whether the edge and handle hinder lips' movement.

(b) *Adjust chair*: In order to avoid patient nausea and vomiting, the clinician should raise chair to make patient's dentition occlusal plane parallel to the horizon. The patient should rinse the mouth to remove the food residue and other objects.

(c) *Liquid and powder blending*: Measure powder and liquid according to product instruction. Put them to rubber cap. Mix quickly along one direction with a plaster spatula. When it becomes smooth and pasty, put it on the tray.

(d) *Impression*: As for some areas, that impression material can't be reached, like deep undercut and buccally gap. Clinicians can use impression material with finger to coat these areas. Pull one side of angulus oris with dental reflector. Put the tray into the mouth in lateral rotation. Make the custom tray in place from back to front. Before impression material is hard, it should be done in a muscle functional setting.

(e) *Check impression*: When the impression solidifies completely, put the tray out. Compare the dentition in the mouth to check whether the dentition and mucosal transition are complete. Small bubblet can be filled by newly mixed impression material. If there's big bubblet, clinician needs to get patient's impression once more. Impression should be perfused with gyp at once.

2. *Working model*

(a) *Clean and disinfect.*

The residual saliva in impression surface will infect the accuracy of gyp model. And it may transfer bacteria. So it must be cleaned before perfused (Fig. 3.25). Besides, it should be disinfected by ultraviolet or ozone (Fig. 3.26). The silastic model should be disinfected by immersion way.

(b) *Perfuse model.*

(i) Measure gyp powder and water according to product instruction. Sprinkle the powder into water. Mix them about 30 s until it becomes smooth and flowing paste. Never add water or powder halfway. It will be better with a vacuum mixer.

(ii) Put the rubber cap on oscillator to shake. To make bubbles go out. Then perfuse gyp from the top of impression. Shake it, and pull gyp constantly until it flows to everywhere of the impression.

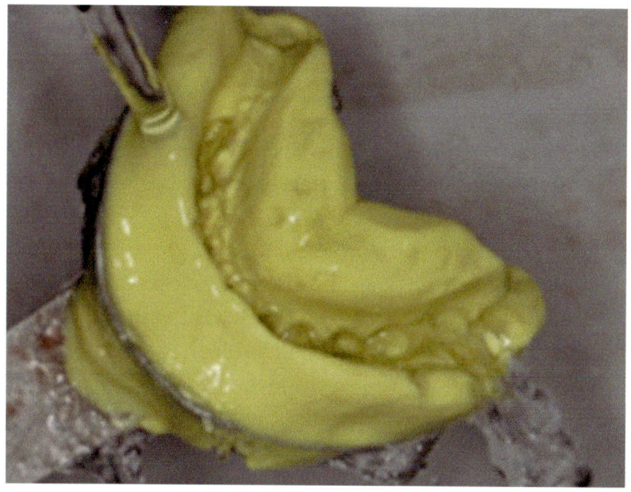

Fig. 3.25 Water cleaning

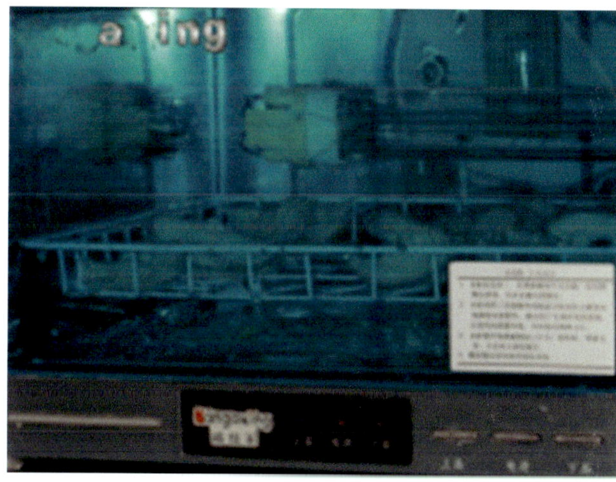

Fig. 3.26 Sterilizing cabinet

(iii) Make base. The thickness of it shouldn't be less than 16 mm.

(iv) Set the model in static about 20 min to make it solidify preliminarily. It will be hardest 2 h later. At that time, the model can be pulled out from impression.

(v) As for working model for removable denture, the record of mucosal transition is very important. The boundary of model should expend to this area.

From now on, all work at the first visit has been done.

The workload is the biggest at the first visit. The most important part is analyzing and designing. According to the steps regularly, clinicians can finish it well organized.

3.2 The Second Visit

3.2.1 Try-In of the Framework

The objective of this stage is to ensure that the framework fits accurately and does not interfere with the occlusion of the natural teeth. Prepare for the next stage-getting bite record.

1. *Put it in place*. Try in the framework according to the insertion pathway designed at first visit (Fig. 3.27). If it can't be wear successfully, induce block area by articulating paper, and wear off them by green sharpening stone.

   Wear off in minor when adjusting block area, especially retention area under guide line, like the tip of clasp. Avoid too much adjustment in case of insufficient retention. In the adjustment process, the bracket should be continuously immersed in cold water to avoid overheating and metal oxidizing.
2. *Adjust occlusion*. The parts in framework influencing occlusal height are generally rest and the arm of clasp cross occlusal surface. Indicate the bite points with occluding paper. Adjust central occlusion first and then protrusive and lateral. If there're frameworks in maxillary and mandible, adjust one by one (Fig. 3.28). At last, check them all. Measure the thickness of metal with caliper when wearing a framework to avoid too thin to break partially.
3. Check after all the wearing process; check whether the framework fits the abutment teeth or not, including the pit of rest, the arm of clasp, tip of clasp, minor connector, anterior lingual panel, and others. The parts adjusted should be polished.

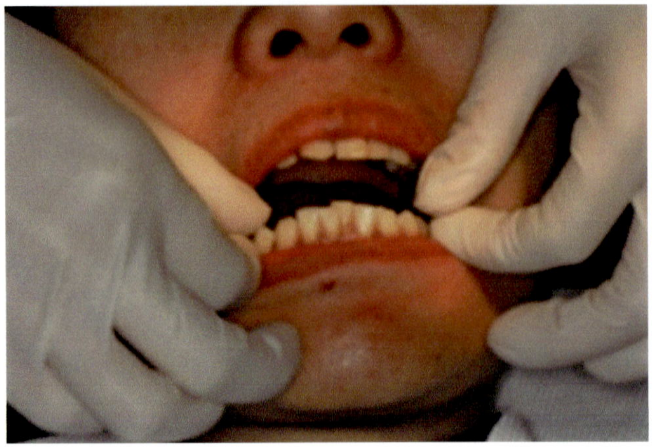

Fig. 3.27 Framework in place

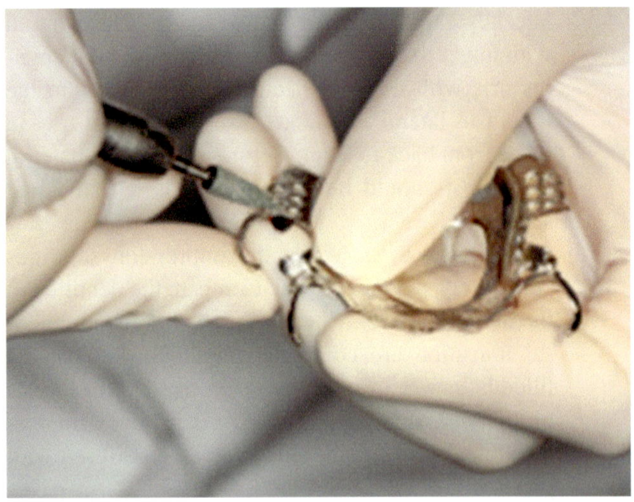

Fig. 3.28 Adjust occlusion

3.2.2 Record Jaw Relation

1. *Few missing teeth*. When a missing tooth is less and maxilla-mandibular relationship is clear, clinicians just need to confirm it on the models.

   The other condition is that even though there are a few missing teeth, vertical distance can be determined, but a unique occlusal relationship can't be found. Now, clinicians can use bite record material like wax or impression material to make patient bite at a central position.
2. *Several teeth missing*. When many teeth missing, like end-free edentulous, the vertical distance can't be determined. Then clinicians need to record occlusal relationship with wax occlusal rim.
   (a) Wetting the surface of working model. Put the framework try-in well in place. Observe the gap between the framework and model.
   (b) Drip wax to the network part at the end of framework with heated wax spatula. Make the flowing wax fill the fitting surface of framework (Fig. 3.29). Ensure to never make wax effect the framework sitting in the right place (no risen and reverse). When there's no obvious gap, clinicians can put it off from the model to fix the interspace. Put it back to the model.

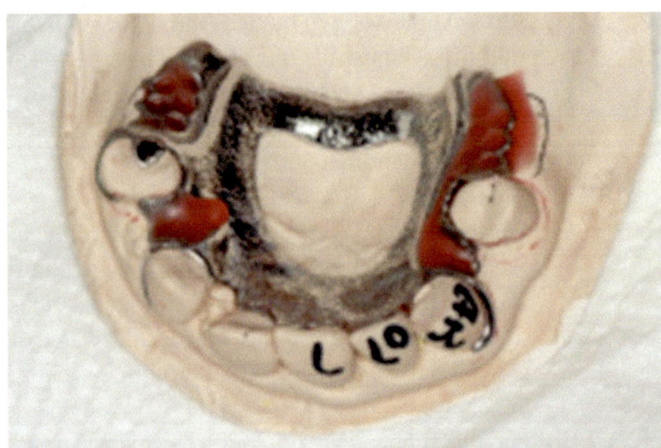

Fig. 3.29 Fill the fitting surface with wax

(c) Heat red wax soft and fold it in 8–10 mm. The length is the same as the edentulous space. The height is about 12–14 mm (Fig. 3.30). Heat the bottle of the wax occlusal rim, and adhere it into the framework (Fig. 3.31). After adhering them, when the wax is still soft, put it into patient's mouth to check whether the height and width are proper (Fig. 3.32) and whether the end of framework influences occlusion. The inappropriate places should be amended as soon as possible.
(d) If the wax hardens, heat the big wax knife to make the occlusal surface of the wax rim soft. Then put it into patient's mouth to bite in a central position.
(e) Put it out to cold water to cold and clean it. Then put it back to the mouth to check the occlusion again. Avoid wax deformation because of cooling.
(f) Most factories and hospitals in China use simple articulators. Other complex semi-adjustable and fully adjustable articulators are in great difference. We won't discuss specifically in this book.

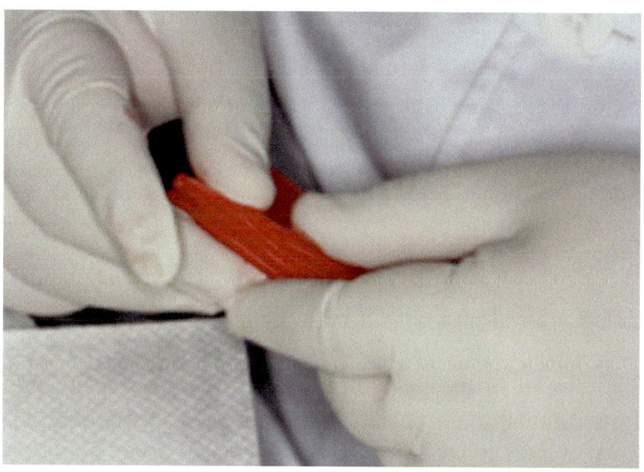

Fig. 3.30 Make wax occlusal rim

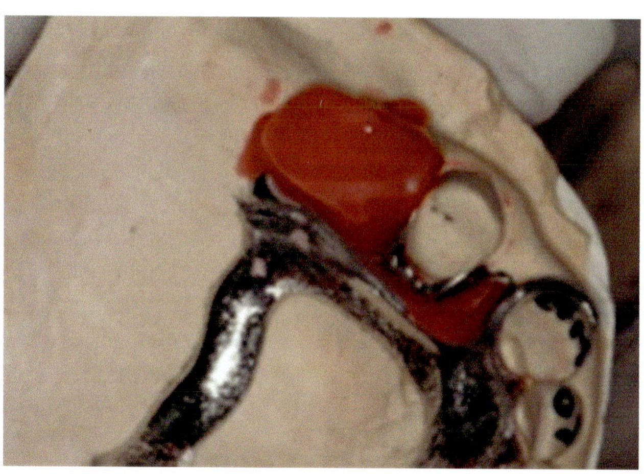

Fig. 3.31 Rax occlusal rim adhered in framework edentulous space

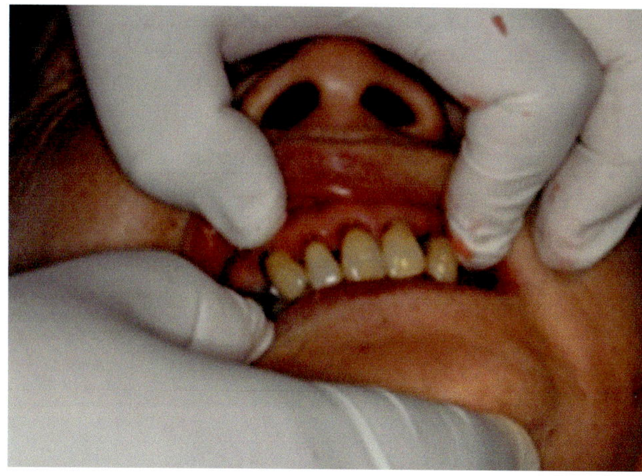

Fig. 3.32 Record occlusal relationship

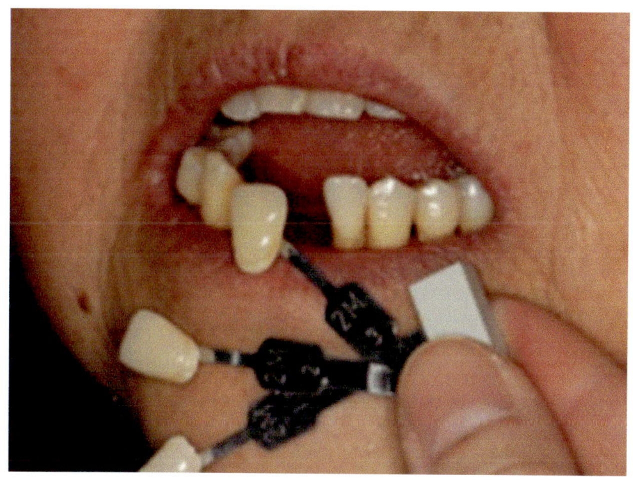

Fig. 3.33 Colorimetric

3.2.3 Design Artificial Tooth

The three elements of artificial tooth design include color, shape, and arrangement. Technician can determine the shape and arrangement of teeth according to the remaining teeth on the model. But the color information can only be recorded by clinician and passed to technician.

When there's no artificial tooth in esthetic area, the artificial teeth design should put function in the first place—only if they were consistent with adjacent teeth and opposite teeth. But the esthetic requirements of the anterior denture are much higher. As fixed prosthetic, artificial teeth need colorimetric. The standard of colorimetric and the transfer of information can reference fixed prosthetics (Fig. 3.33).

When there are more anterior missing, and there's no enough information, clinician can not only design it based on the remaining teeth but also consider the natural color changes, the color of the skin, personal preferences, aging, the transparency of tooth decreases, the saturation increases and the pigmentation becoming yellow.

With the development of material technology, artificial teeth can also simulate the different levels wrapped around like natural teeth. Color and texture are more realistic. To achieve a better esthetic effect, the technician can also carry out surface resin dyeing on artificial teeth, like veneering porcelain in fixed prosthetic to increase the simulation of resin teeth (Figs. 3.34, 3.35, and 3.36).

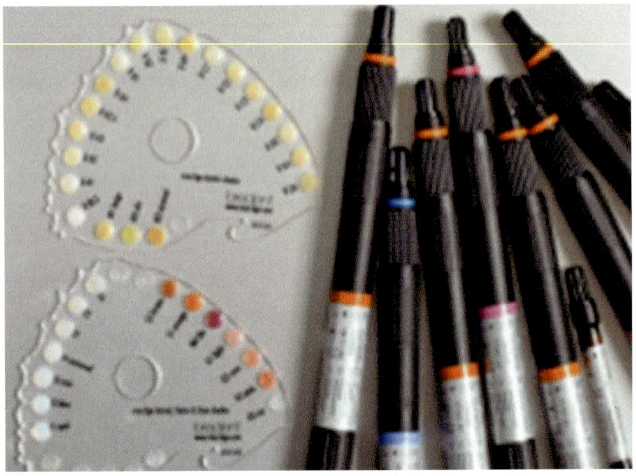

Fig. 3.34 Simulation material

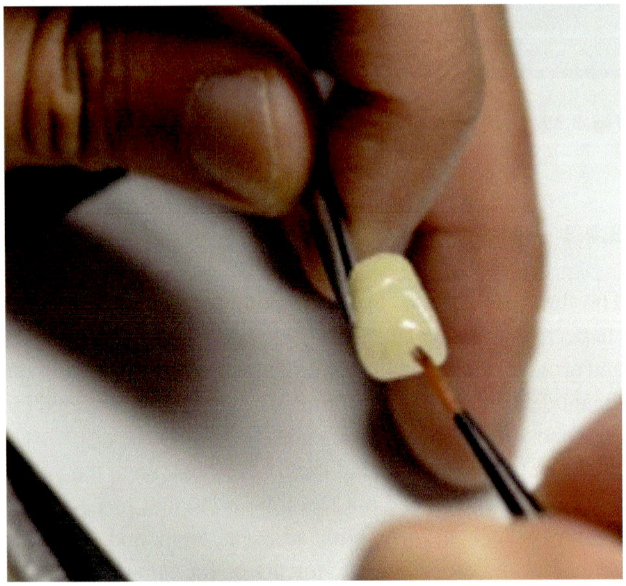

Fig. 3.35 Groove simulating

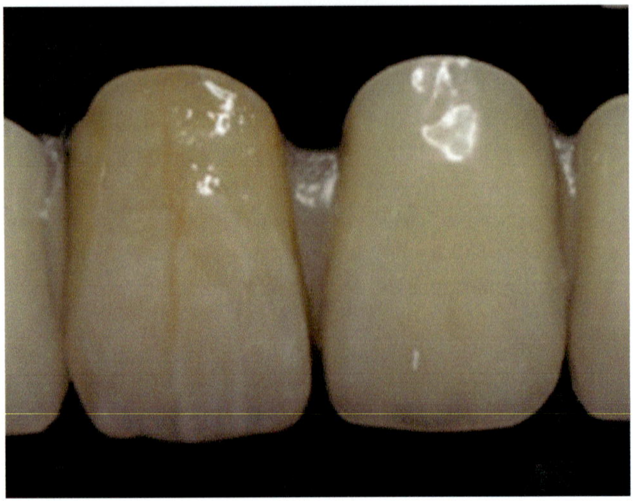

Fig. 3.36 The comparison of esthetic and normal artificial teeth

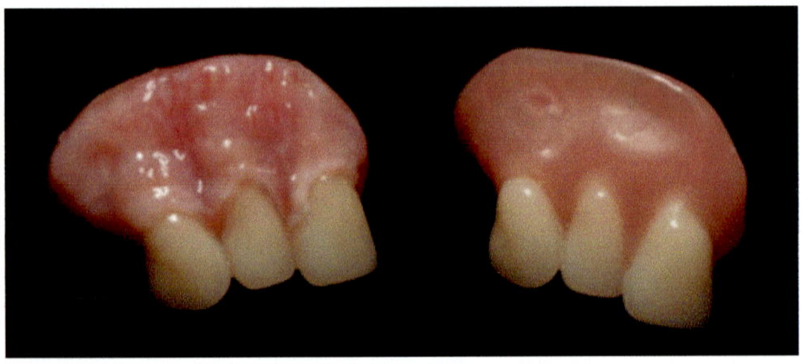

Fig. 3.37 Comparison of esthetic and normal base

3.2.4 Design Base

The design of the base includes two elements: color and form. Similar to artificial teeth, technician can simulate gingival margin and root form by referencing adjacent gingival tissue on working model. But the color of the base can only be recorded and transferred by clinician.

1. *Red-white esthetic effect*. Two completely different objects tied together will give people a visual impact. At the same time, they can highlight their characteristics. A strong contrast between red gingival and white teeth can deliver a message of health and vitality. That is what we call "red-white aesthetic effect." The color relationship between gingival and teeth is not simple red-white contrast, but a color progression, hierarchy of light, and dark.
2. *Blood effect*. Despite the coordination of color and surrounding soft tissue, the best choice for an esthetic base is simulate resin, which has a certain bionic effect with resin fiber similar to red blood (Fig. 3.37).

3.3 The Third Visit

If clinicians carry out everything according to the operating process strictly, it will be easier to wear the denture at last.

3.3.1 Adjust Position and Occlusion

1. Before wearing the denture, the clinician should check whether there's a sharp boundary or bump.
2. Modified resin base mainly. Check if the patient has tenderness. Coat methylrosanilinium in the alveolar ridge. Put the denture in place. Then put it out to modify coloring area slightly. Still follow the principle of "less amount many times."
3. Check whether the denture has set in a place completely, including the fitness between clasp and abutment teeth and fitness between base and mucous.
4. Modify the overlong boundary of the base (Fig. 3.38).
5. Adjust occlusion with articulating paper. If they're all dentures in maxillary and mandibular, clinician should modify them one by one. The sequence is tooth support, mixed support, and mucous support.

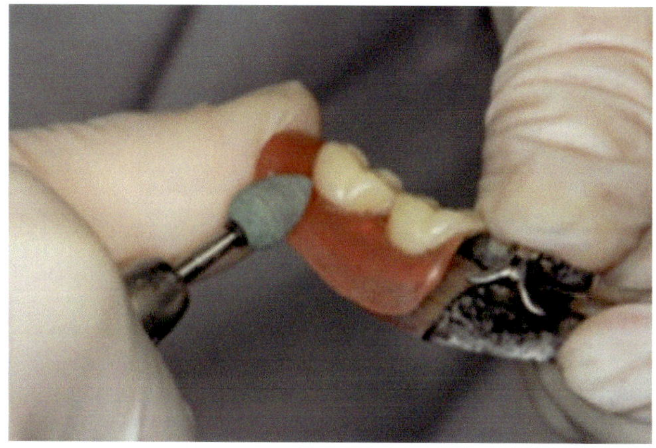

Fig. 3.38 Modify denture

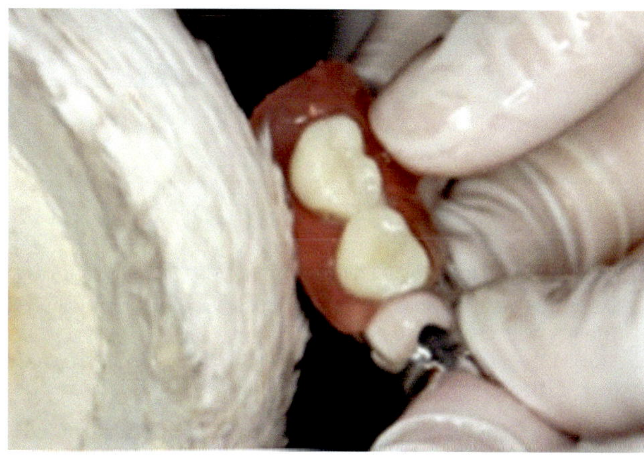

Fig. 3.39 Wear and polish

3.3.2 Grind and Polish

The denture must be polished by a cotton wheel after grinding (Fig. 3.39). Clean the signet of articulating paper.

3.3.3 Clinician's Advice

Practice speaking first after wearing dentures. Overcome foreign sensation generally. Start eating liquid food like porridge when speaking fluently. When there's no problem eating liquid food, begin to eat solid food. Never bite hard stuff. Removable denture can't compare with natural dentition. The restoration of occlusal efficiency is limited. Be patient.

After eating, put off the denture to flush with a soft toothbrush. Everywhere should be brushed. Remove denture before going to bed at night. Never wear it when you sleep but soak it in cold water or denture cleaning tablets.

Never modify the denture by yourself. Go to the doctors as long as you feel uncomfortable. Go back for review every half year (Fig. 3.40).

> Make everything as simple as possible, but not simpler.
> Albert Einstein

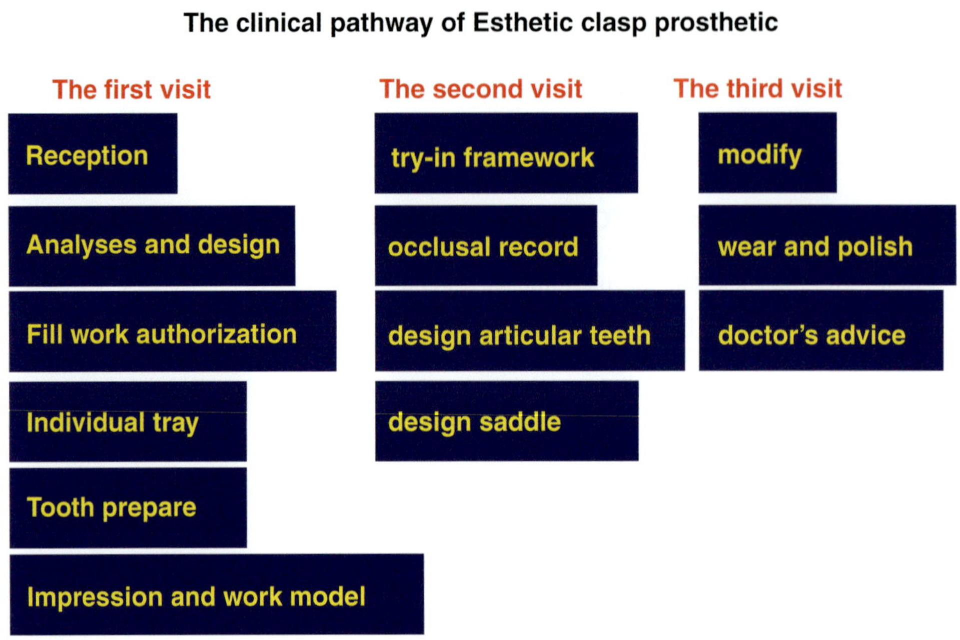

Fig. 3.40 The clinical pathway of esthetic clasp prosthetic

References

1. Alan BC, Glen PM, David TB, et al. McCracken removable partial prosthodontics. Zhang FQ, translated, 11 ed. Beijing: People's Military Medical Publishing House;2007.
2. Aras MA, Chitre V. Direct retains: esthetics solutions in the smile zone. J Indian Prosthod Soc. 2005;5(1):4–9.
3. Shi B. Practical series of clinical stomatology//removable denture restoration. Wuhan: Hubei Science and Technology Press; 2003.
4. Rodney D. Stewart's clinical removable partial prosthodontics. Batavia: Quintessence; 2008.
5. Alan B. McCracken's removable partial prosthodontics. St. Louis: Elsevier Science Health Science div; 2004.
6. Beaumont AJ. An overview of esthetics with RPDs. J Quintessence Int. 2002;33(10):747–55.
7. Yu HY. Rehabilitation design of aesthetic removable denture. Chin J Pract Depart Stomatol. 2012;5(2):72–4.

Digitalization in RPD

4

In the past, the restoration was fabricated entirely by hand, and the work of clinicians and technicians was sharply divided, while the success and esthetic of the restoration depended on the technician's skill and experience. The overall quality of restoration varies because of great technical dependence and the lack of communication between clinicians and technicians. With the rapid development of digital technology, the integration of CAD/CAM (computer-aided design/computer-aided manufacturing) technology with medicine and stomatology has greatly changed the production process of dental prostheses. At present, with the powerful function of CAD software, every link of the restoration design can be visualized by computer, and the design of complex and varied removable partial frameworks can be entirely completed on the computer.

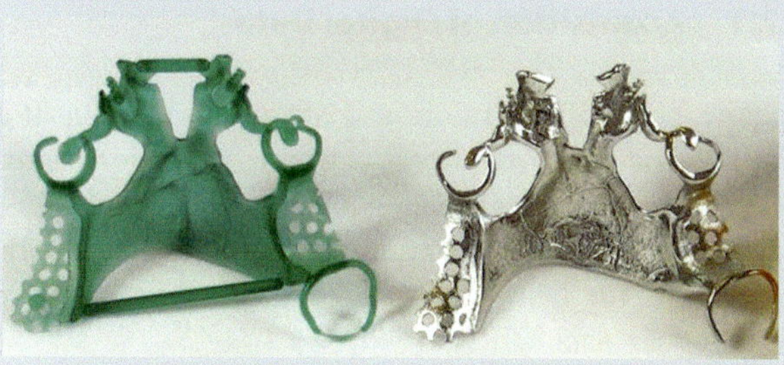

4.1 Introduction

Digital dental prosthodontics, referring to the process that clinicians and technicians participate in, to collect, analyze, and transmit the oral and facial digital information and to design and fabricate the restoration with the help of digital facilities and software, has good repeatability of operation and predictability of result, beneficial to quality supervision and risk management of the process and to the standardization and unification of clinic and laboratory. Therefore, the application of digital technology in dental prosthodontics is not limited to the digital information collection and CAD/CAM of the definitive restoration, but throughout the whole process of oral prosthesis; it should also include preoperative simulation analysis software, for example, Digital Line-plane Design (DLD) of West China Hospital of Stomatology, Digital Smile Design (DSD), 3Shape Smile Design, and so on, and digital recording and transmission of the design.

The application of digital technology in RPD can be roughly divided into three processes: design, transmission, and realization. The process of design includes the personalized RPD design developed by clinicians according to the situation of patients and designed by the RPD decision system. The process of transmission includes that the clinical design is transmitted from the clinician to the technician through dental laboratory work authorization or working chart, and the two-dimensional clinical design is transmitted to a three-dimensional gypsum cast and refractory model; it also includes that the physical design is transmitted to the digital design utilizing digital scan and design software (i.e., the process of CAD). The process of realization includes elaborate and accurate tooth preparation under the microscope in the clinic and transformation from virtual design to physical object (i.e., the process of CAM) in the laboratory.

Digital technology can be applied to design, transmission, and realization of RPD. For patient-requiring RPD, the clinical RPD decision system (RD Designer) will provide optional plans according to their conditions, which will be transmitted to the laboratory after optimization of clinicians, where two types of transformation will accomplish before delivery, from physical cast to digital data and then from virtual design to final restoration.

With the development of technology as well as the support of national policies, the application of digital technology in stomatology is wider than ever before, not only in the field of dental fixed denture where digital technology has

H. Yu, *Digital Removable Partial Denture Technology*, https://doi.org/10.1007/978-981-19-7923-1_4

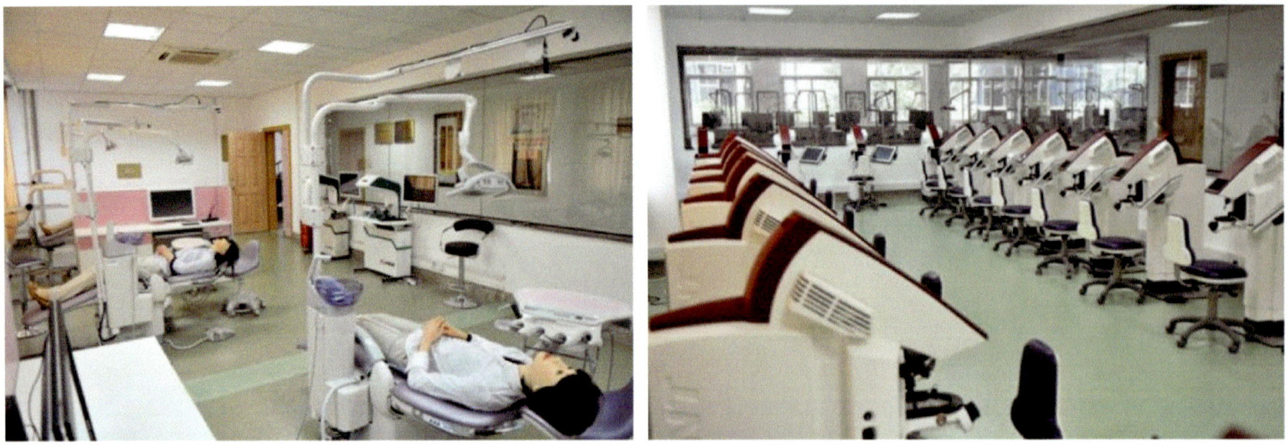

Fig. 4.1 virtual simulation teaching laboratory

achieved remarkable results but also in the field of RPD; digitalization in RPD adopts a series of fast and efficient digital processes including the digital acquisition of oral and facial information, digital design, and digital production, improving the quality of RPD effectively and the efficiency of the clinicians and technicians and reducing the cost time and frequency of the patients' visit. The digitized data is convenient for storage, exchange, and transmission, avoiding physical space occupation and material waste. It is convenient for patients to check the previous information in the later visit and convenient for clinicians and technicians to carry out the repeatable production in the later period. Nonetheless, there are some deficiencies at present such as the high cost of software and equipment, lack of intuition, and perception of the process of design and production compared with the conventional.

Digital technology has been widely applied in clinical practice, as well as in education. At present, the application of RPD in education is mainly in the teaching of the school and the instruction of the laboratory. In order to adapt to the development of digital technology, colleges and laboratories have set up courses to introduce digital technology in dentistry and have equipped with the digital scanning system, digital design software, digital production equipment, etc. Based on the fundamental theory of RPD, teachers explain how to operate the software and equipment and then assist in operation practice, letting the students have a deeper understanding of the digital process and operation. Students learn to design by themselves to solve different problems by means of 3Shape or EXOCAD software, to guarantee a combination between theory and practice. Digitalization makes teaching vivid, practical, shared, and open, modifying and enriching the teaching content, keeping pace with the times, improving students' ability of autonomous learning, expanding their innovative thinking, and fully arousing their enthusiasm and interest in learning.

West China College/Hospital in Stomatology, Sichuan University, has set up a virtual simulation experimental teaching center on the basis of the digital 3D virtual oral anatomy practice platform, the digital virtual training system of oral skills, and the oral medical simulation robots (Fig. 4.1), providing students with advanced digital equipment for their study and research. It is believed that, in the future, more and more new materials and equipment will be put into clinical practice and teaching to promote the continuous development of digital technology.

4.2 Digital Design Terminology

4.2.1 Acquisition of Digital Data

Acquire necessary position, and shape information of the maxillofacial region, dentition, and bite registration based on the principle of image and photoelectric information by means of the digital processing system. It is an important prerequisite for fabricating the good prostheses to obtain accurate scan data.

There are lots of errors during the traditional process of impression taking and cast pouring, such as incomplete and blurry impression, bubbles in impression, shrinkage of impression materials, impression deformation, cast deformation, bubbles on the surface of the cast, wear of the cast, errors generating when duplicating cast several times, and damage of cast or death. Some irreversible operations in the laboratory may result in loss of oral information.

The acquisition of a digital model can be divided into direct method and indirect method: direct method refers to oral scan and maxillofacial scan while indirect method to digital scan of cast and impression.

Direct Method

Combined with optical and electronic technology and computer image recognition and processing technology, the acquired optical signals are converted into electronic signals that can be recognized by the computer through the corresponding scanning equipment, and the physical objects are converted into virtual information. Thus, a 3D digital model is acquired (Figs. 4.2 and 4.3).

At present, the main operating principles of intraoral scanning are as follows:

1. *Confocal microscopy* adopts the mode of scanning layer by layer, with high data clarity, good detail reproduction ability, and high scanning accuracy but with low scanning speed; representative products are iTero (Cadent, Israel), 3D Progress (MHT, Italy), and TRIOS (3Shape, Denmark).
2. *Triangulation of light*, including linear laser scanning technology, structure light scanning technology, three-dimensional photographic technique, and so on, is characterized by fast scanning but needs humidity isolation and spraying powder according to the requirement of equipment; representative products are CEREC Bluecam (Sirona, Germany) and its improved version Omnicam, Bluescan (A.T RON3D, Austria), IOS FastScan (IOS, USA), MIA3D (Densys3D, Israel), and DirectScan (HINT-ELS, Germany).
3. The *active wave front sampling* technology is represented by Lava COS (3M, USA) and the latest True Definition Scanner.

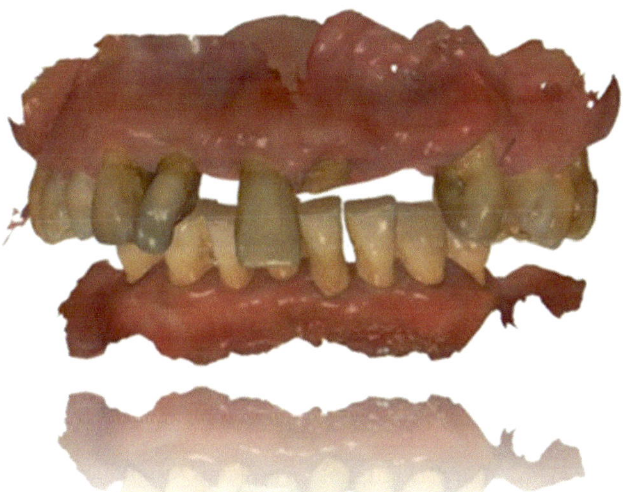

Fig. 4.2 Intraoral scan

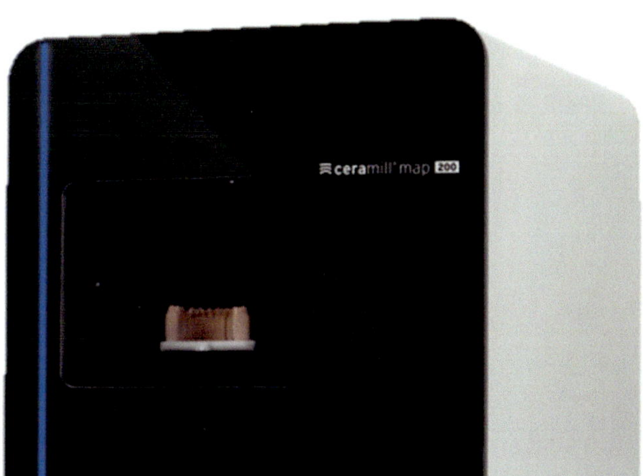

Fig. 4.3 Facial scan

Some intraoral scanners (e.g., 3M Lava COS) need to spray powders on the teeth before scanning to increase the number of reference points for system recognition, but it's important to note that it will lead to abnormal scan morphology of some sites due to uneven distribution of powders, and patient's discomfort makes it difficult to keep a stable head position, which may negatively affect the precision of and reduce the reliability of the scan data. TRIOS (3Shape, Denmark), widely used clinically, whose accuracy is 5 μm, can reflect the color and shape characteristics of soft and hard tissue.

Introduction to Some Common Intraoral Scanner

1. *CEREC system*

   Based on triangulation of light, whose basic principle is that a beam of light that is sent to the surface of the tooth and reflected back to the charge-coupled device for imaging, due to the uneven light reflection on the surface, would affect the accuracy of information collection, a kind of opaque powder was sprayed on the surface of the teeth to improve the quality of information collection. Files containing collected information are transmitted through CEREC Connect in a proprietary format to CEREC MC and CEREC in Lab, terminals supported by Sirona, meaning that CEREC is a closed system.
2. *TRIOS system*

   Based on confocal microscopy and ultrafast optical sectioning technique combined with a special optical path oscillation system, the system can automatically recognize the change of the object's focus plane and keep the relative position between the scanner and the scanned object fixed. The acquisition speed is up to 3000 images per second, reducing the scan error. TRIOS outputs 3D graphics which becomes a digital impression with the method of image collection and combination construction. TRIOS is an open system, namely, files can be exported in an STL format, compatible with other CAD/CAM system. 3Shape also provides mobile terminals, allowing the digital impression to be displayed on mobile phones or tablets to patients, doctors, and technicians, and also provides true color scanning, so it is very convenient for communication among the doctors, patients, and technicians.

3. *Lava COS system*

   Developed by 3M company, based on active wave front sampling, Lava COS is a semi-open system, which means that in most cases the system transmits files on proprietary platforms in a proprietary format, which can be recognized by a specific CAD software and CAM equipment to design and to fabricate the restoration, but it's still compatible with other software.

4. *iTero system*

   Based on the principle of confocal microscopy, the data obtained by the system is of high definition, good detail expression, and high scanning accuracy, but the scanning speed is relatively slow because of the layer-by-layer scanning mode. Using red laser as the light source, the iTero system captures all the structures and materials in the mouth through parallel confocal scanning, without the need to spray the powder on the teeth. The iTero system is an open system in which data is transmitted in an STL format and is compatible with software that accepts the STL format.

5. Common maxillofacial scanning equipment: 3dMD scanner (USA), FaceScan scanner (Germany), etc.

FaceScan, based on structured light technology, consists of two digital cameras, a structured light projector and scanning software. Structured light works like this: several strips of black and white are projected onto the face or object for 3D reconstruction, which will be captured by the camera, and the software then automatically reconstructs the surface. Finally, a highly accurate 3D reconstruction of the face or object is obtained. iTero can be used to obtain 3D digital data from the surface of complex objects quickly and accurately.

Main characteristics of the 3dMD dynamic face system include the following:

1. Easy to use.
2. The scanning process is fast, taking approximately 5 s, requiring the scanned object to remain stationary.
3. High sensitivity, high resolution. Color, black and white output format, with 640 × 480 and 1280 × 1024 resolution camera lens.
4. Can be adjusted according to the light/surface conditions.
5. Acquisition of texture.
6. Support varieties of output formats.

The accuracy of oral scan and face scan, used to acquire patients' information, is affected by the following factors:

1. Scanning equipment factors: scan accuracy, scan speed, match degree, etc.
2. Operator technical factors: operation angle, operating method, etc.
3. Patient factors: patient compliance, oral environment, open degree, space in the mouth

Indirect Method

In vitro, the model or impression is converted into an editable 3D virtual model by means of an extraoral scanner. Currently, the commonly used model scanning systems include 3Shape, Dental Wings, Sirona, Girrbach, Wieland, and so on, and the accuracy can reach up to 15 μm.

4.2.2 Digital Analysis

Digital analysis refers to the process that clinicians analyze and process patients' digital photos by means of 2D or 3D software preoperatively, combining the treatment plan, to obtain the result expected by both doctors and patients, beneficial to the communication between doctors and patients before the implementation of the irreversible operation, improving the quality of diagnosis and treatment process. The software used for digital analysis includes DSD (Digital Smile Design), DLD (Digital Line-plane Design), and Tooth Assistant (Fig. 4.4).

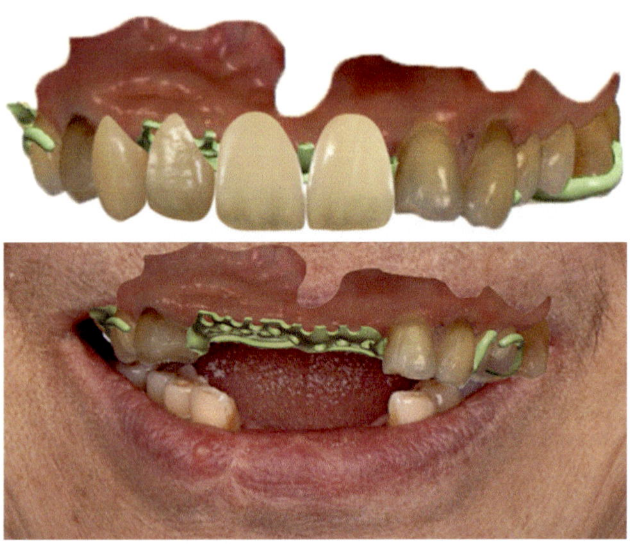

Fig. 4.4 Simulation by Tooth Assistant

4.2.3 Computer-Aided Design (CAD)

The CAD software of removable denture mainly includes SensAble (SensAble Technologies, USA), dental system (3Shape, Denmark), Ceramill (AmannGirrbach, Germany), etc. Each has its own advantages, but the design procedures are similar:

1. Determine the path of insertion, and block out undesirable undercuts.
2. Adjust the wax pattern, and reserve the space for retaining clasp.
3. Build meshwork patterns, major connector, minor connector, occlusal rest, and clasp.
4. Add wax virtually to simulate the shape of rugae, and build tissue stops and retention pins and other auxiliary structures.
5. Add the support, and finish design (Fig. 4.5).

The traditional way to fabricate the framework is to obtain the manual wax pattern first, where there are human errors and limitations in design. With the help of CAD software, each part of the digital framework can be added, subtracted, deleted, hidden, and modified freely. In addition, the virtual articulator can be used to simulate the mandibular movement of different patients as soon as possible through adjusting the technique parameters, which could obtain more accurate RPD. In the process of digital design, we should pay attention to the combination of theory and practice and design reasonable and effective prostheses according to different cases.

4.2.4 Import and Arrangement

For additive technology systems (laser sintering and 3D printing) and subtractive technology systems (milling), supports are added to the structures before submitting the finished design (Fig. 4.6). Appropriate supports of adequate strength are required to stabilize the RPD framework. Also, during manufacturing, it prevents movement and (or) dissipates heat away from the finished part of framework during manufacturing. After that, files can be sent to a production machine.

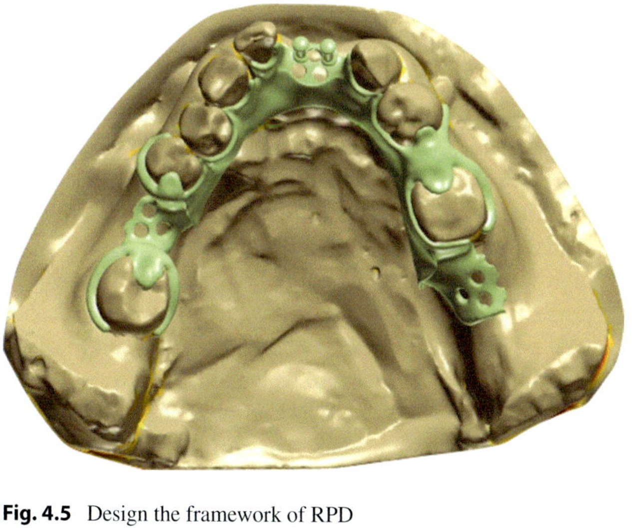

Fig. 4.5 Design the framework of RPD

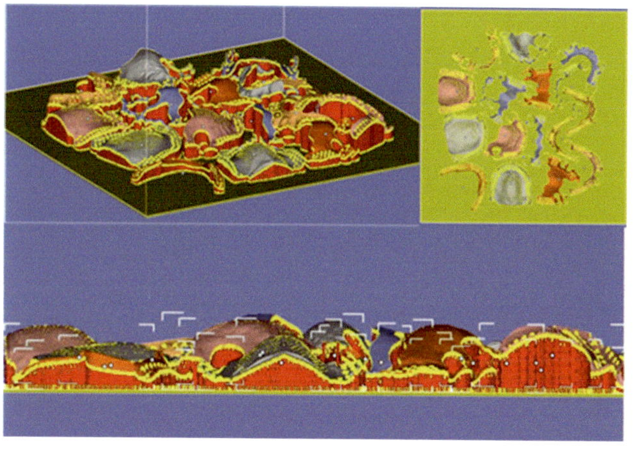

Fig. 4.6 Arrangement of frameworks

4.2.5 Computer-Aided Manufacturing (CAM)

CAM can be divided into subtractive manufacturing and additive manufacturing (AM). The details are as follows:

1. *Subtractive manufacturing*

   Subtractive manufacturing refers to a technology that selectively removes materials from a blank block or disc by means of mechanical milling, chemical treatment, discharge processing, laser processing, etc. Computer numerical control (CNC) milling system is the most widely used in prosthodontics, whose advantage lies in high accuracy, high smoothness, no need for too much post-processing, numerous kinds of materials that can be processed, good internal homogeneity, etc.; nevertheless, the material waste of this method is large, which can't be used to process nested, hollow-out, and other complex structures.

2. *Additive manufacturing*

   Additive manufacturing, in contrast to subtractive manufacturing, is a method with which to fabricate objects by stacking and accumulating materials layer by layer, also known as rapid prototyping or 3D printing. It can be used to process complex structures, saves materials, and increases production efficiency, but high cost and rough surface are disadvantages of this method. Available materials include metal (cobalt-chromium alloy, pure titanium, etc.) (Fig. 4.7), resin, and wax.

   Additive manufacturing has many different molding methods, which can be divided into three categories according to the different status of raw materials.

LaserCUSING® Processing materials	CL 20ES	stainless steel (1.4404)
	CL 31AL	aluminum (AlSi 10Mg)
	CL 41TIELI	titanium alloy (TiAl64V ELI)
	CL 42 TI	Grade II pure titanium
	CL 50WS	hot processed steels (1.2709)
	CL 91RW	stainless hot processed steel
	CL 92PH	precipitation hardening stainless steel (17-4PH)
	CL 100NB	nickel alloy (Inconel 718)
	CL 101NB*	nickel alloy (Inconel 625) *
	CL 110CoCr*	CoCr casting alloy (F75) *
	remanium star® CL	CoCr casting alloy (Dentaurum, Germany)
	rematian® CL	titanium alloy (Dentaurum, Germany)

Fig. 4.7 Materials can be processed by LaserCUSING® (Concept Laser, Germany)

The first kind is liquid, processed by means of stereolithography (SLA), which is mainly used to fabricate the working model of the intraoral scan and the implant guide.

The second kind of materials is lamellar or filamentous, which can be processed through laminated object manufacturing (LOM), fused deposition modeling (FDM), electron beam fuse molding, and plasma beam fuse molding.

The third kind is powder material, which can be processed by selective laser melting (SLM), selective laser sintering (SLS), laser engineered net shaping (LENS), and electron beam selective melting (EBSM). Among them, SLS technology, which is widely used, is mainly used to fabricate wax and resin patterns, metal restorations and guides, etc., while SLM technology is mainly used to fabricate metal restorations.

In the next part, some common metal additive manufacturing technologies are described:

(a) *Selective laser melting (SLM)*

Selective laser melting (SLM) technology was proposed by Fraunhofer Institute (German) in 1995, and the first SLM equipment was launched by MCP Hek company (German). SLM technology uses high power density small spot laser beam and high precision powder spreader, which forms without heating powder and melts powder layer by layer by high-energy laser during the forming process, forming metallurgical bond directly.

(b) *Selective electron beam melting (SEBM)*

ARCAM company (Sweden) proposed selective electron beam melting (SEBM) technology in 1994 and launched the first equipment EBM S12 in 2002. SEBM technology preheats the metal powder to 600~700 °C before manufacturing, which reduces the cooling rate of metal powder to improve stability of that, and then uses high-energy and high-speed electron beam to selectively bombard metal powder to make it melt into shape.

(c) *Laser direct metal deposition (LDMD)*

Laser direct metal deposition (LDMD) was first proposed by Sandia National Laboratory in the 1990s, but different research institutions call this technology differently: laser engineered net shaping (LENS) of the University of Michigan, direct laser fabrication (DLF) of Birmingham University in the UK, laser rapid forming (LRF) of Northwestern Polytechnical University of China, etc. During the forming process, the powder is gathered on the working plane through the nozzle, and the laser beam also gathers at the point; two points coincide to make it melt powder and then get an accumulated cladding solid by movements of workbench or nozzle. LDMD can print high melting point metal directly, while the diameter of focused laser spot is usually over 1 mm; the dimensional accuracy and surface roughness of parts manufactured by LDMD technology are not ideal.

(d) *Selective laser sintering (SLS)*

Selective laser sintering (SLS) was first proposed by Carl Deckard who came from the University of Texas at Austin in the USA. Based on the metallurgical mechanism of liquid phase sintering, the powder material is partially melted, and its solid core is retained during the process of forming. The powder is densified by subsequent solid-phase particle rearrangement and liquid-phase solidification and bonding. SLS technology is suitable for titanium and titanium alloy, cobalt-chromium alloy, stainless steel, nickel-titanium alloy, etc., and it should be used under an inert gas environment like argon or nitrogen with CO_2 laser; both one-way and two-way scanning are available. SLS technology has a relatively high rate of material consumption; besides, it can also process without support. However, powder material won't be melted entirely due to the semisolid-liquid-phase sintering mechanism, which will lead to some process defects of parts such as high porosity, low density, poor tensile strength, and high surface roughness. The viscosity of solid-liquid mixture is usually high in the semisolid forming system of SLS, and the fluidity of fused materials is poor; therefore, there will be a unique metallurgical defect of the SLS process called balling effect. Balling effect not only will make higher surface roughness but also will make it hard to spread powder over the surface of sintered layer and even will hinder the subsequent process.

(e) *NanoParticle Jetting (NPJ)*

XJET (Israel) launched a metal 3D equipment of NanoParticle Jetting (NPJ) in 2016. The technique mixes nanoscale metal particle into adhesive forming metallic ink. The metallic ink is sprayed out and printed by a special nozzle, and the adhesive is evaporated at high temperatures after molding, leaving the metal part for manufacturing. The printing speed of NPJ is as five times as that of common laser printing with high-dimensional accuracy and excellent surface quality, while the temperature resistance of NPJ is lower than that of other printing metals.

(f) *Inkjet 3D printing/binder jetting (3DP/BJ)*

Inkjet 3D printing/binder jetting (3DP/BJ) was proposed by MIT in 1993, which belongs to Indirect Metal 3D printing. 3DP/BJ ejects the adhesive according to the CAD design and bonds the metal powder layer by layer. Next, the adhesive volatilizes under the high-temperature irradiation, and the parts are manufactured by sintering after printing. This technology is a variant of material spraying technology, generally using a water-based adhesive. 3DP/BJ technology can form in different materials without adding support and has simple back disposal, so it makes it possible to print complex parts. Some equipment can realize large format forming without large-scale distortion, but having lower precision than SLM.

(g) *Atomic diffusion additive manufacturing (ADAM)*

A metal 3D printer Metal X adopting ADAM technology was introduced by Markforged in September 2017, which belongs to indirect additive manufacturing. This technology mix metal powder and resin adhesive to form silk material. The machine prints out the "green mold" after enlarging CAD file and then sinters it after resin removal to make the final parts consistent with CAD file. The metals that can be used in Adam technology include Ti6Al4V, copper-base alloy, 316L stainless steel, etc. The density of parts reaches 95~99%. The mass production of parts can be realized by using Adam technology but spend long preparation time.

A prosthesis can be manufactured in different techniques; metal 3D printing technology and wax molding technology are mainly used in activity restoration:

(i) *3D printed metal*

SLM uses a laser to selectively melt and sinter metal powders layer by layer to acquire the desired three-dimensional shape. The whole process includes the establishment of CAD model, data processing and sending, powder laying, melting and sintering, and post-processing.

(ii) *3D printed wax and resin patterns* (Fig. 4.8)

At present, wax molding technology is mainly divided into two types:

Stereolithography appearance

Stereolithography appearance (SLA) was patented by Charles Hull in 1984 and commercialized by 3D Systems, which is widely recognized as one of the most deeply researched and earliest 3D printing methods in the world. This technology takes the photosensitive resin liquid as the raw material, which is solidified and superimposed one by

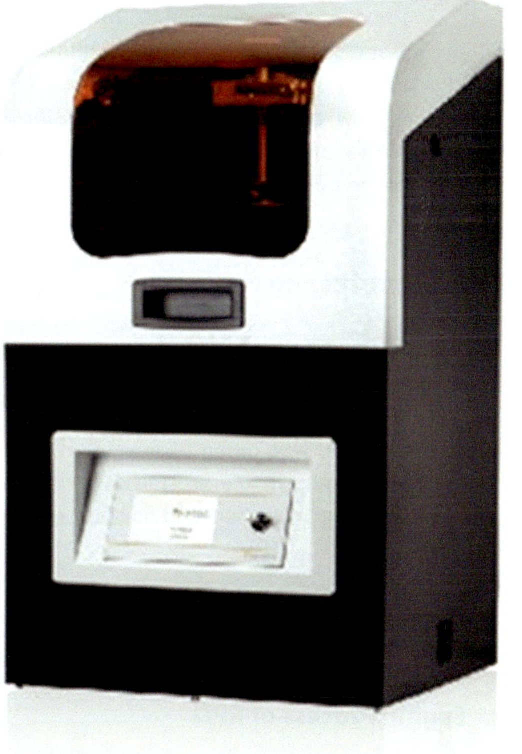

Fig. 4.8 3D printed wax patterns

one thin layer by the ultraviolet laser beam controlled by the computer to generate the three-dimensional solid model. Its advantages lie in high precision as well as accurate and smooth surface. The representative company is 3D Systems.

Light curing molding technology based on digital light processing

Digital light processing (DLP) and inkjet printing, based on DLP, have developed rapidly and attracted wide attention due to its high precision and low price. However, it is difficult to complete large format printing work. The representative company is BEGO.

There are always defects and pinholes in traditional process such as investment and casting. Digital 3D printing technology can effectively avoid the bubbles, cracks, and shrinkage deformation, switching to automated production mode to simplify production process, with high precision, less waste of materials, improved quality of restorations, etc. The framework of RPD requires materials with high strength, good ductility, and good processability to ensure enough retention force and no deformation, preventing plates from crack and reducing the volume of prostheses. Cobalt-chromium alloy (Co-Cr alloy) is now commonly used to print the frameworks of RPD, due to its good mechanical properties and corrosion resistance.

4.2.6 Post-processing

The printed metal prostheses need to be retrieved and subjected to post-processing following manufacturer instructions to eliminate the thermal stress generated in SLM process, to prevent the generation of adverse deformation, and to ensure the quality of the prostheses. They are then separated from the supporting base and finished and polished in several steps.

4.3 Digital Design Principles

4.3.1 Digital Process of RPD

1. *Prosthodontic plan*

   Clinicians make the individual prosthodontic plan according to the intraoral situation of patients and draw the framework components on the work authorization, indicating the insertion path of the framework, key points of design (e.g., illustrate parts that can't be displayed on the work authorization due to dimensional restriction, especially the direction of roach clasp and minor connectors); materials, which should be strong enough to guarantee the strength of structures such as split major connector of stress breaker design and short retainer arm of esthetic clasp and which should be replaced with other metal materials or nonmetallic materials such as PEEK and PEKK when patients are allergic to metal; and other auxiliary structures (e.g., number and location of retention pin).

2. *Digital forecast*

   Collect patient's digital photographs of different angles or 3D face scan data preoperatively, forecast the result through DLD, and show patients 2D and 3D prosthodontic plan to obtain the consent.

3. *Acquisition of digital model*

   Kennedy class III arches of patients can be scanned through the intraoral scanner, such as TRIOS. However, the final impressions should be made in rubber base materials for Kennedy class I, II, and IV arches and then either scanned directly or poured into stone master casts that are subsequently scanned using an extraoral scanner, such as 3Shape D800 or E3, to acquire the digital model.

   Kennedy class III arches are usually restored by tooth-supported RPD without special consideration of the tissue situation of edentulous areas, and intraoral scan data can meet the need. Nonetheless, functional impressions should always be made for Kennedy I, II, and IV class arches, which can't be acquired through the intraoral scanner. In addition, application of the intraoral scanner will be subjected to restrictions when the range of opening is small and the vestibular groove is shallow.

4. *Computer-Aided Design (CAD)*

   The Digital Workflow of RPD Through 3Shape Dental System

   (a) Determine the insertion path, and block out undesirable undercuts virtually (Fig. 4.9).
   (b) Trim the wax pattern to reserve space for retentive arms of clasps (Fig. 4.10).
   (c) Build the virtual meshwork in the edentulous areas according to the design drawn on the model, and adjust the distance between the crest of the cast and the bottom of the meshwork if necessary (Figs. 4.11, 4.12, 4.13, and 4.14).
   (d) Build the virtual major connector, and adjust the position and shape of the edge (Fig. 4.15).
   (e) Draw the virtual clasp, occlusal rest, and minor connectors three-dimensionally, and adjust technical parameters such as width and thickness (Fig. 4.16).
   (f) Build virtual retention pins and other auxiliary structures, and simulate the shape of rugae in the maxillary RAD if necessary (Figs. 4.17 and 4.18).

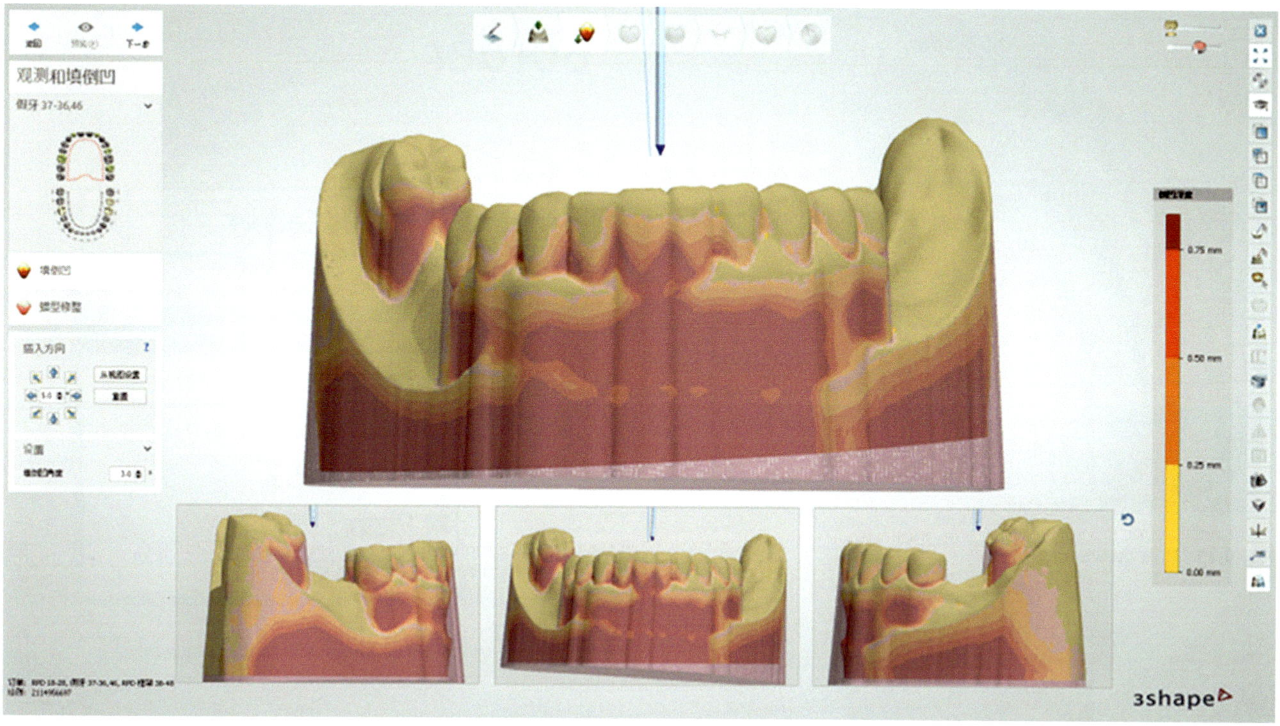

Fig. 4.9 Determine the path of insertion and block out the undercuts virtually

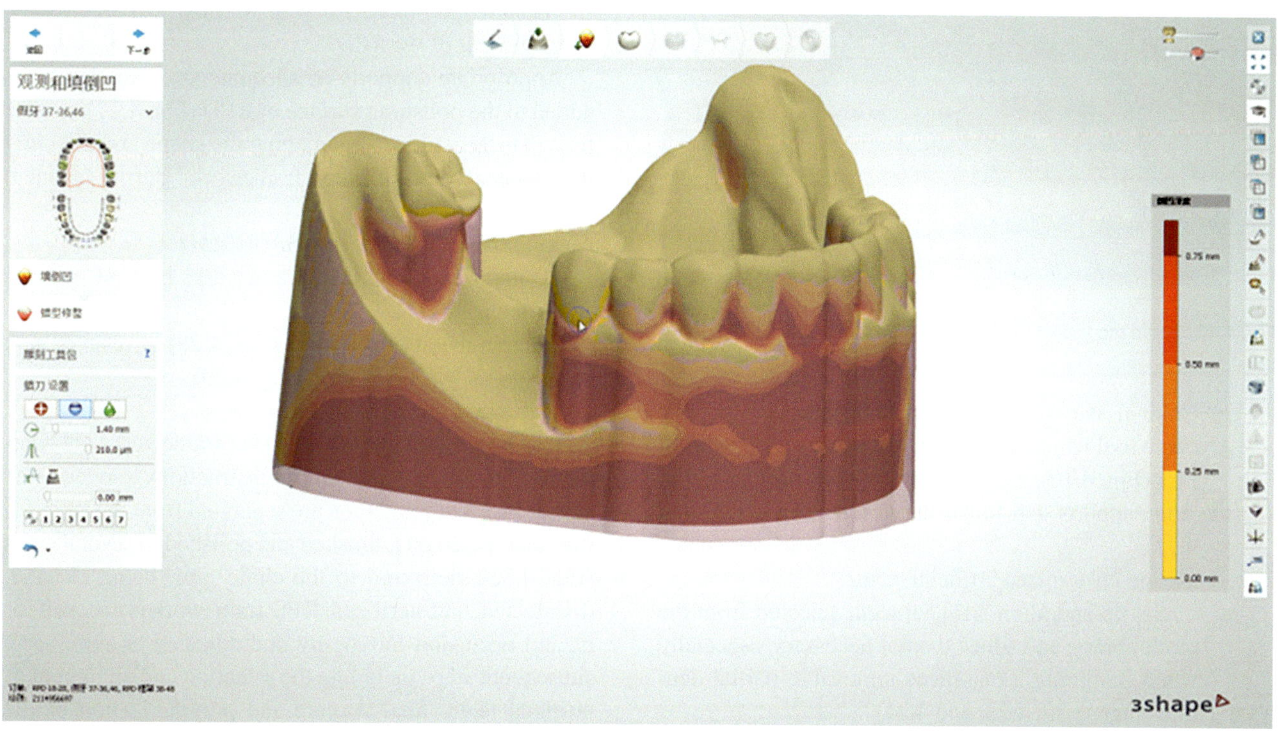

Fig. 4.10 Reserve the space for clasp retentive tips

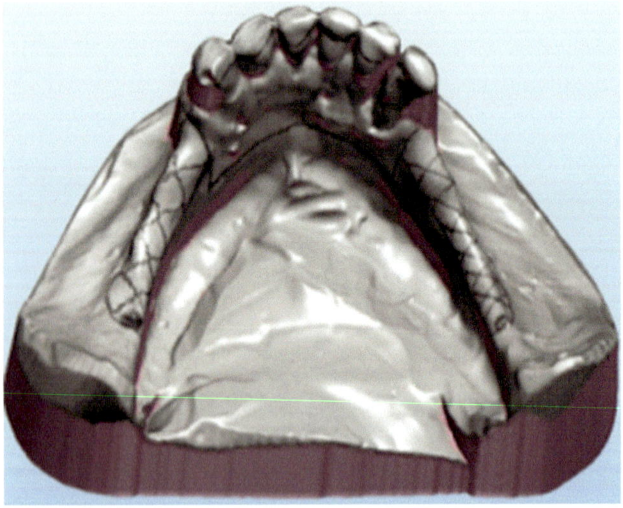

Fig. 4.11 Plan drawn on the cast

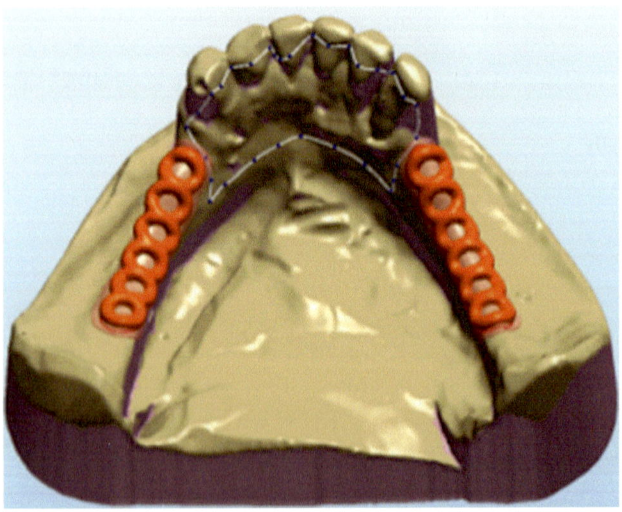

Fig. 4.12 Build the virtual meshwork pattern

(g) Build tissue stops, and draw finish lines using the curve tool which utilizes default and customized profiles (Fig. 4.19).

(h) Add supports and finish the design (Figs. 4.20 and 4.21).

(i) Design customized artificial teeth.

Set up and align artificial teeth selected from the tooth library, and adjust them if necessary, especially when designing a one-piece removable partial denture (Figs. 4.22, 4.23, and 4.24).

(j) Design digital dental base.

Adjust the shape of the customized base when designing a digital complete denture or one-piece removable partial denture (Fig. 4.25).

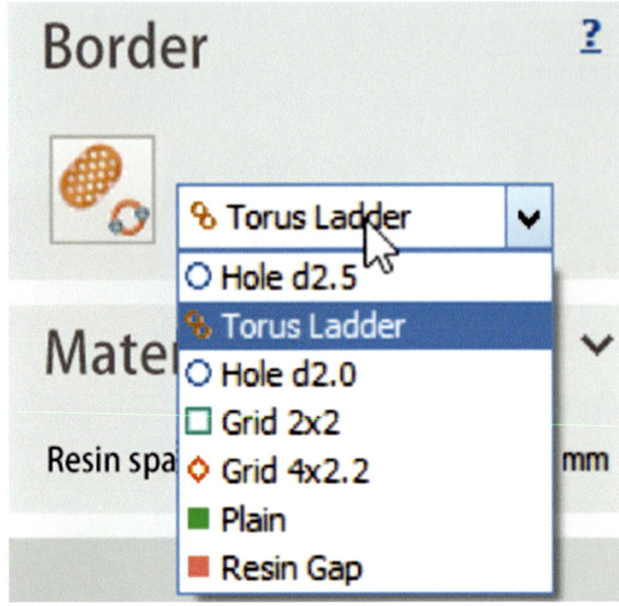

Fig. 4.13 Adjust technical parameters of the meshwork

(k) Design the one-piece RPD.

Combine all components through the Boolean operation function of the software after the completion of the framework, artificial teeth, and base to design one-piece RPD (Fig. 4.26).

5. *Arrangement of the RPD*

Appropriate supports of adequate strength should be added to the polishing surface of RPD (Fig. 4.27), not the tissue surface, to avoid damaging the shape and affecting the adaptability of the framework during manual grinding.

6. *Computer-Aided Manufacturing (CAM)*

(a) Obtain metal or PEEK frameworks by CNC milling system.

(b) Obtain metal frameworks (Fig. 4.28) or resin or wax patterns by 3D printing (Fig. 4.29).

7. *Post-processing and Subsequent Steps*

In the case of 3D printing, metal frameworks are heat-treated following manufacturer instructions to release the stress (Fig. 4.30) and then are separated from the supporting base (Fig. 4.31), finished and polished in several steps (Fig. 4.32), delivered to the clinic after being cleaned, disinfected, and sterilized. RPD framework is checked for fit and occlusion intraorally and adjusted as necessary; subsequent steps including the selection and alignment of artificial teeth, final wax-up and polymerization of the base, finishing, and polishing are in similar manners used for traditional RPD. However, there's no need to be subjected to post-processing for milled metal and PEEK frameworks.

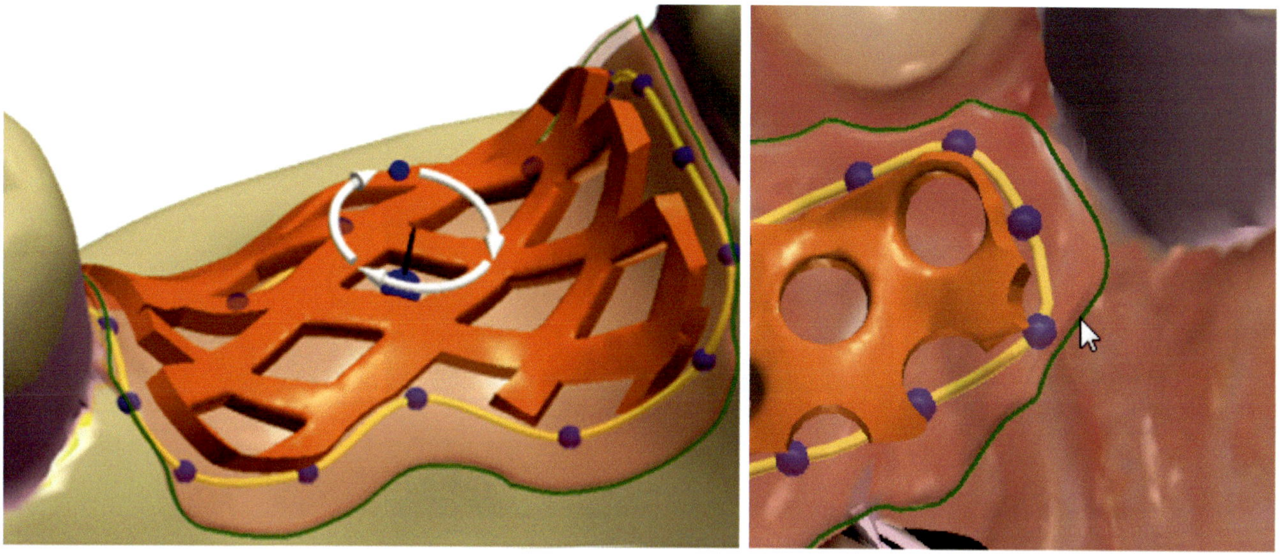

Fig. 4.14 Different shape and size of the meshwork

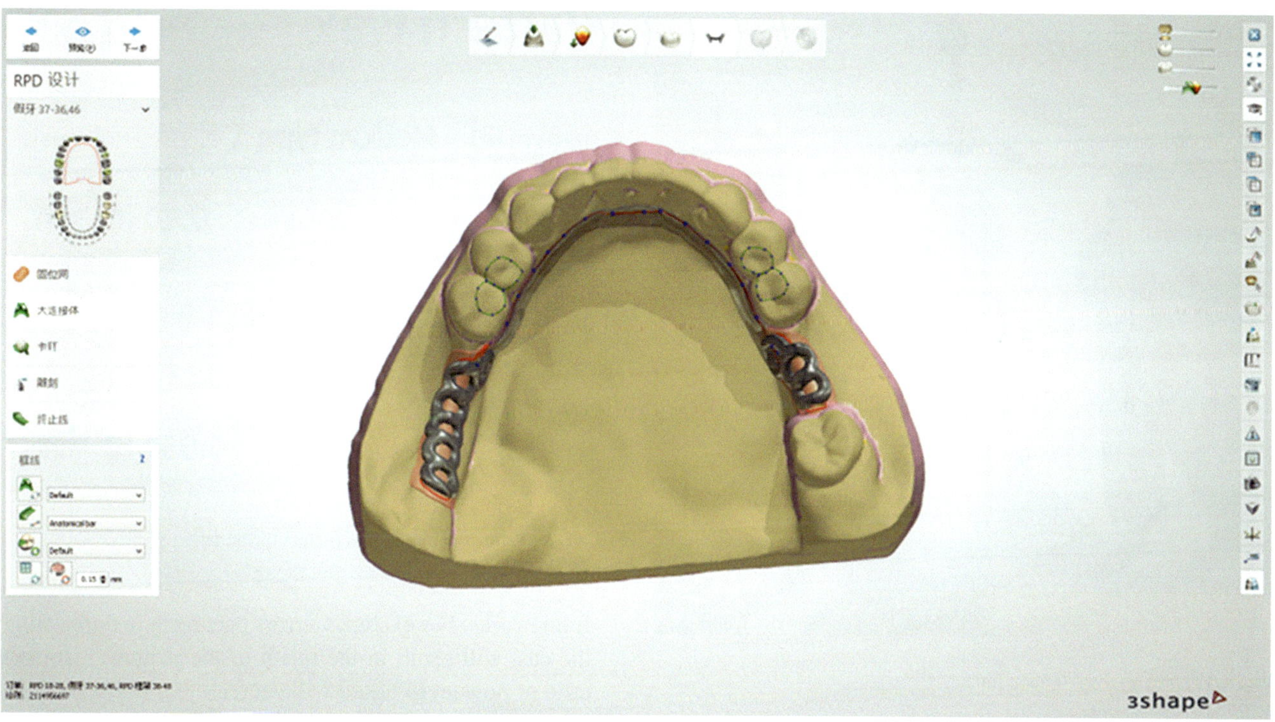

Fig. 4.15 Build the virtual major connector

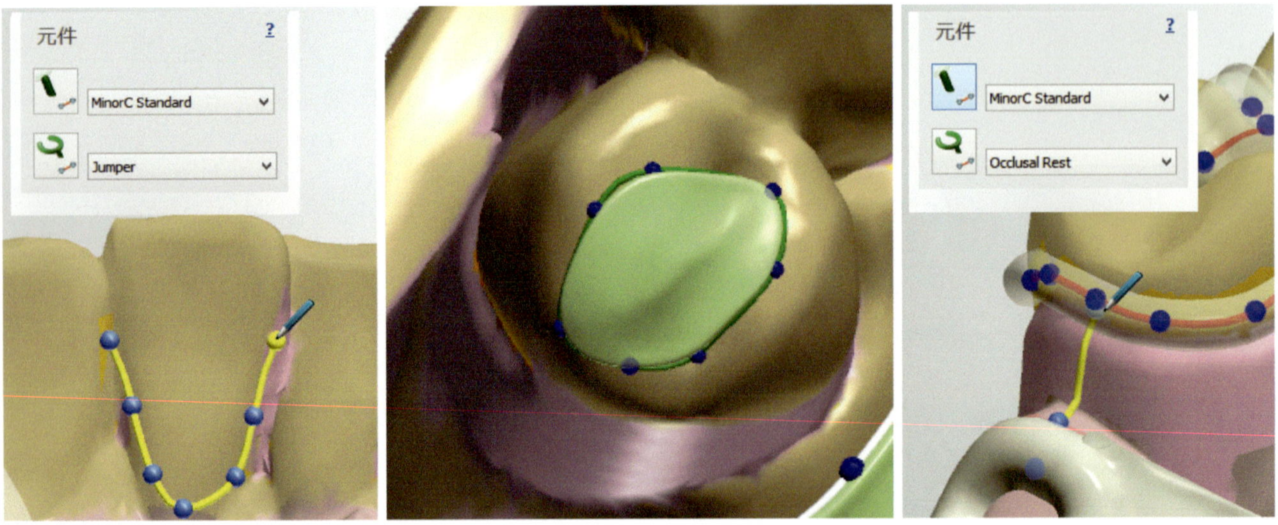

Fig. 4.16 Draw the clasp, rest, and minor connector three-dimensionally

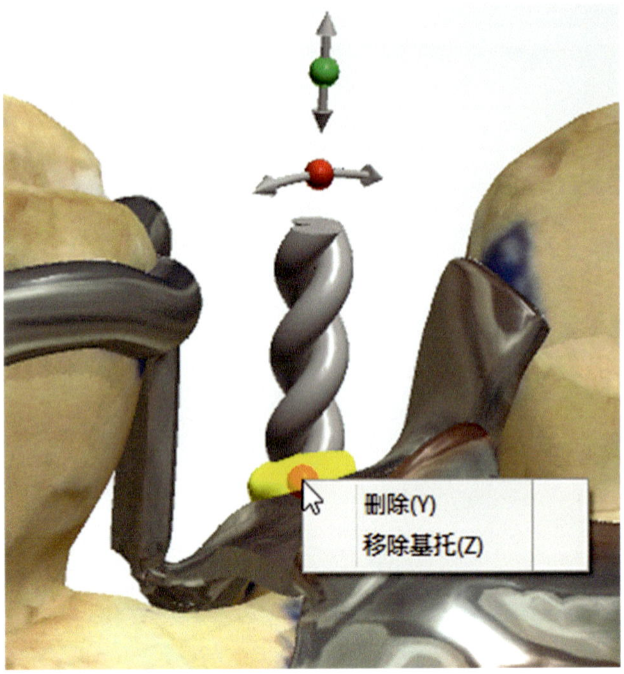

Fig. 4.17 Set up the retentive pin

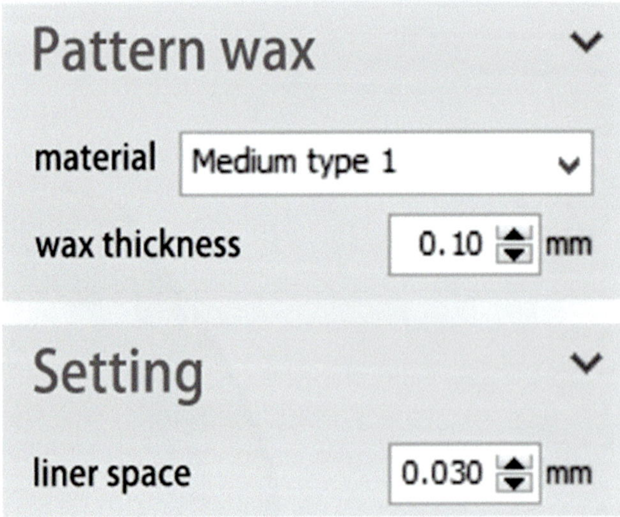

Fig. 4.18 Adjust technical parameters of the wax

The 3D printed wax (Fig. 4.33) or resin pattern is then cast conventionally using lost-wax technique (Fig. 4.34), and subsequent procedures are the same. It's worth noting that the wax or resin pattern should be invested and casted together with the refractory model to reduce the possibility of deformation.

Compared with 3D printed and milled metal frameworks, there is a traditional workflow of spruing, investing, burnout, and casting from 3D printed resin or wax patterns to the final metal framework, which is complex and has many human errors decreasing the quality of frameworks. For example, errors occurring in duplicating the cast will result in the misfit of the pattern; incorrect ratio of powder to liquid will decrease the strength of the investment, and then it will be prone to cracks during casting or generate the wear debris and contaminate the alloy; the mismatch between the expansion rate of the investment and the alloy may result in the misfit of frameworks; mixture of old and new alloys results in the uncertain expansion rate; selection of the investment is complicated; improper setting of sprues and storage pool will result in incomplete casting.

8. *CAD/CAM of the Custom Tray*

Based on the digital primary model, firstly determine the path of insertion, block out undesirable undercuts, and lay thin layers of virtual wax on relief areas

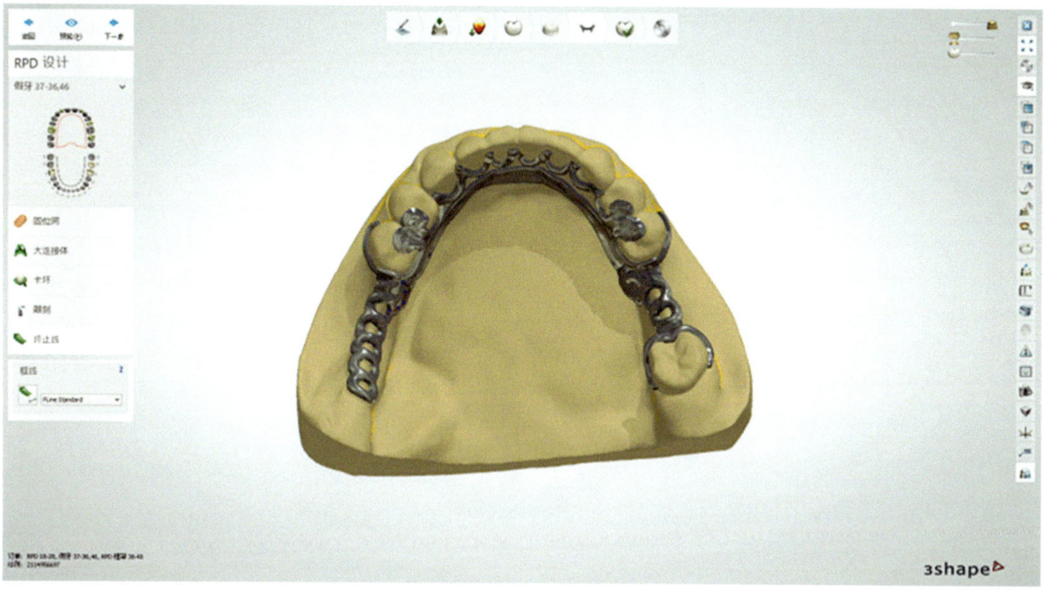

Fig. 4.19 Draw the outer finish line

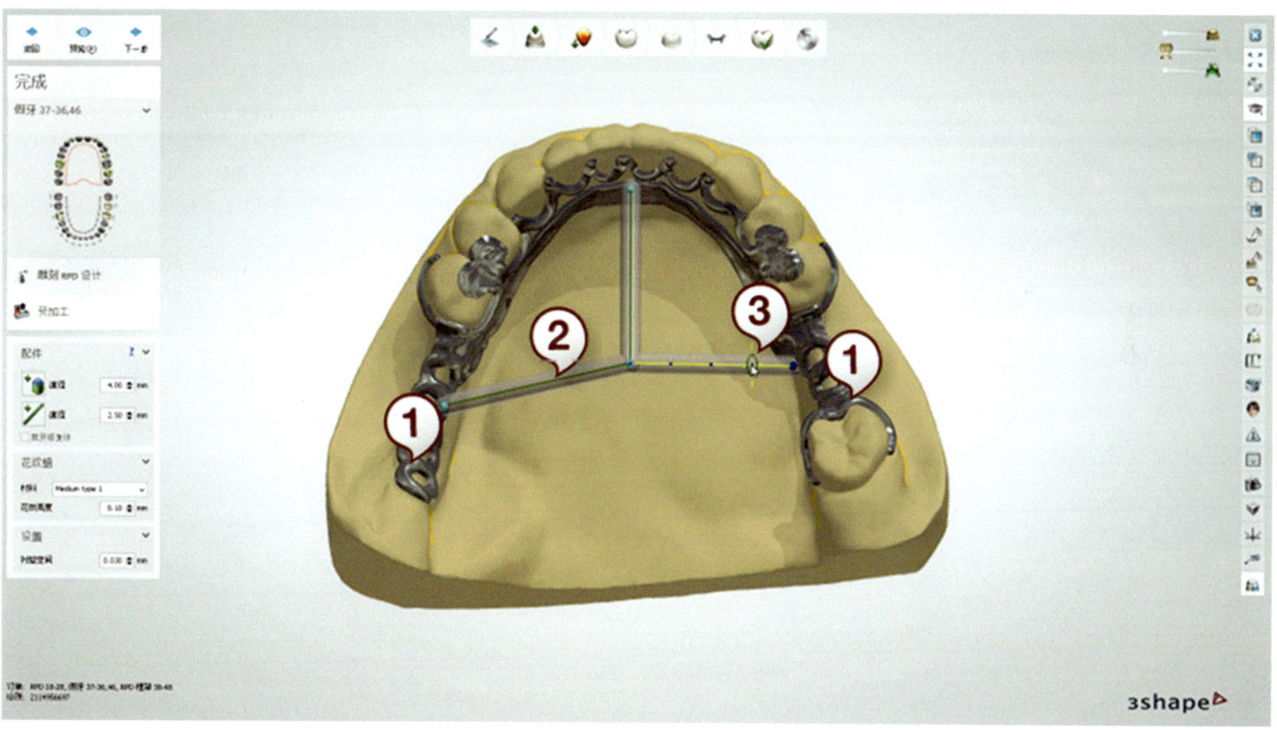

Fig. 4.20 Add appropriate supports to structures

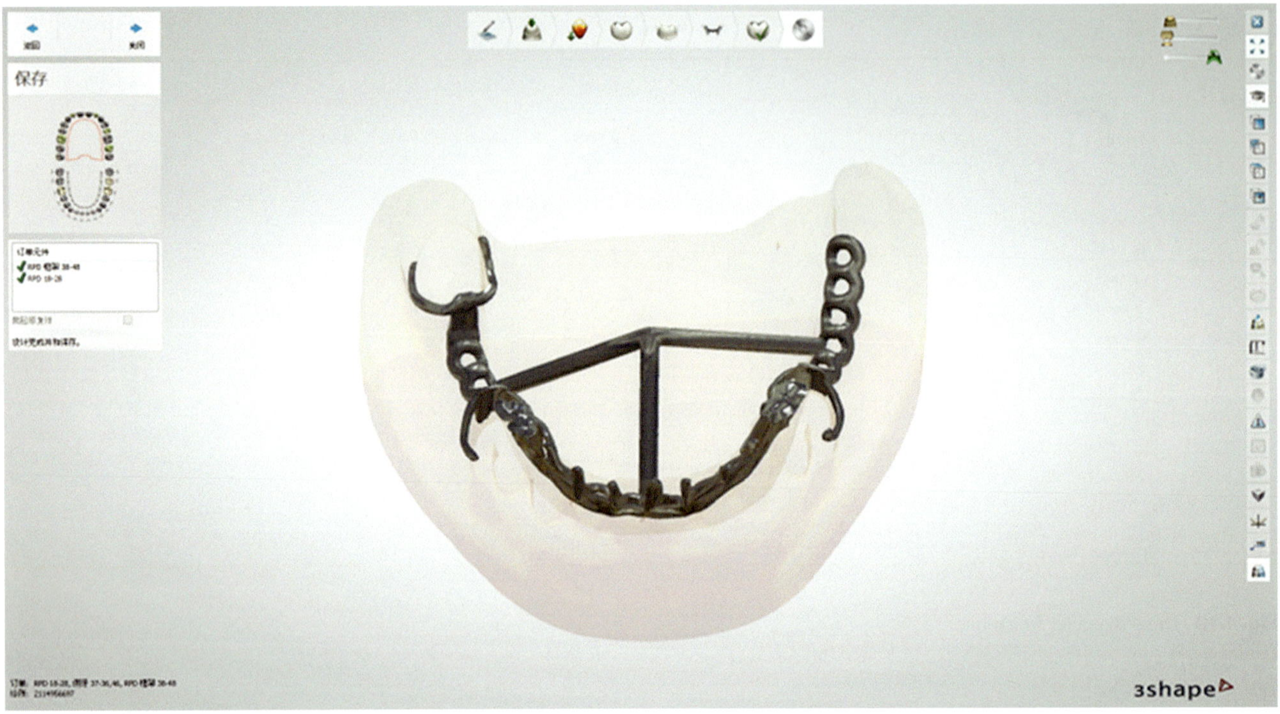

Fig. 4.21 Finish the design

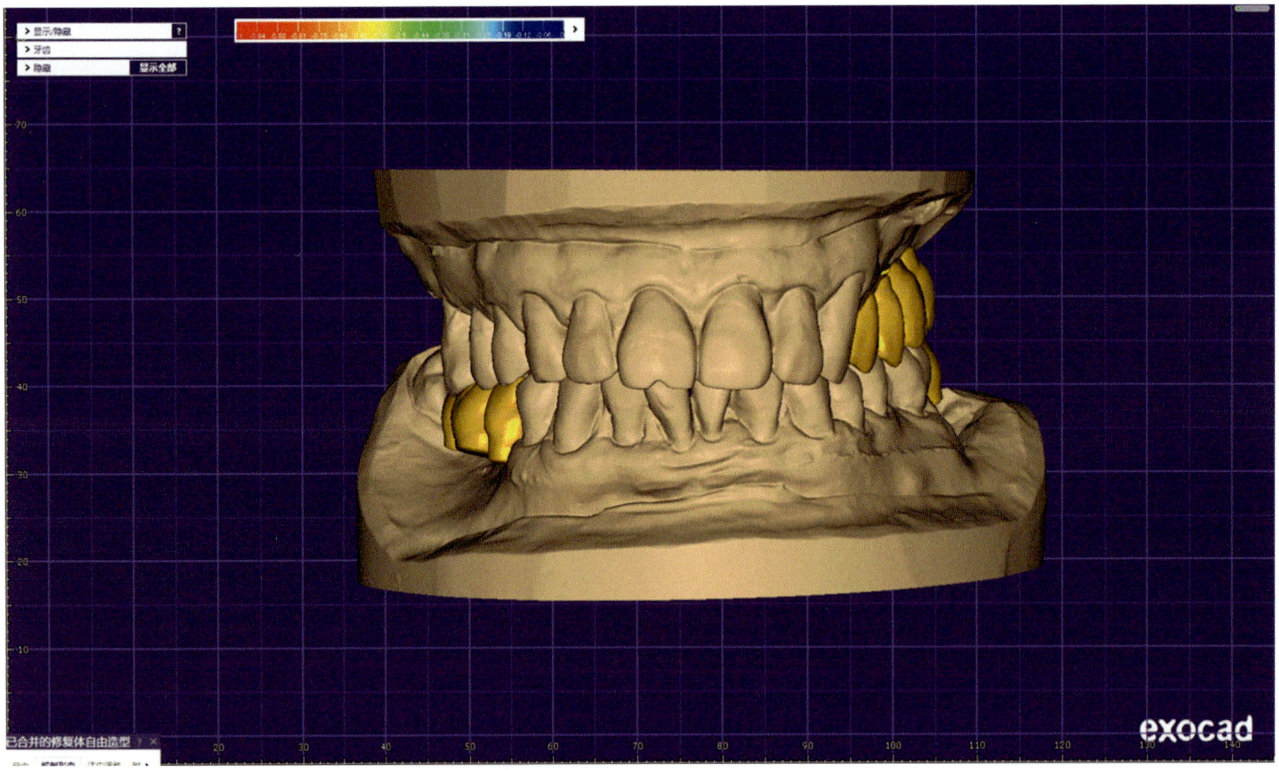

Fig. 4.22 Select and align the artificial teeth from tooth library

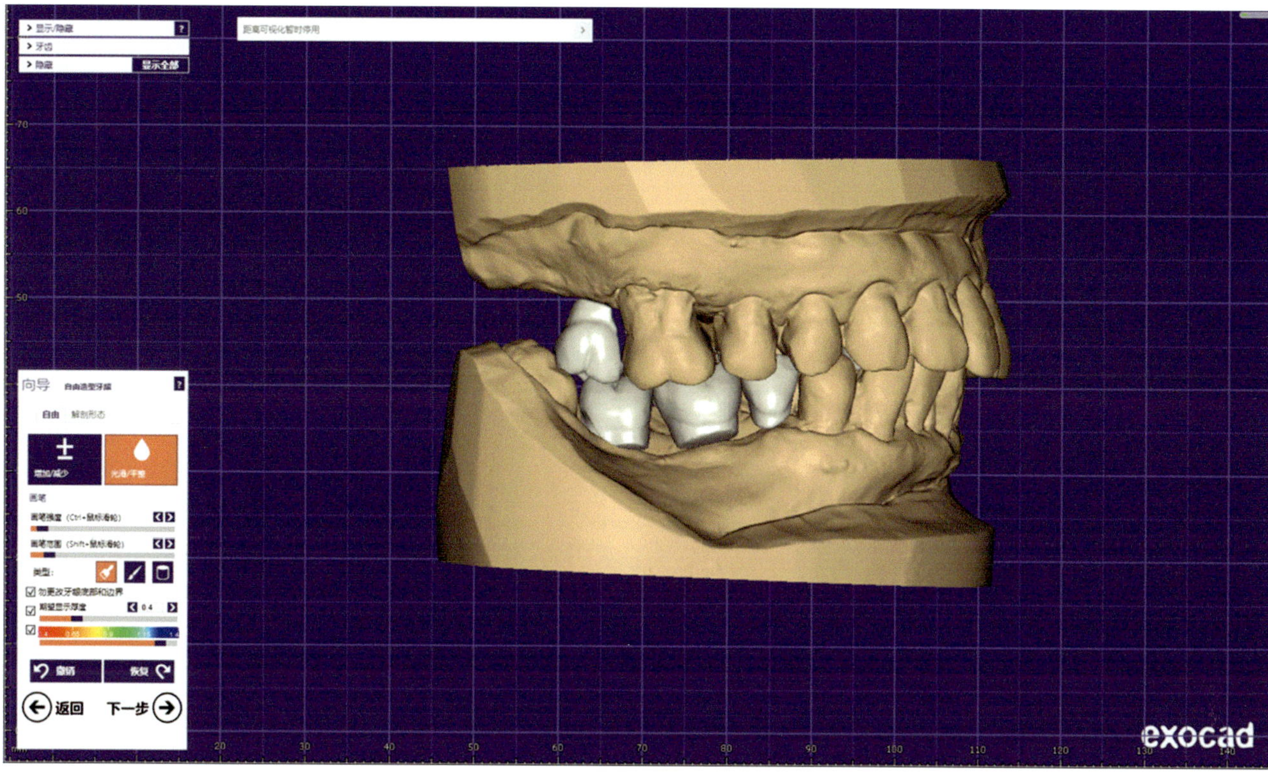

Fig. 4.23 Adjust the shape of the artificial teeth as needed

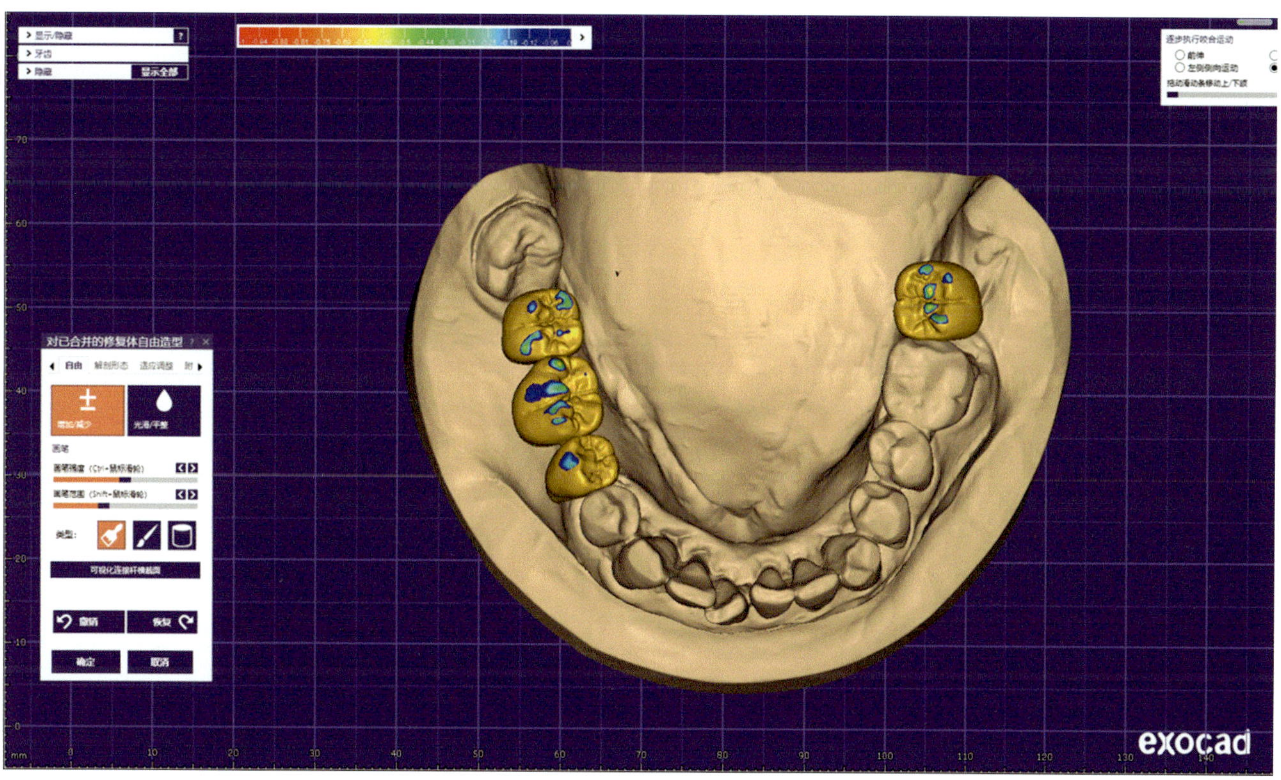

Fig. 4.24 Occlusal adjustment

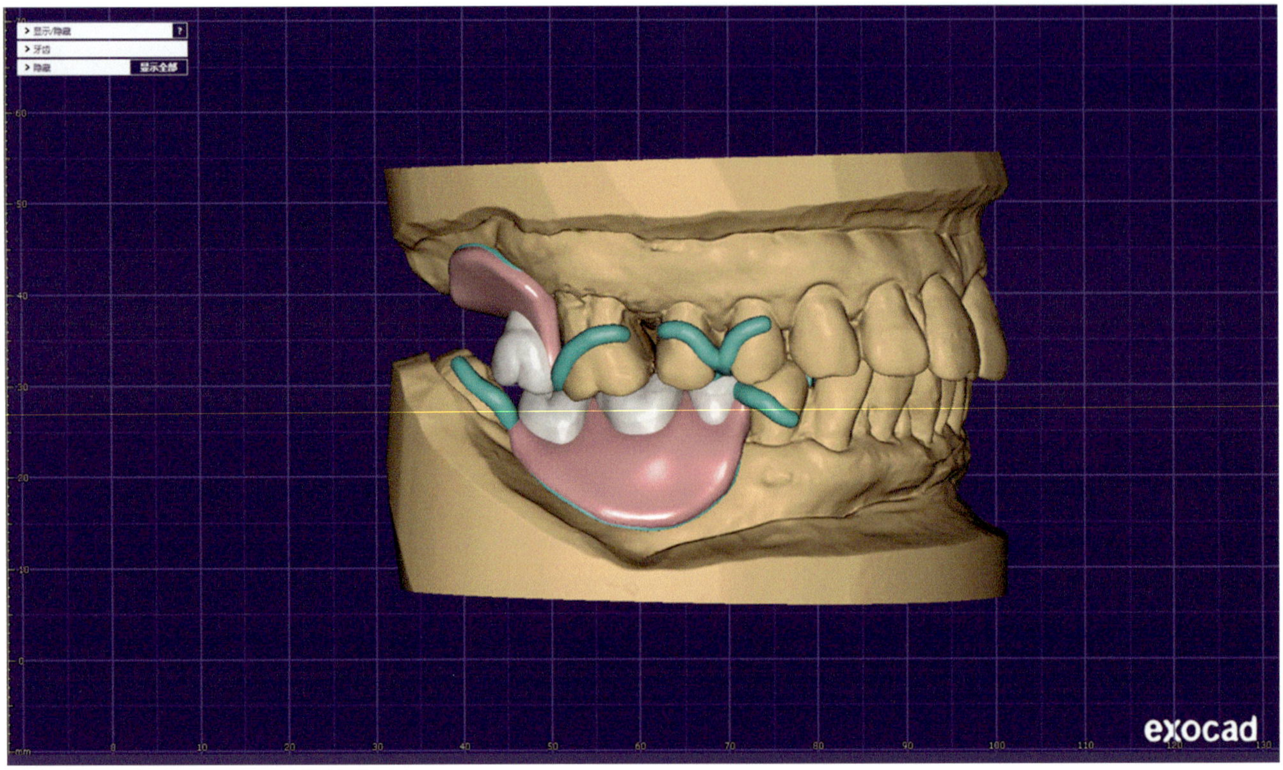

Fig. 4.25 Design the base of RPD

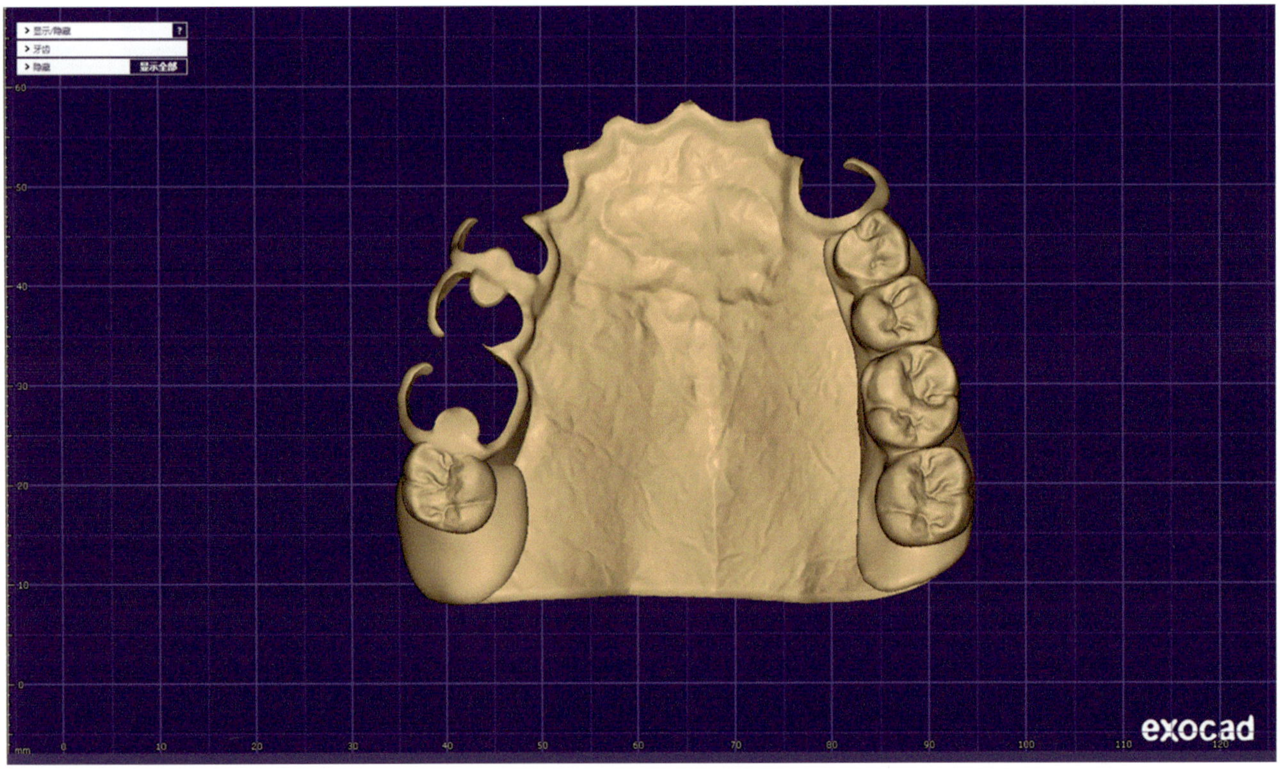

Fig. 4.26 One-piece RPD

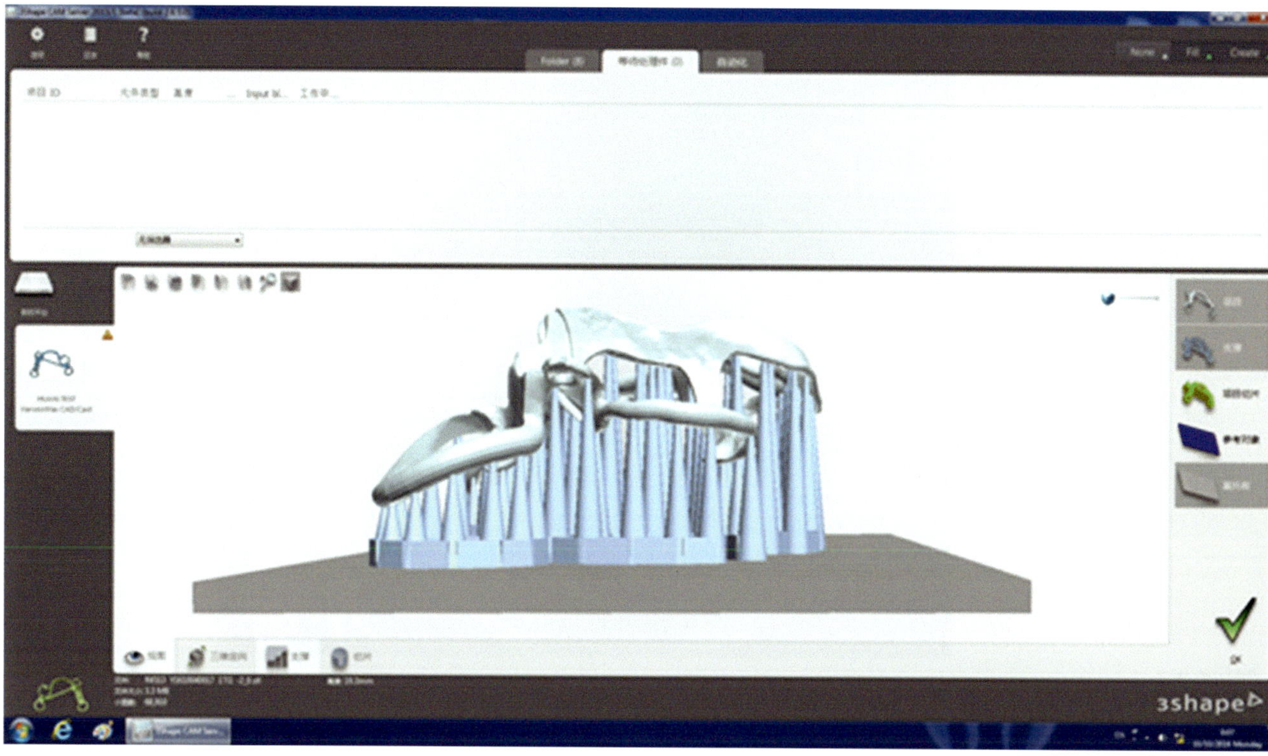

Fig. 4.27 Add supports to structures

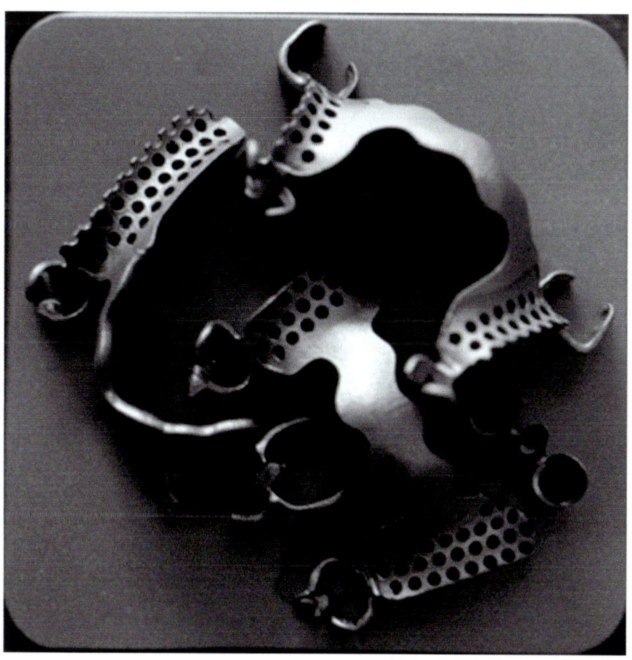

Fig. 4.28 3D printed Co-Cr framework

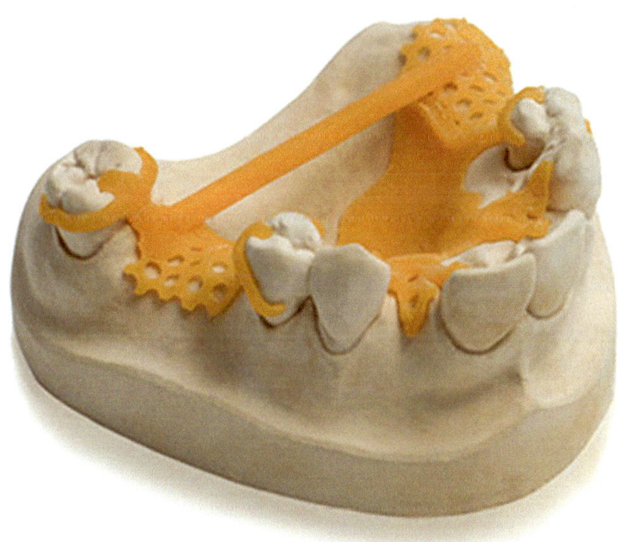

Fig. 4.29 3D printed wax pattern

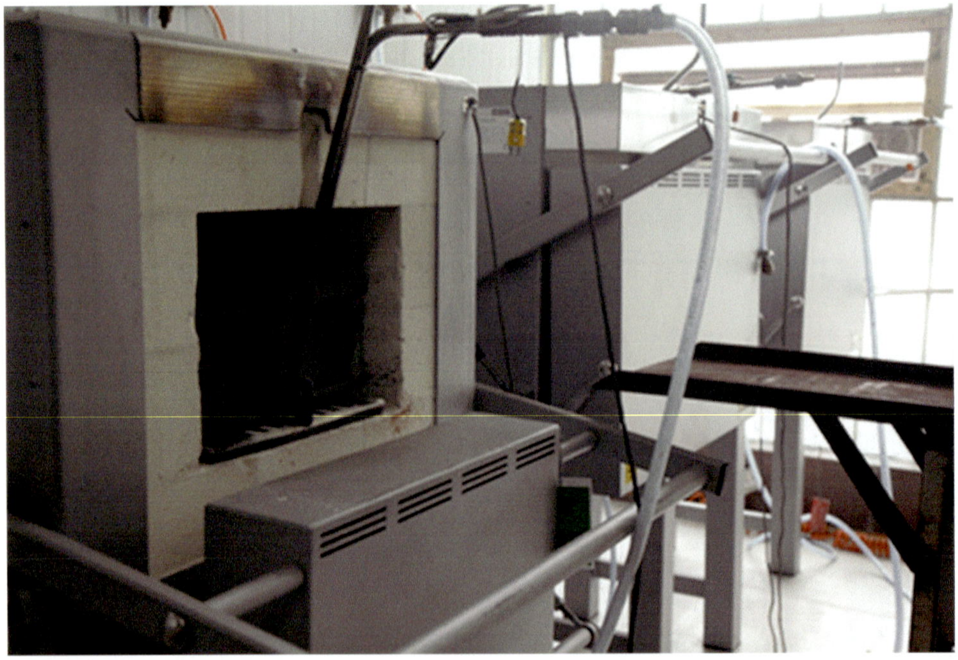

Fig. 4.30 Post-processing for stress release

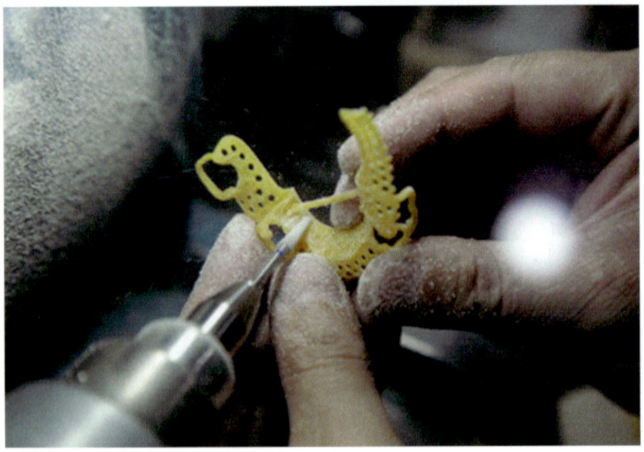

Fig. 4.31 Manual removal of supports added to 3D printed wax patterns

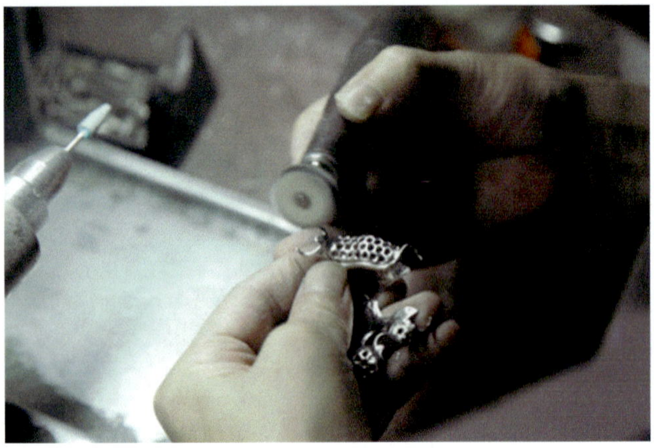

Fig. 4.32 Polish the 3D printed framework

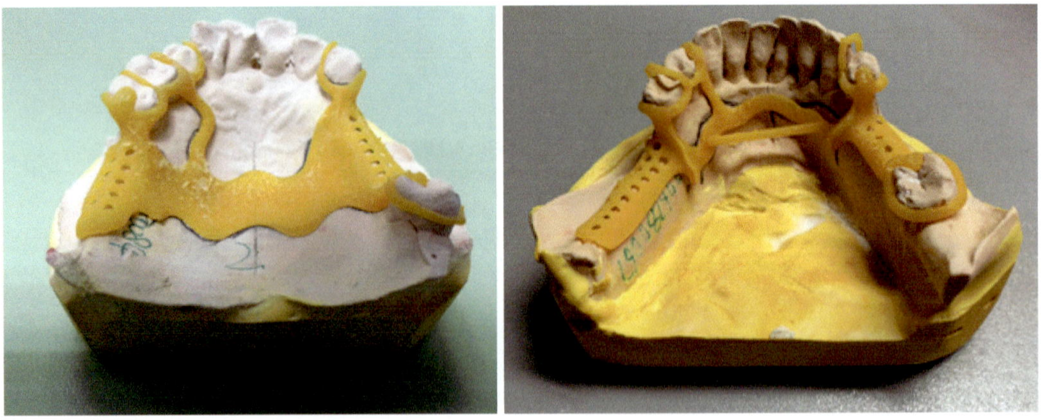

Fig. 4.33 3D printed wax pattern of the framework

(Fig. 4.35); then determine the extension range (Fig. 4.36) and the thickness to generate a tray with preliminary shape; finally design the handle (Fig. 4.37), and perforate the tray virtually according to the actual needs. Export the data after completion (Fig. 4.38), and print the tray using the resin printer.

4.3.2 Comparison of Digital and Traditional Frameworks

The conventional workflow, including making primary and final impression, making and trimming primary and final casts, waxing, investing, casting, finishing, and polishing of

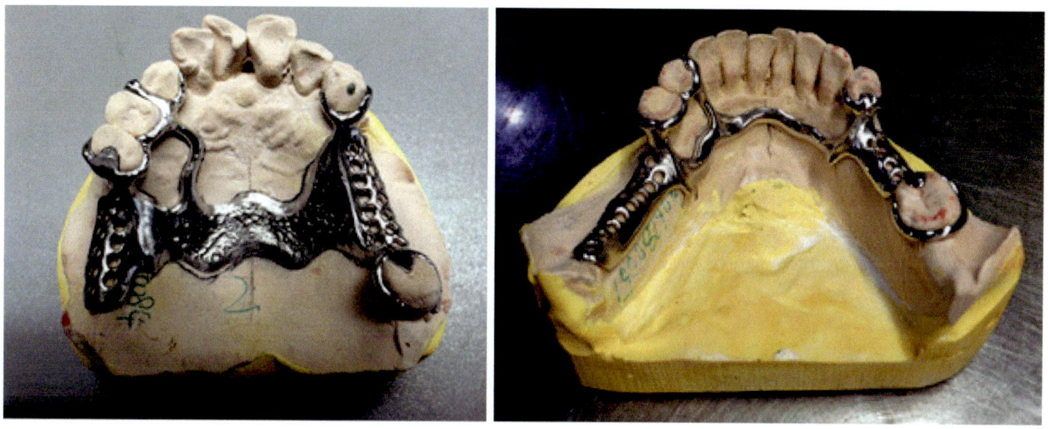

Fig. 4.34 Cast metal framework by lost-wax technique

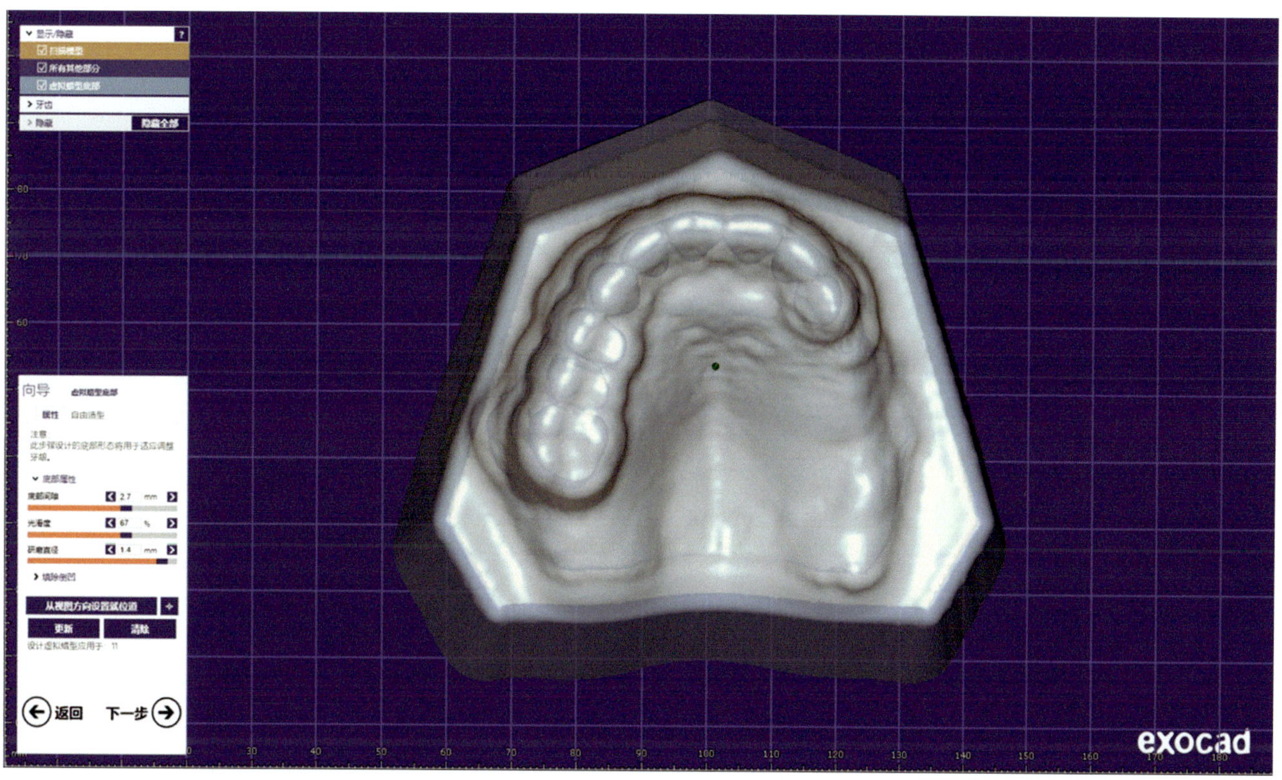

Fig. 4.35 Primary model with relief and blockout of undercuts

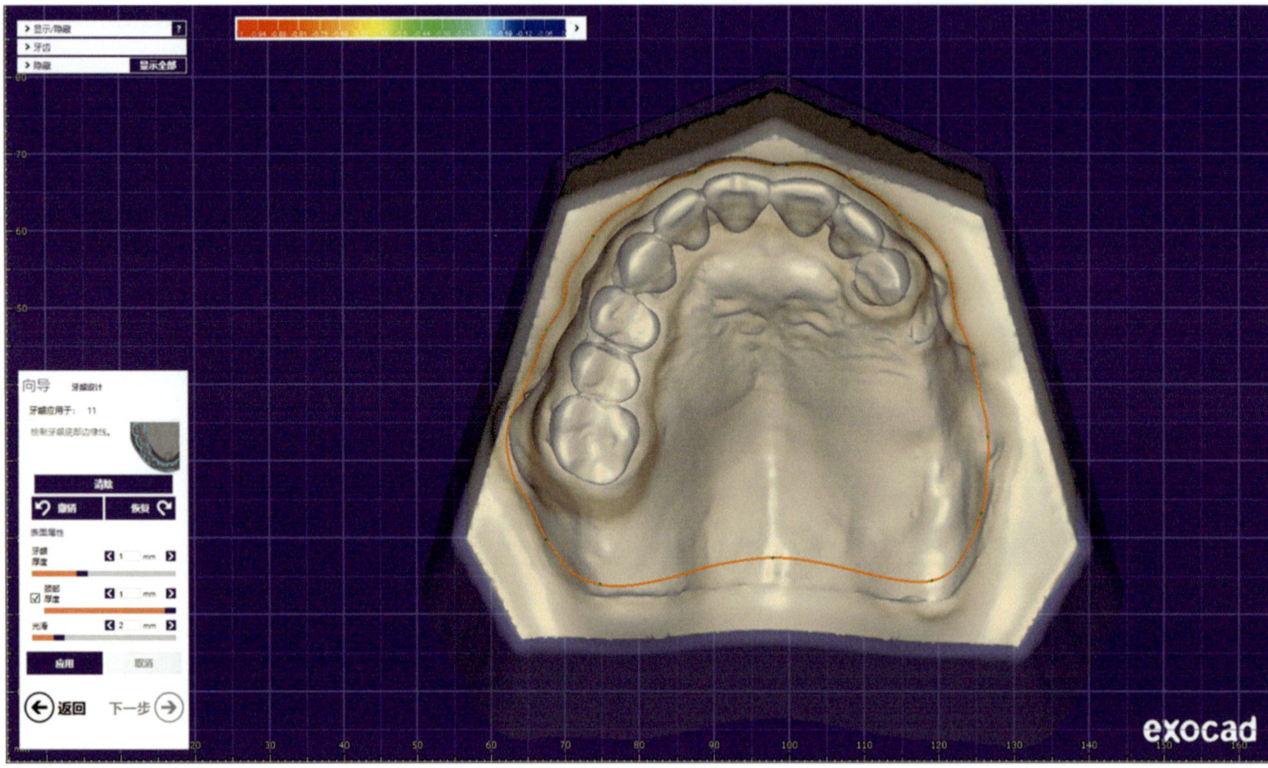

Fig. 4.36 Draw the expansion range

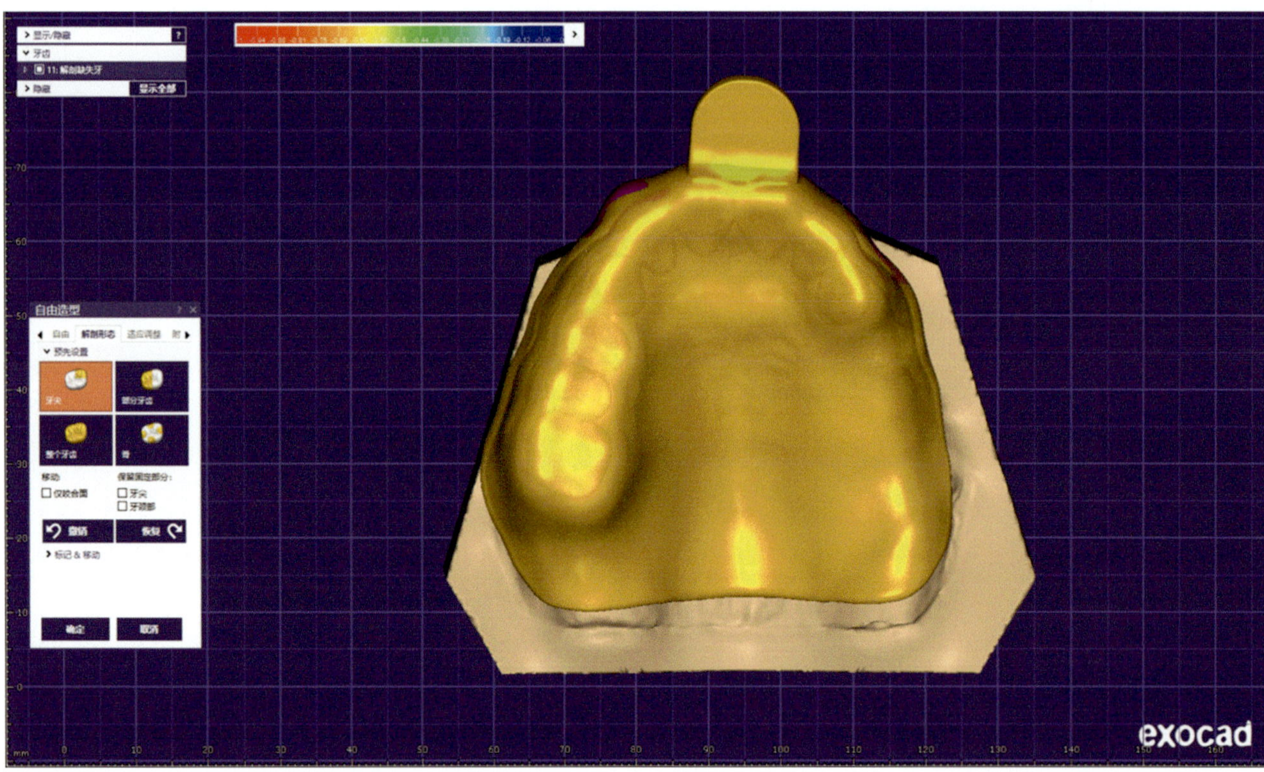

Fig. 4.37 Generate the preliminary shape and add the handle

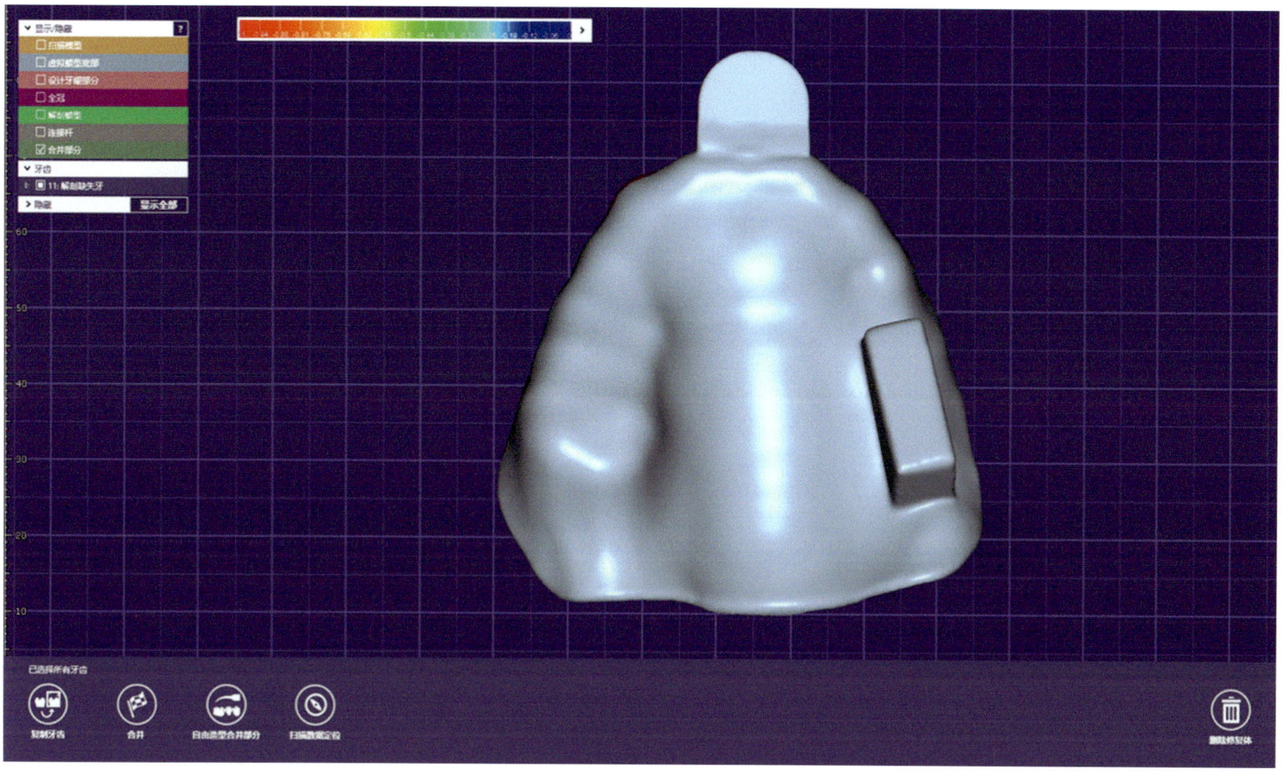

Fig. 4.38 Finish the design

the framework, mainly relies on the theoretical knowledge and operation experience of doctors and technicians and lacks the technical stability and objective standards, which is apt to generate errors in the production process, resulting in a series of problems such as the misfit of the framework, casting failure, and materials waste.

In the digital design, build the virtual structures of RPD three-dimensionally such as meshwork patterns, major connectors, minor connectors, clasps, and the finish line through CAD software, and print or mill the metal framework, or wax or resin sacrificial patterns by means of CAM equipment.

1. *Clinical analysis and design*

   The traditional design process of RPD consists of surveying, blocking out of undercuts, duplicating to form the refractory cast, waxing up, and so on (Fig. 4.39). Survey the cast fixed on the platform of the surveyor, and determine the path of insertion and undesirable undercuts that then will be blocked out. The traditional framework is made manually using prefabricated wax patterns for clasps, connectors, palatal coverage, and so on. The size of the clasp limited by wax patterns is relatively fixed.

   In the digital design workflow, the first step is to acquire the digital arch information through intraoral or extraoral scanners, and the second is to design the framework virtually by means of proprietary software, through which the insertion path of the framework can be adjusted and undercut areas of the abutment, presented by the color strips on the right side, will change accordingly, which can assist in the selection of the most suitable insertion path that will be indicated by the blue arrow (Fig. 4.40). After determining the path of insertion, undercuts will be blocked out automatically using red wax (Fig. 4.41), and some wax in retentive areas, where the tip of the retentive arm of the clasp contact with the abutment (Fig. 4.42), should be removed, leaving appropriate depth of the undercut.

2. *Process of fabrication*

   Table 4.1 shows the clinical failure rate of the cast framework, with a total of 30,618 dentures. Within 18 months, 89 of the 5076 pieces of pure titanium framework broke, with a failure rate of 1.75%. Among the 25,542 cobalt-chromium alloy framework, 146 pieces broke, and the failure rate was 0.57%. The clasp is the most common fracture location for both pure titanium and Co-Cr frameworks.

   Due to human errors and casting defects in traditional framework fabrication, the quality of prostheses will be affected to some extent. Some scholars have made statistics on the casting defects of cast Co-Cr frameworks (Table 4.2). According to literature reports, among the 258 clasps of 90 cast Co-Cr frameworks, 111 clasps have casting defects, accounting for 43% of the total. The

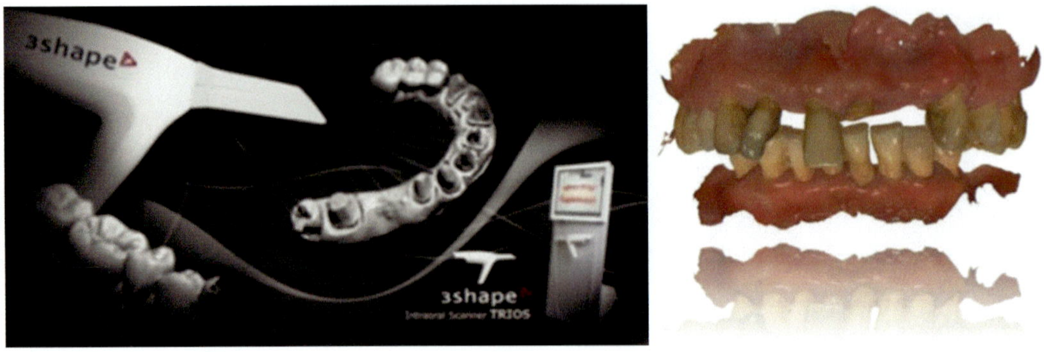

Fig. 4.39 Traditional design and fabrication procedures of cast frameworks

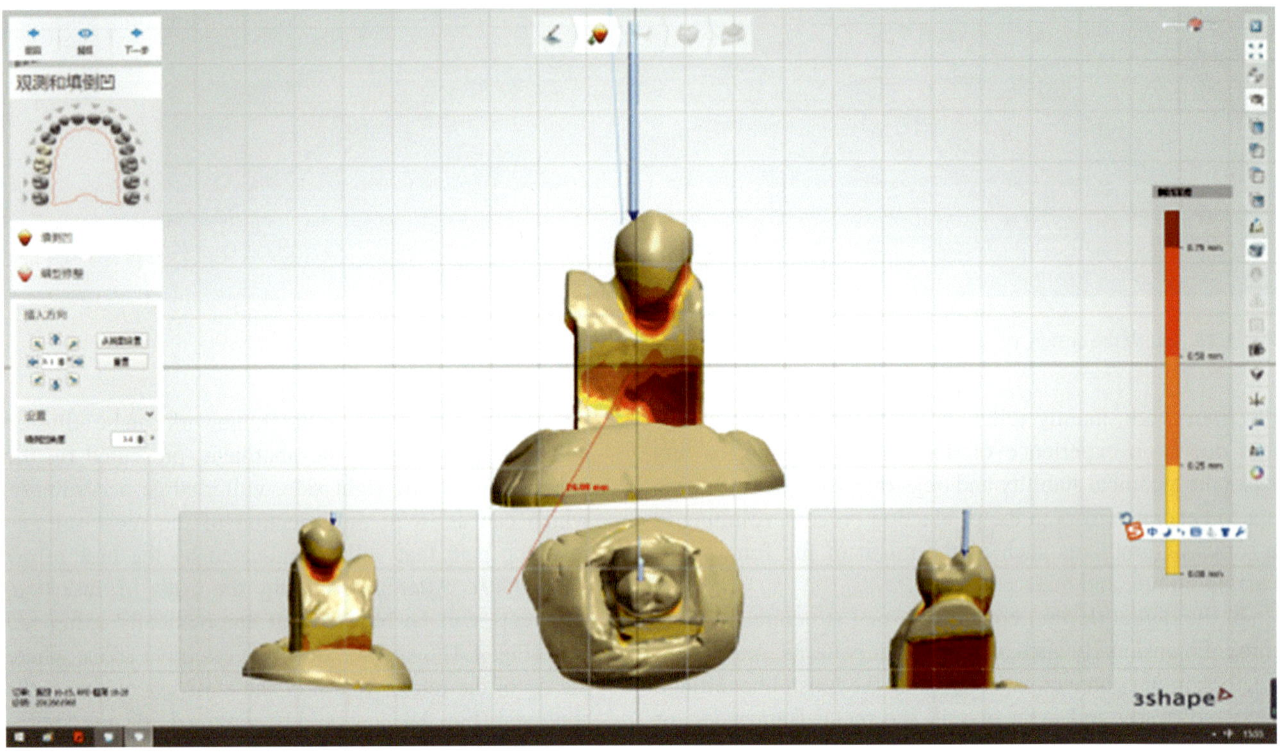

Fig. 4.40 Adjust the path of insertion

number and proportion of defects in each part of the clasp are shown in the following table. It can be seen that the casting defect rate of the occlusal rest is the highest, reaching 24.18%.

Table 4.3 shows the number and prevalence of casting defects. It can be seen that among the 90 frameworks, 12 of them have no casting defects, 26 of them have 1–2 casting defects, and 16 of them have extensive defects.

Compared with traditional frameworks, 3D printed metal frameworks have obvious advantages:

(a) Net formability. There're almost no wasted metal powders, and unused materials can be recycled.
(b) Superior design and geometric flexibility. Enable producing a complex 3D design and geometries, especially suitable for metal frameworks.
(c) No micropore, high density, and high precision.
(d) A variety of materials can be used for dental applications, such as Co-Cr alloy, titanium alloy, etc.
(e) Reduce the fabrication step of molding and shorten the production time.

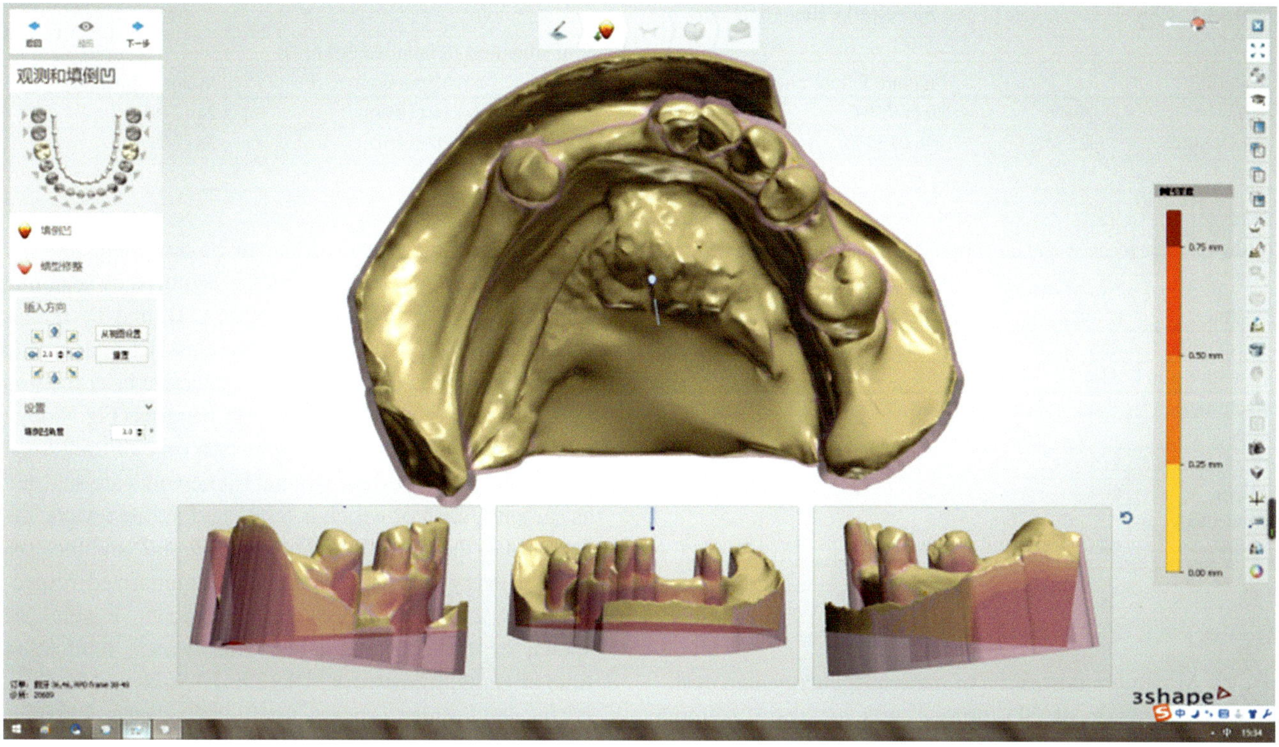

Fig. 4.41 Block out undesirable undercuts

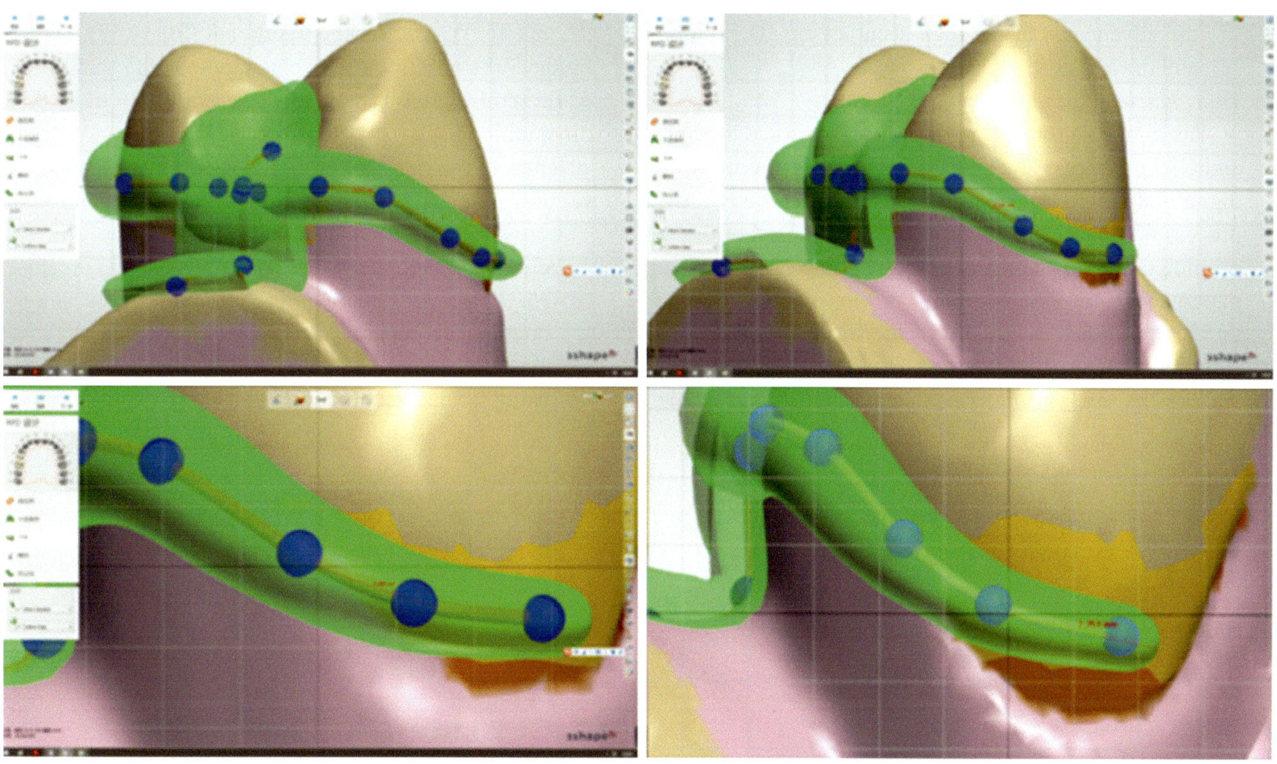

Fig. 4.42 Draw the virtual clasp three-dimensionally and the retentive tips are placed in the undercuts

Table 4.1 Clinical failure rate of cast frameworks after 18 months

			Rates of situations in failure cases n(%)		
Materials	n	Fracture failure rates n(%)	Clasp	Minor connector	Major connector
Ti	5076	89 (1.75%)	49 (55%)	16 (18%)	24 (27%)
Co-Cr alloy	25542	146 (0.57%)	88 (60%)	20 (14%)	38 (26%)

Table 4.2 The location and proportion of casting defects

Casting	No. of castings studied	No. of castings defects	Percentage
Clasp units	258	111	43.00
Retentive arm	334	31	9.28
Reciprocal arm	326	28	8.58
Occlusal rests	215	52	24.18
Minor connector	204	43	21.07
Major connector	90	18	20.00

(f) Maximum utilization of materials, energy, and cost.

Advantages of 3D printed wax or resin patterns (Fig. 4.43):

(a) The framework is also designed digitally, reducing human errors associated with manual wax-ups.
(b) Low cost of the equipment and effectively combining the advantages of the high accuracy of 3D printing and the low cost of casting.

3. *Time, efficiency, and workflow*

The digitalization of frameworks is composed of CAD and CAM process. The CAD process refers to collecting digital data by 3D scanner and designing, and the CAM process is to fabricate the framework by means of direct printing of the metal or casting of the printed wax or resin patterns (Fig. 4.44).

The traditional procedure of the framework includes steps of making impression, pouring into plaster cast, waxing up, and casting. But in semi-digital and whole digital workflow, frameworks can be designed virtually based on the digital model, which is acquired by scanning the gypsum cast for Kennedy class I, II, and IV arches and by intraoral scan for Kennedy class III arches, and then be fabricated directly through selective laser melting (SLM) or cast from 3D printed wax patterns (Fig. 4.45).

To compare the average production time of traditional and digital frameworks, 20 metal frameworks are selected as samples, each of which is fabricated in three ways, the traditional, the semi-digital, and the digital, and the cost time of every step is recorded and summarized respectively by the same experienced technician. Results are shown in the following table. The average fabrication time of single framework is 4.12 h, 10.56 h, and 20.85 h, for the semi-digital process, traditional process, and digital process, respectively (Fig. 4.46).

From the perspective of the average cost of a framework, we can see that the average cost of the framework is 54.95 yuan for the semi-digital, 95.05 yuan for the digital, and 45.05 yuan for the traditional (Fig. 4.47). Digital frameworks cost about twice as much as the traditional, while semi-digital frameworks cost only 22% more than the traditional.

Thus, the advantages of digital RPD are as details:

(a) *Repeatability*: Conducive to the quality control of prostheses and standardized management of the clinic and laboratory.
(b) *Predictability*: Facilitating communication among doctors, technicians, and patients.
(c) *Resource integration*: Facilitating the efficient application of new technologies and equipment.

Table 4.3 The number and prevalence of casting defects on cast frameworks

No. and status of specimens						
No. of castings studied	No castings defect	One casting defect	Two castings defect	Three castings defect	More than three castings defect	Generalized castings defect
90	12	26	26	18	8	16

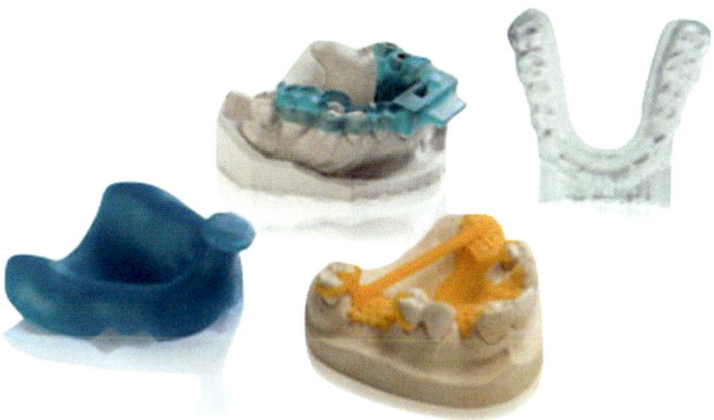

Fig. 4.43 3D printed resin patterns

(d) *Process integration*: Facilitating the integration of each link and avoiding errors in the information transmission.
(e) *Efficiency* improvement: Streamlining operations
(f) *Environmentally friendly* Computer-aided design and computer-aided manufacturing (CAD/CAM) replacing the traditional process of waxing up, investing, and casting, greatly improving the working environment of technicians.

However, there are still problems to be solved in digital RPD at present.

(g) *Equipment*: The precision and accuracy of the existing equipment still need to be further improved, so as to make more precise prostheses. There are still shrinkage holes in the printed metal. In addition, the printing time is long, and the printing rate needs to be increased.
(h) *Materials*: There're only two main kinds of digital dental alloys for printed RPDs, Co-Cr alloy and Ti alloy, needing to develop more kinds of metal powders.
(i) *Cost* At present, most of the equipment and materials are imported, and the cost of the whole digital process is relatively high. It's necessary to develop equipment and materials independently to reduce the cost of digital production and make it more widely used.

Digitalization in RPD refers to a series of digital process, done through the computer, including the evaluation of the patient's anatomy physiology, the design of the prosthesis, the impression of arches, and the precise production of the prosthesis, making the prosthesis a perfect work of art. With the continuous development of new materials and technologies, the aim is to optimize the digital operation and to reduce the cost, developing from powder spray to no powder spray, from rough to precise, from complex to intelligent, from slow to fast, from manual to automatic, from big to small, and from more to less.

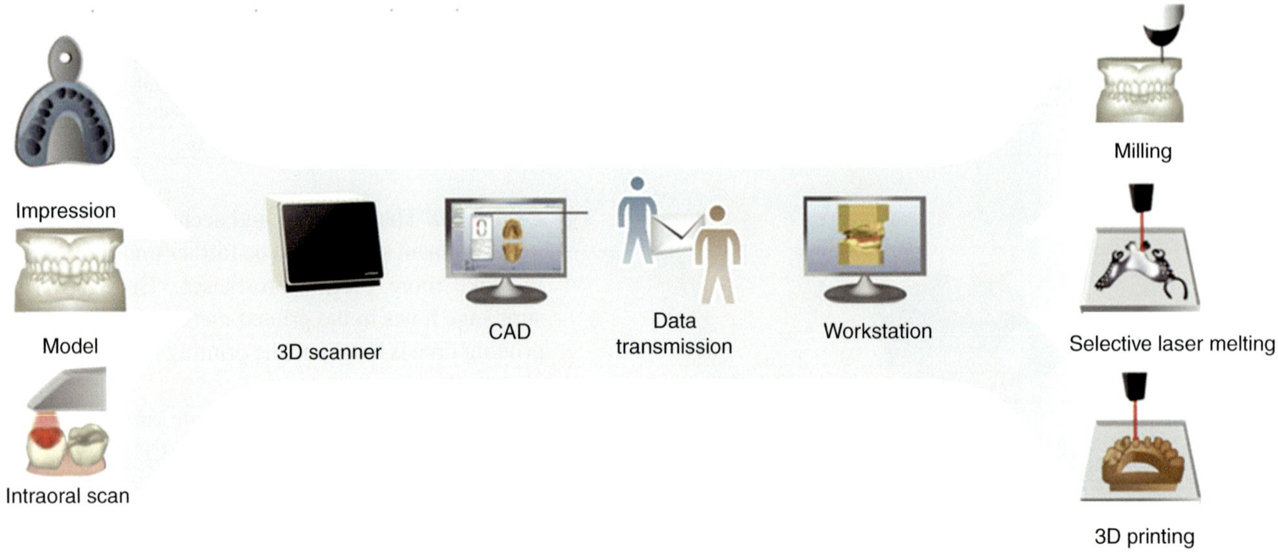

Fig. 4.44 Digital workflow of the framework

Fig. 4.45 Process comparison of cast and digital esthetic frameworks

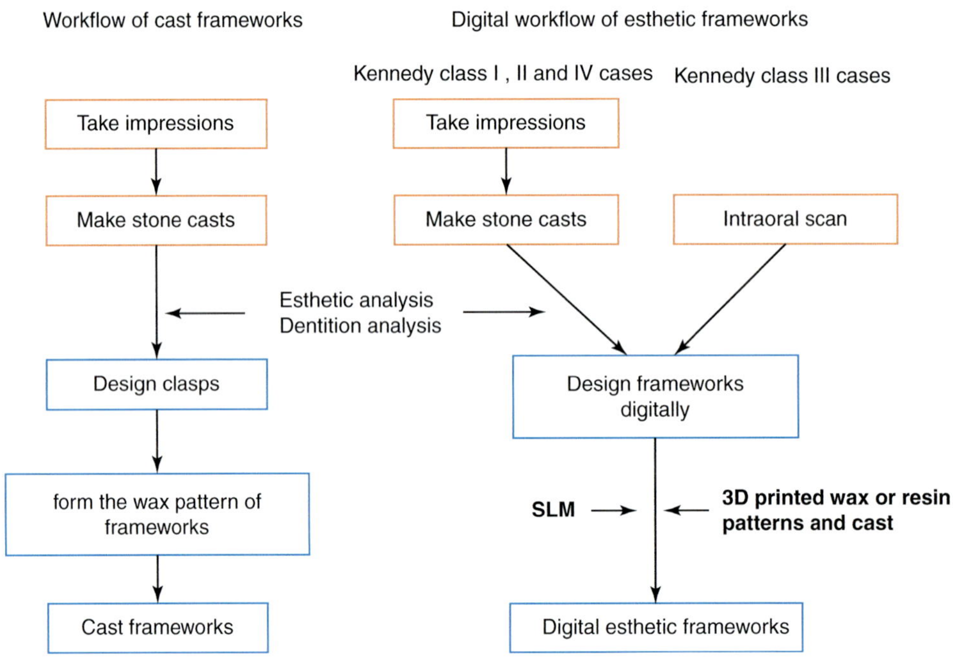

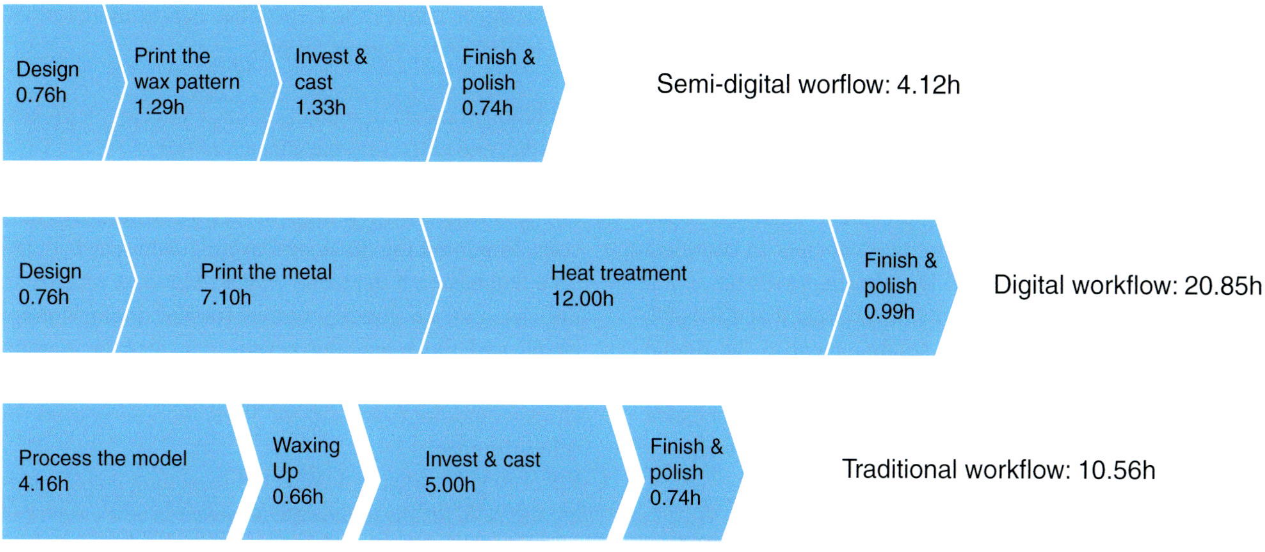

Fig. 4.46 Average production time of cast frameworks and digitalized frameworks

Fig. 4.47 Cost of a framework fabricated by three different techniques

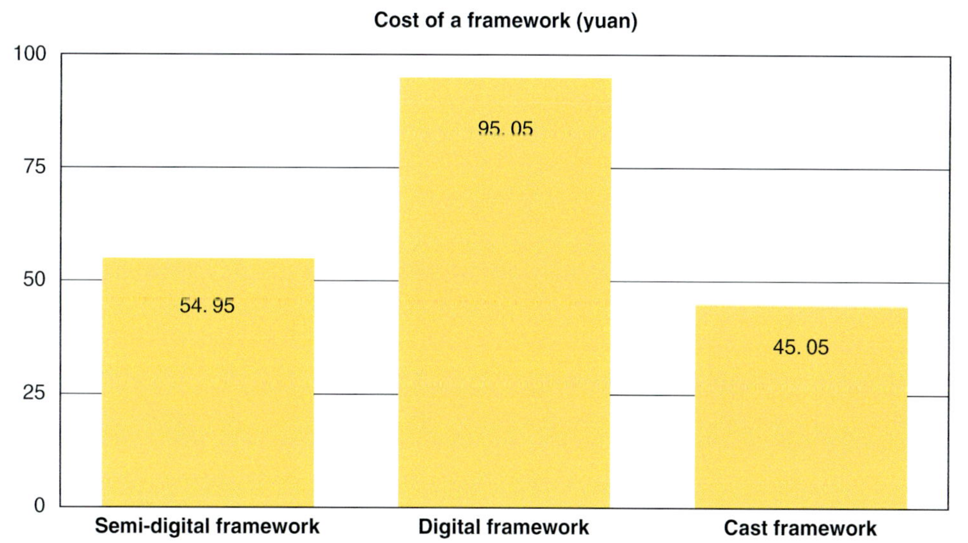

4.4 Application of RD Designer Software in RPD

4.4.1 RD Designer

RD designer is a clinical decision support system software for removable partial dentures in prosthetic dentistry. It can be applied in clinical practice to assist doctors to complete the design of frameworks of RPD according to the basic oral conditions of patients and to provide a standard and feasible delivery path of the plan. It is a supplement to the digital process of RPDs. In addition, it can also be applied to the analysis and design of virtual cases in teaching to enhance the combination between teaching and clinical practices.

4.4.2 Working Principles of RD Designer

Case-based reasoning (CBR) is an important reasoning method in the field of artificial intelligence. It gives the solving process and result of the new problem through the retrieval and match of previous cases. Rule-based reasoning (RBR) system, also known as a production system, connects rules in series through logical relations and draws the required conclusions through logical derivation. Combination of RBR and CBR, playing their respective advantages, uses rules to guide case retrieval and to achieve the goal that the cases should be as few as possible and as relevant, similar or matching as possible to the target cases.

RD designer applies the CBR-RBR hybrid model to the design of RPD. Steps are as follows:

1. Obtaining the data of medical cases, carrying out preprocessing, and extracting the characteristics.
2. Performing CBR case retrieval on the test data.
3. For test cases with a high degree of similarity, it is considered that the most similar medical records in the case database are the same as the diagnosis results, so the case can be directly output for the doctor's diagnosis, and the reasoning results can also be output. For the test cases with low similarity, the most similar cases cannot be found, so the RBR module is used for rule inference.
4. Recording the diagnostic effect of reasoning results, adding the valid results to the case database as new cases, and updating the decision tree rules of RBR module.

4.4.3 Digital Workflow of RD Designer

1. *Create a case*. Select missing teeth according to the edentulous areas of the patient (Fig. 4.48).
2. *Preliminary judgment*. The software will judge the alternative plans preliminarily based on the situation of edentulous areas, for example, elastic dentures will be suggested firstly when a few anterior teeth are lost.
3. *Preliminary scheme*. The software will recommend the optimal plan and the alternatives according to the rules (Fig. 4.49).

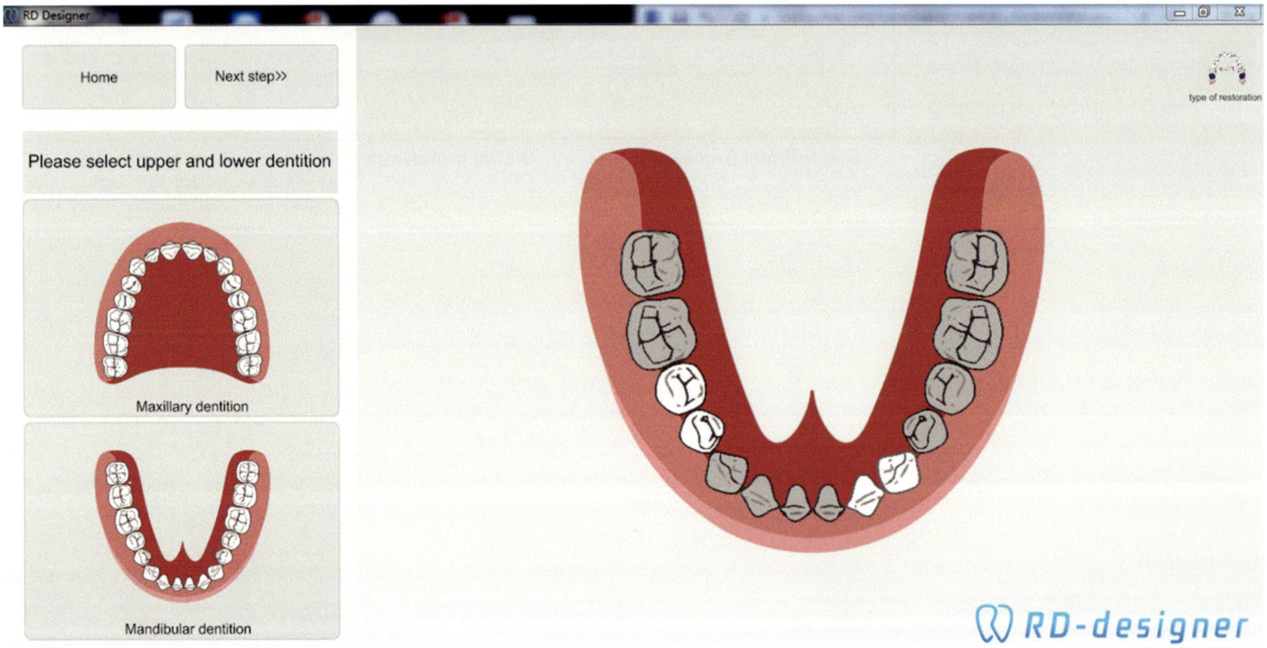

Fig. 4.48 Software interface of creating a case

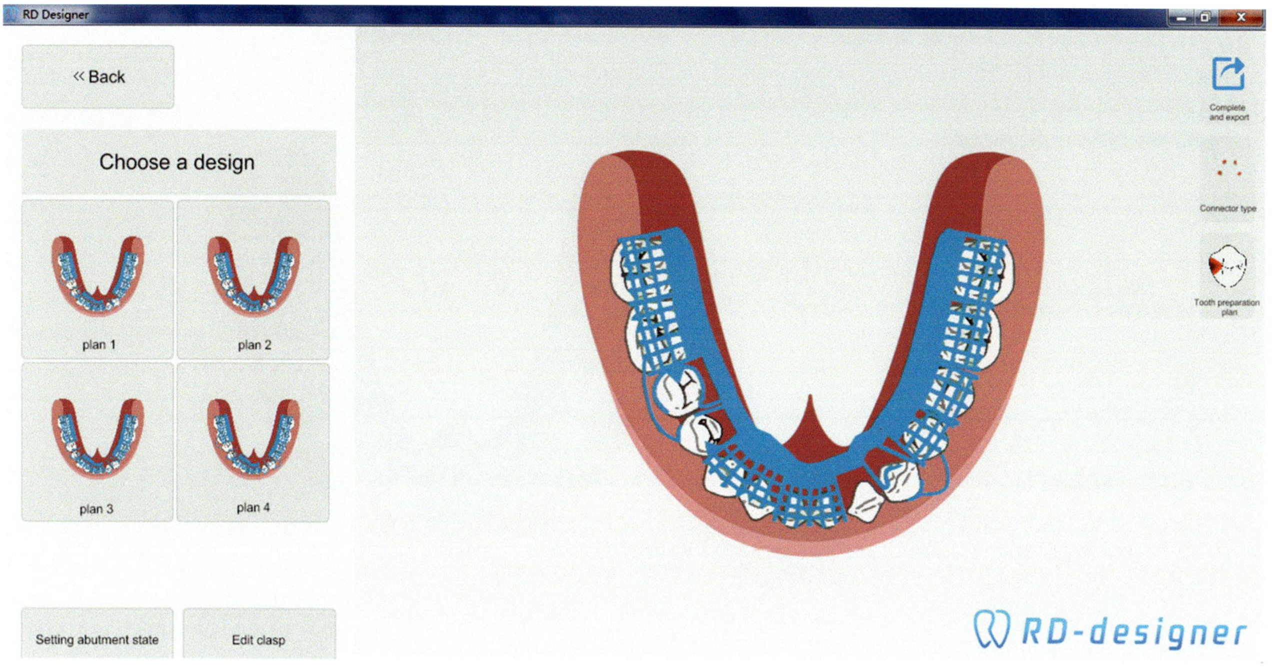

Fig. 4.49 Software interface of preliminary scheme

4. *Secondary scheme*. The software will adjust the primary plan automatically according to the abutment situation of looseness and tilt (Fig. 4.50).
5. *Customized adjustment*. Clinicians are allowed to replace clasps and connectors with alternatives according to the personalized situation of the patient (Fig. 4.51). The design of the framework will be completed primarily.
6. *Analysis of load*. The software will analyze the stress of the designed framework while functioning according to the law of fulcrum line and plane, providing certain reference for the rationality of the framework.
7. *Guidance of tooth preparation*. The preparation plan of rest seats and guide planes will be generated according to their locations by the software (Fig. 4.52). Finish the design of RPD.

4.4.4 Future of RD Designer

1. Optimizing the database through deep learning based on of big data
2. Increasing the dimension and combining with the intraoral scan to display the esthetic result digitally and immediately
3. Facilitating the linkup of RD designer and CAD/CAM software and importing editable STL files to avoid errors in transmission from 2D to 3D

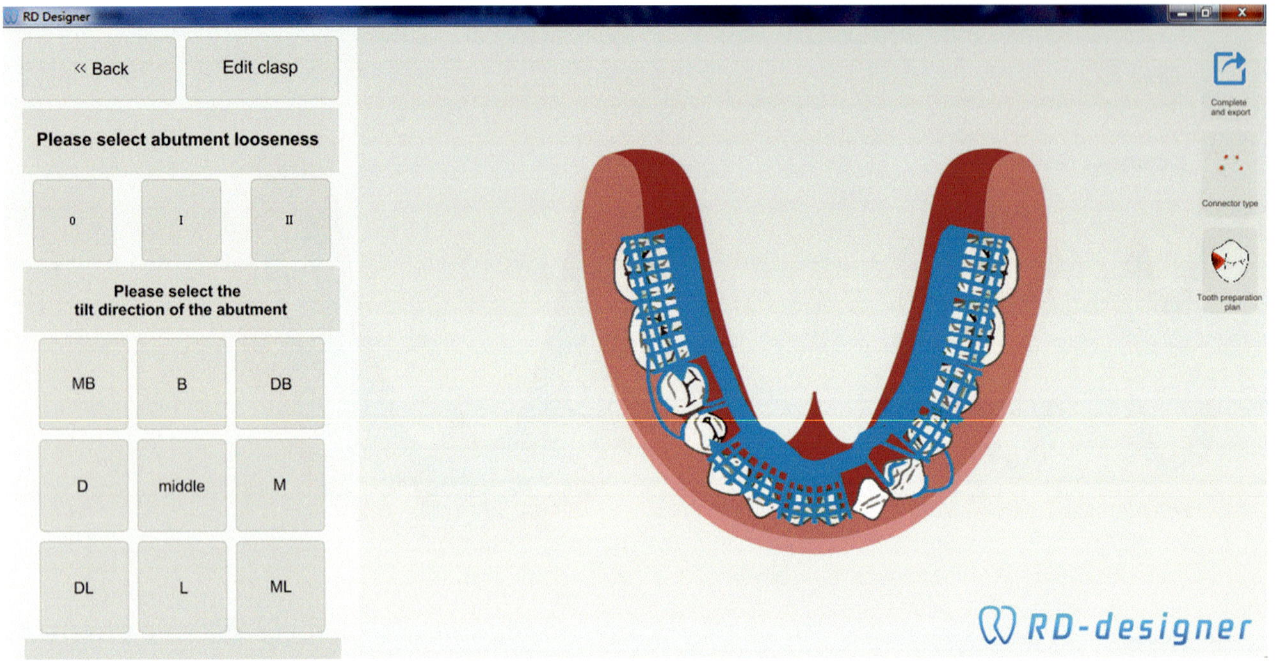

Fig. 4.50 Software interface of secondary scheme

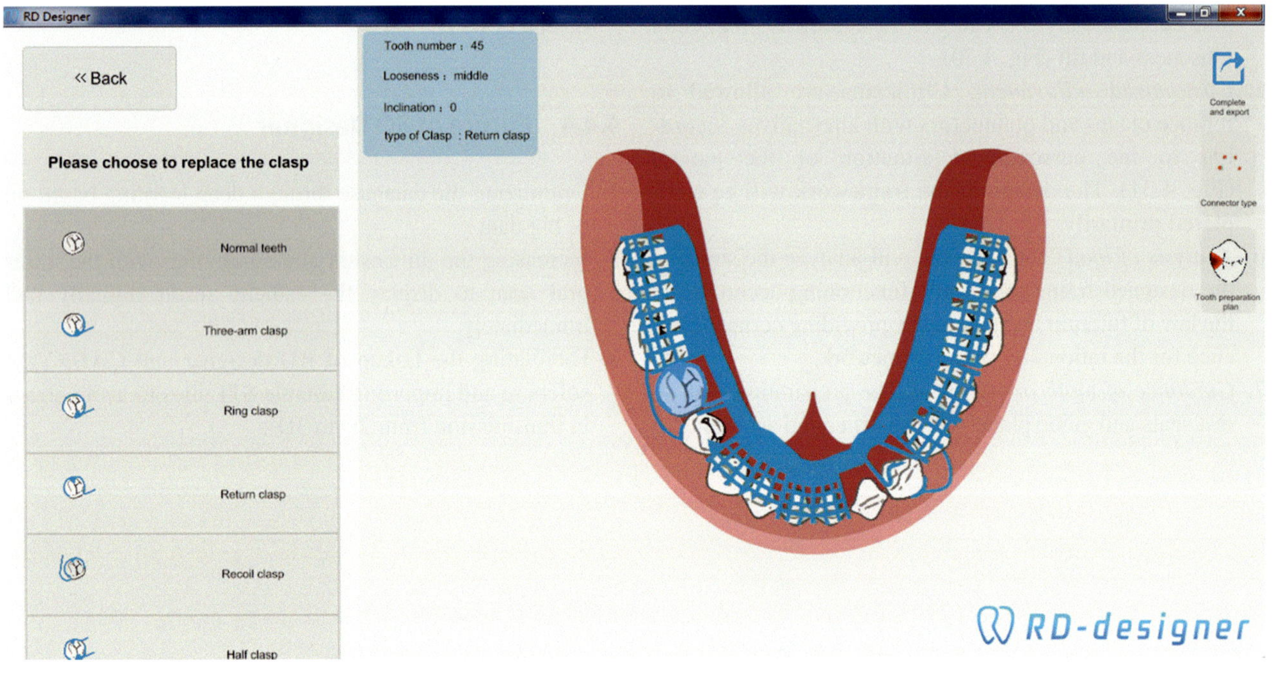

Fig. 4.51 Software interface of customized adjustment

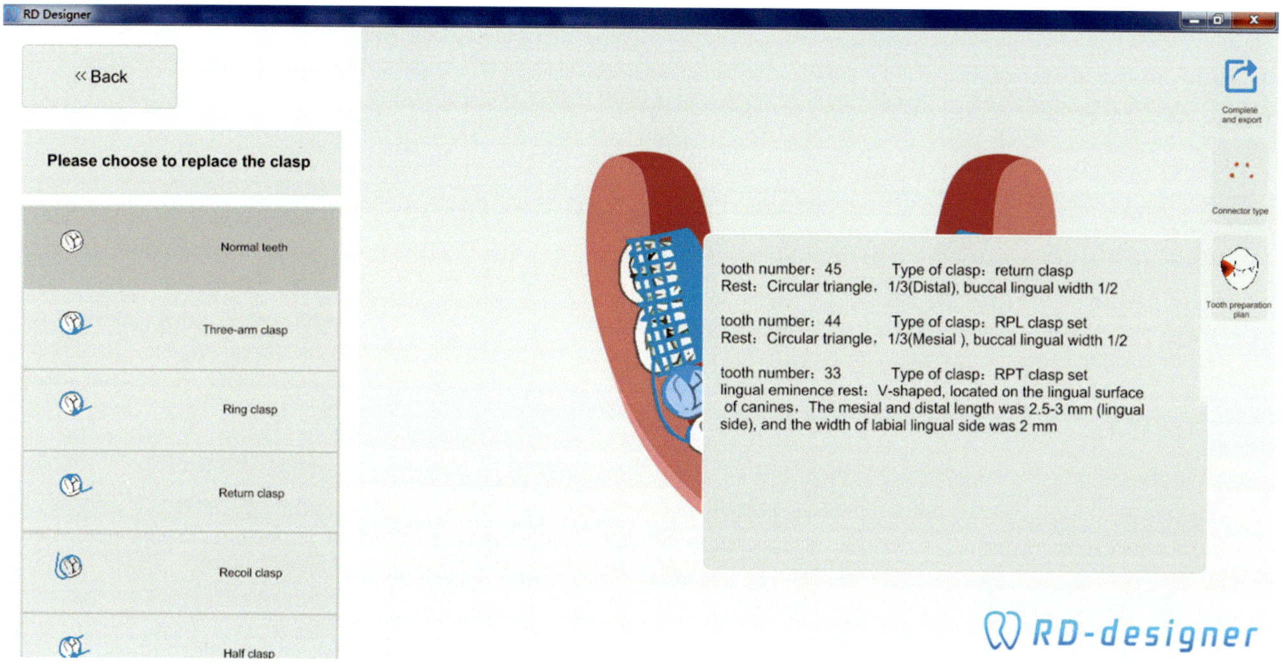

Fig. 4.52 Software interface of guidance of tooth preparation

DLD (Digital Line Design): Esthetic Analysis and Design

5

The digital frameworks of RPDs are divided into ordinary digital frameworks of RPDs and high esthetic digital frameworks of RPDs. For ordinary digital frameworks of RPDs, esthetic analysis and esthetic design are needed, and for high esthetic digital frameworks of RPDs, DLD esthetic prediction section is added. As a feature of the design of digital frameworks of RPDs with high esthetics, the esthetic prediction section is the necessary step for the comprehensive restoration of clinical cases. E-clasp (esthetic clasp) is our original concept, and clasp design, which integrates the esthetic analysis and design (DLD) concept into RPD design, is an innovation of it that makes metal invisible. It is realized in a digital way, and the production is completed by many kinds of CAD/CAM methods, such as in-mouth, model scanning, digital design, 3D printing, and so on.

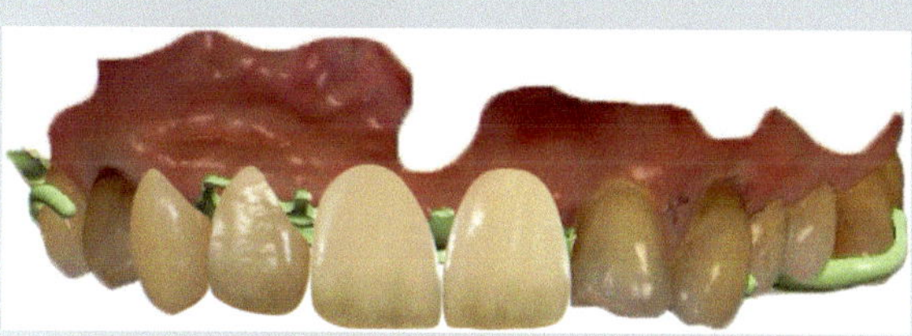

The esthetic clasp can achieve the effect of invisibility through ingenious design, bringing the patient a smile without metal exposure. However, RPD generally uses finished artificial teeth to arrange teeth, and most of the finished artificial teeth lack personalized features, and it is difficult to match the color of natural teeth, let alone simulate the fine structure of the surface of natural teeth [1]. If patients have high esthetic requirements and choose RPD for restoration, they can choose comprehensive restoration, such as movable fixed combined restoration (e-clasp ceramic type or all-ceramic type). This high esthetic digital frameworks of RPDs, like fixed esthetic restoration, can be predicted by DLD esthetics [2].

DLD esthetic prediction's four characteristics:

1. Effective doctor-patient communication
2. Design of noninvasive prostheses
3. Making wax-up appearance
4. Intuitive scheme determination

The following is a case of digital RPD's DLD esthetic prediction process:

5.1 Esthetic Analysis

First, use an intraoral scanner to obtain patients' information, Peng's upper and lower dental arch information (Figs. 5.1 and 5.2).

The intraoral scanner can be used to scan Kennedy class III of dentition defect patients with anterior and posterior teeth. However, if the missing teeth are excessive or it is a Kennedy class I or II dentition defect, the effect of intraoral collection is not ideal because of the mobility of soft tissue, so it is not recommended to use intraoral scanners. You can first take a plaster model and scan it with a model scanner.

After collecting the facial photos of the patients, the esthetic analysis (Fig. 5.3) was carried out. The patient belongs to the middle and high smile line, the exposure of the anterior teeth is relatively large when smiling (Fig. 5.4), and the second premolars can be seen in both upper and lower jaws.

Determine the tooth position of the esthetic area as follows: A5–B5 or C5–D5.

H. Yu, *Digital Removable Partial Denture Technology*, https://doi.org/10.1007/978-981-19-7923-1_5

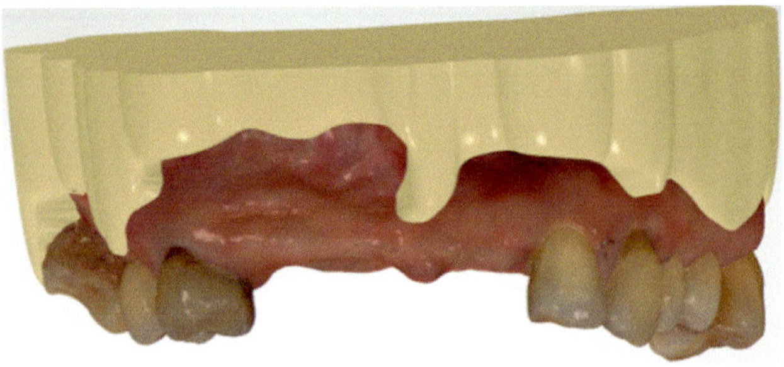

Fig. 5.1 Intraoral scanning of the maxillary model

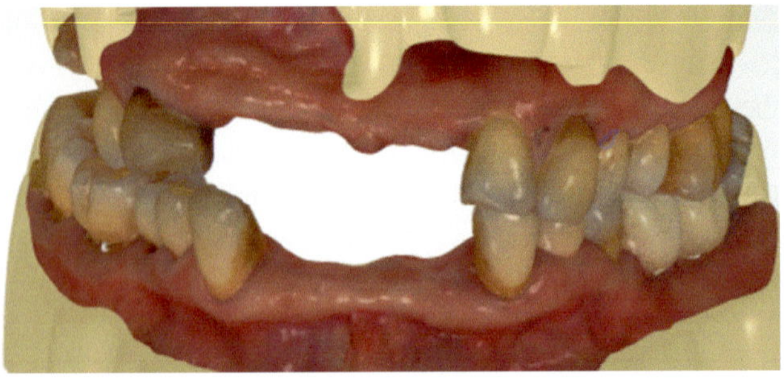

Fig. 5.2 Intraoral scanning of the occlusal model

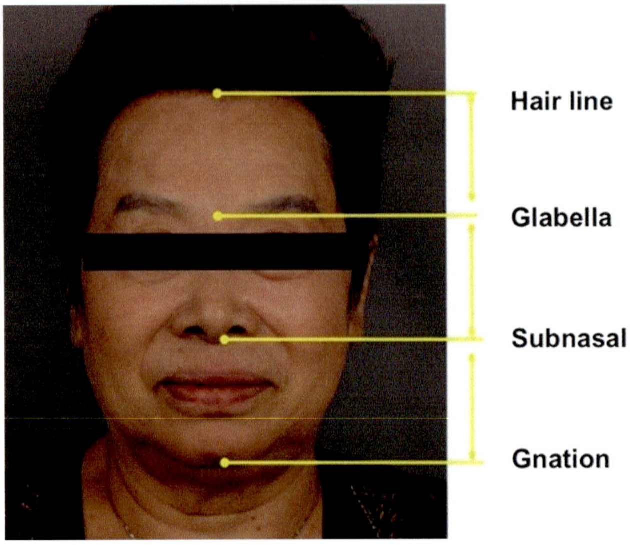

Fig. 5.3 Facial analysis

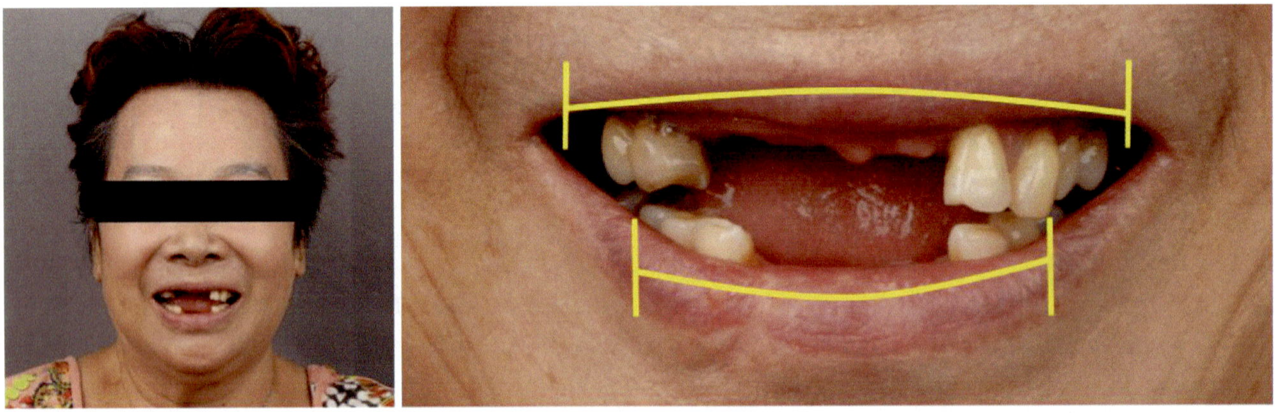

Fig. 5.4 Smile analysis

Through dentition analysis, the situation of missing teeth was defined: A1–3, B1–2, C1–2, or D1–2.

Preliminary determination of esthetic abutment teeth: A5, A7, and B6 (Fig. 5.5).

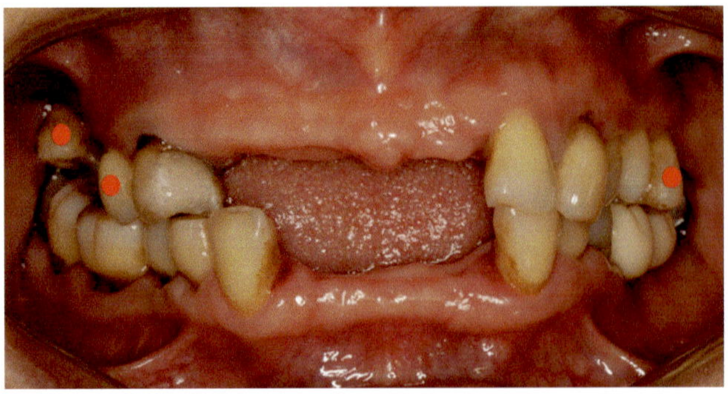

Fig. 5.5 Dentition analysis

5.2 Preliminary Design of the Digital Frameworks of RPD

DLD esthetic prediction's four processes (Fig. 5.6):

1. E-clasp digital design
2. DLD facial fitting design
3. Personalized tooth shape and color design
4. Making wax-up appearance

5.2.1 E-Clasp Digital Design

In order to compare the effect, we made two designs. The common design (Fig. 5.7) is to put the normal length C clasp on A5 and the gap clasp on B4 and B5. Put a three-arm clasp on A7.

The esthetic design (Fig. 5.8) is to place the C clasp with a short cheek retainer on A5 and the traditional clasp on B6. Due to the tight bite, the B6 is not designed to support it. The inclination of B6 to the buccal side is more obvious, so the clasp position will be higher [3].

The scaffolds of the two designs are completed in the design software.

Now, we can see the buccal view of the two designs (Figs. 5.9 and 5.10). The common design is that the abutment is placed in the front, and the clasp length is long, which is easy to expose the metal.

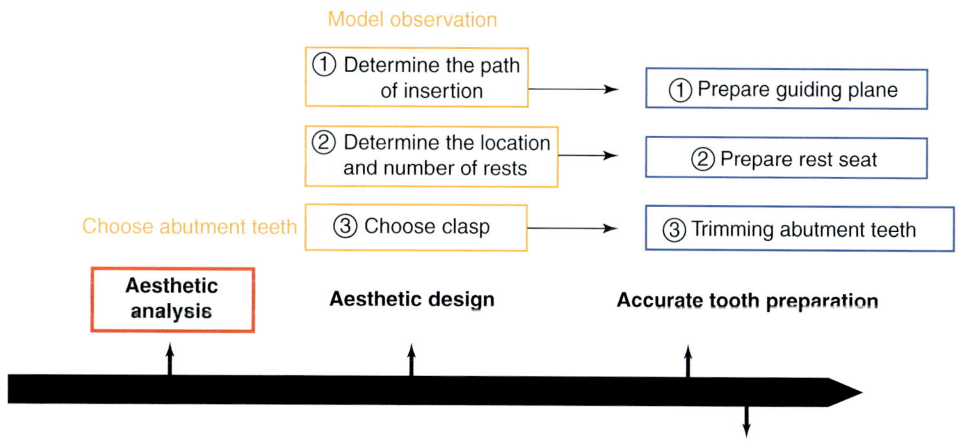

Fig. 5.6 The digital frameworks of RPD design process

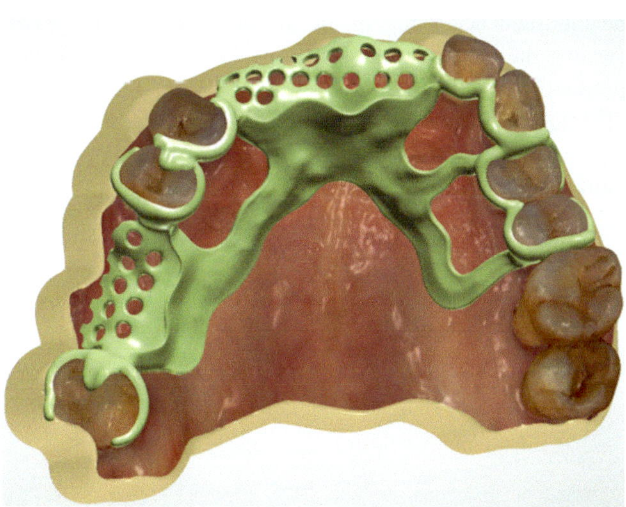

Fig. 5.7 Common design (occlusal view)

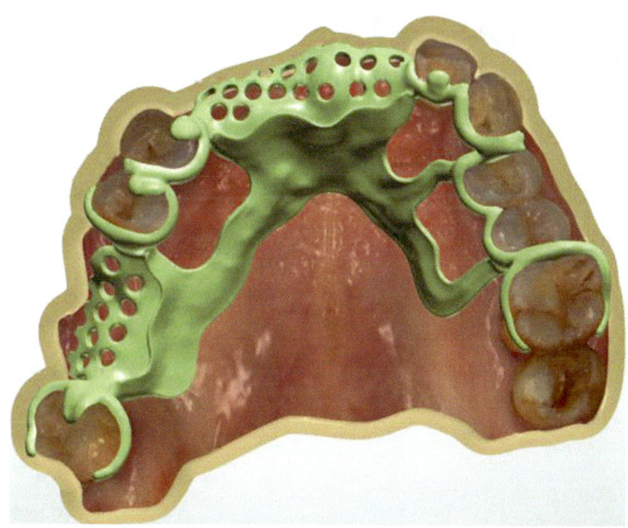

Fig. 5.8 Esthetic design (occlusal view)

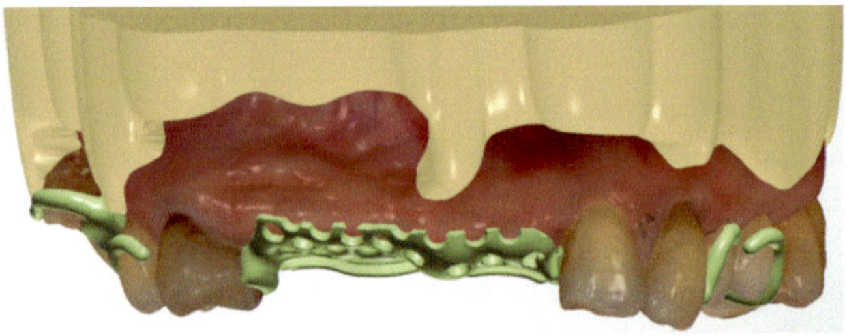

Fig. 5.9 Common design (buccal view)

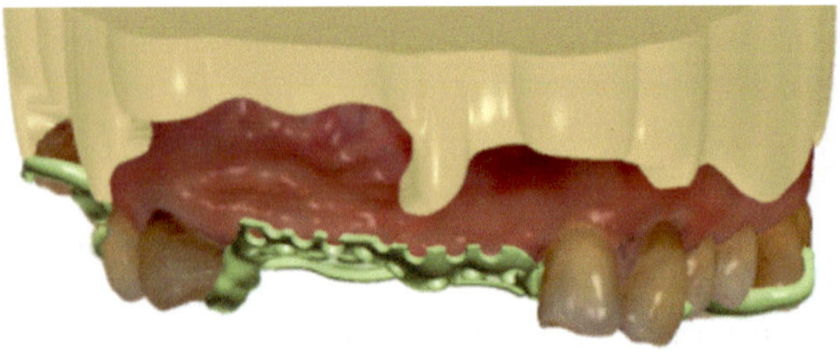

Fig. 5.10 Esthetic design (buccal view)

5.2.2 DLD Facial Fitting

The fitting of the intraoral photo and the designed digital frameworks (Fig. 5.11) can be implemented in the PS software. The results of the common design we look after fitting. The clasps in areas A and B are at risk of exposure.

If we take a look at the results of facial photo fitting, we can see that the clasps on B4 and B5 have been exposed and the esthetic effect is not good (Fig. 5.12).

This is the effect picture of the esthetic design of facial fitting. You can see that in contrast, there is no clasp exposure in the range of A5–B5, while the normal corner shadow should cover the clasp part of B6 exposed. Compared with the two schemes, the esthetic design has a better effect. After communicating with the patient, the patient chooses to use the second esthetic design (Fig. 5.13).

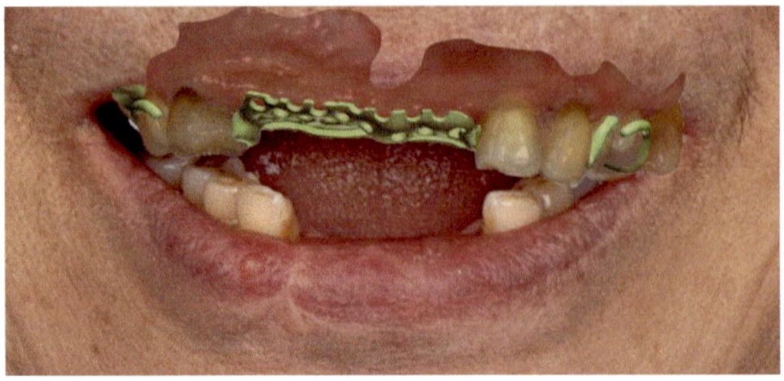

Fig. 5.11 Fitting with intraoral photo

5.2.3 Personalized Tooth Shape and Color Design

The facial fitting photo and the digital frameworks of RPD are used to operate, and the tooth shape prediction is realized by using the Beauty Tooth Assistant software (Fig. 5.14).

5.2.4 Making Wax-Up Appearance

According to the esthetic design of the tooth shape that the patients were satisfied with, we made the esthetic wax-up, which needed to replicate the parameters of the original design and tried it on in the patients. After the trial, it could be modified according to the actual situation (Fig. 5.15). Finally, the wax-up was used to guide the final restoration production (Fig. 5.16).

After the oral trial, the patient was satisfied with its shape, and the esthetic forecast was completed. The e-clasp framework design was determined, and the esthetic wax shape was completed, which can guide the final restoration (Fig. 5.17).

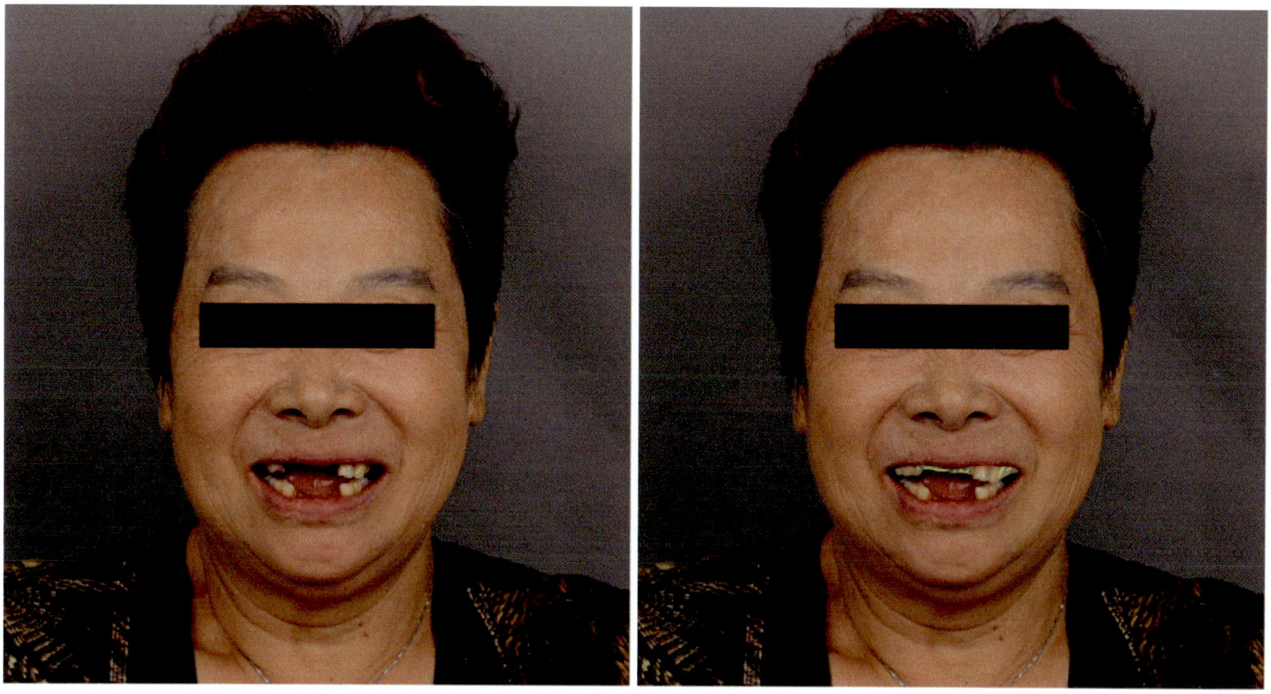

Fig. 5.12 Facial fitting according to common design

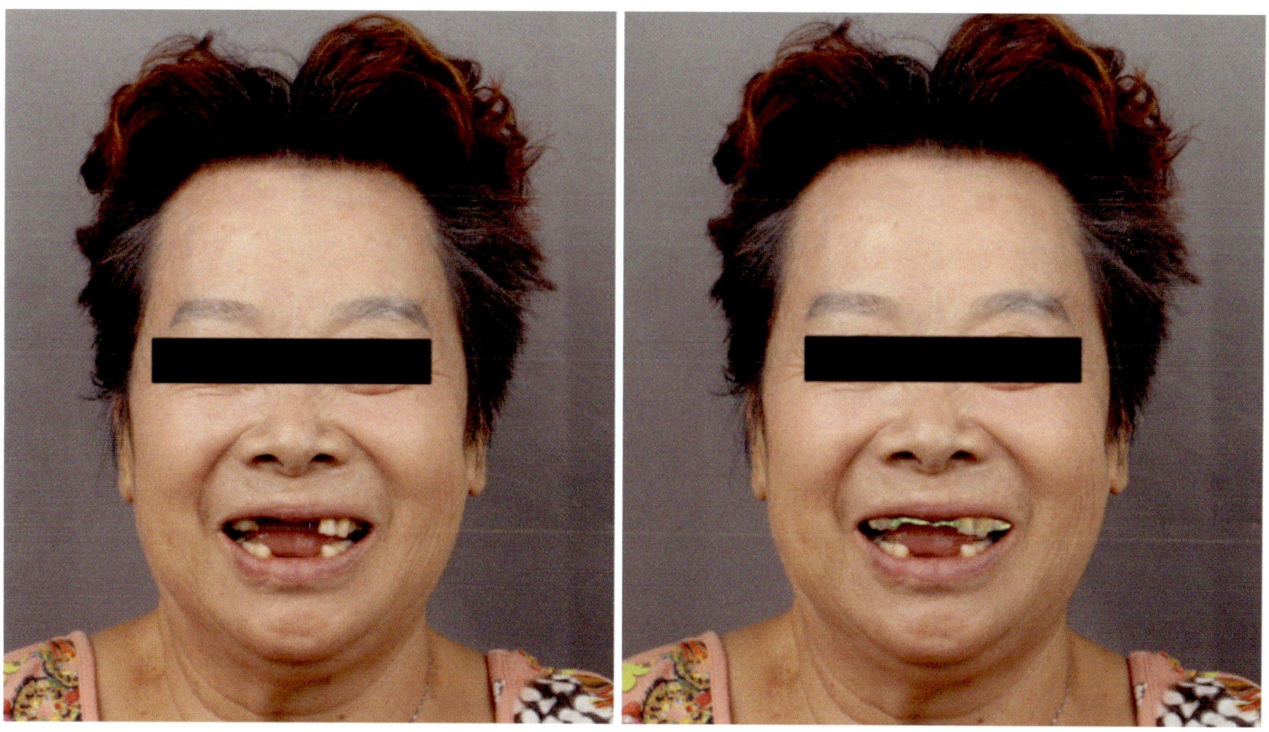

Fig. 5.13 Esthetic design and facial photo fitting

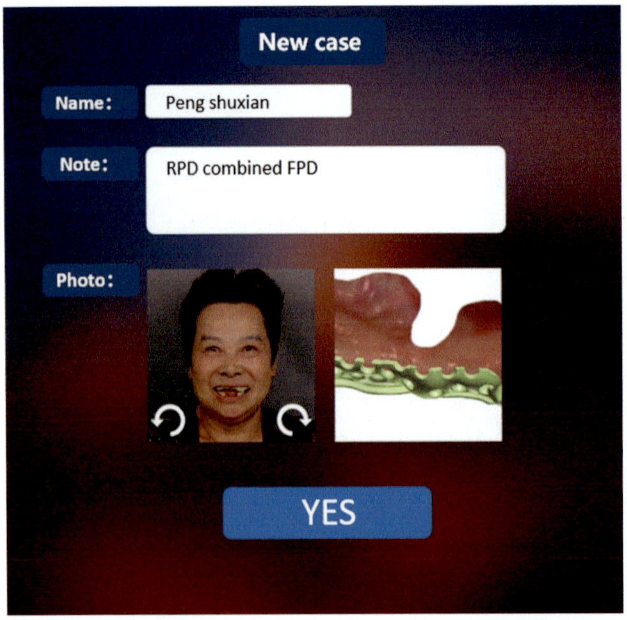

Fig. 5.14 Interface of Beauty Tooth Assistant

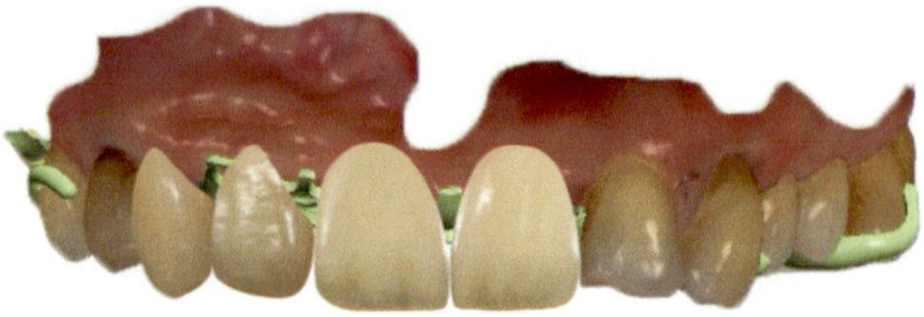

Fig. 5.15 Tooth shape prediction

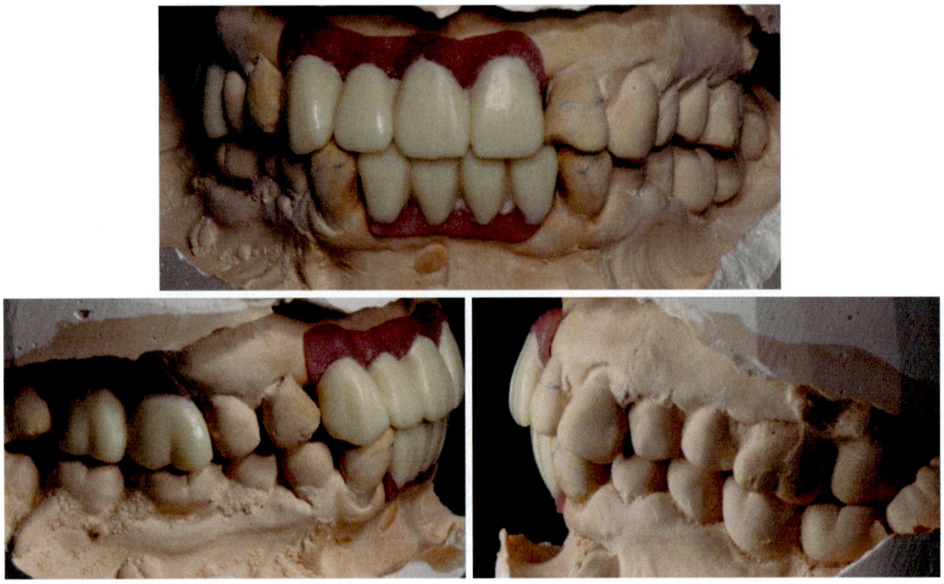

Fig. 5.16 Wax-up appearance

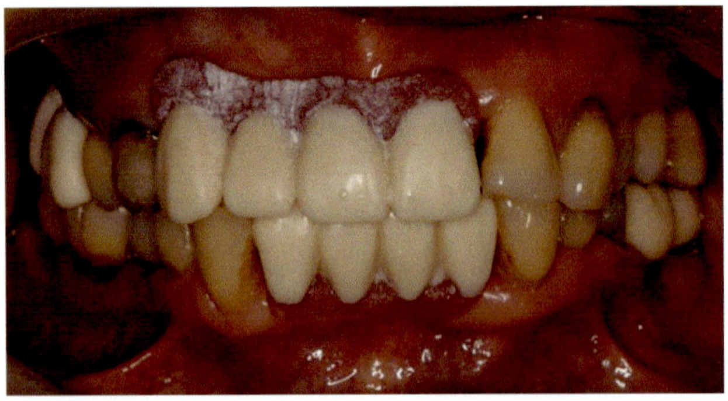

Fig. 5.17 Trying on the wax appearance

5.3 Accurate Tooth Preparation

Apart from the conventional tooth preparations discussed in Chap. 3, such as the rest seat and wrought wire clasp groove, tooth preparations such as guide plane and insertion path adjustment are often required in complex RPD cases. In the past, these more complex tooth preparations have always been highly dependent on visual experience and have poor accuracy, which not only affects the efficiency of clinical work but also affects the final restoration effect of RPD. Therefore, complex tooth preparation of RPD urgently needs better and more accurate solutions to improve the quality of treatment.

With the development of digital technologies, a novel guide plane adjustment scheme under the guidance of a digital template will be introduced as followed, mainly using the HX-04 bur independently developed by the author's team based on TRS theory (Fig. 5.18):

1. Determine the insertion path.

   In EXOCAD, determine a proper insertion path. Then, place a cutting plane (20 × 20 × 0.2 mm) in the insertion path to determine the proximal surface to be removed (Fig. 5.19).
2. Design the major structure of the template.

   The thickness of the template is designed to be 2.5 mm, and the extensions are designed to more than three teeth in a total of two sides of the missing tooth space (Fig. 5.20).
3. Design the starting point and terminus of the bur.

   Construct the digital HX-04 bur in SolidWorks software according to its actual size.

   Align the starting point and the terminus of the bur according to the cutting plane in Geomagic Wrap software (Fig. 5.21).

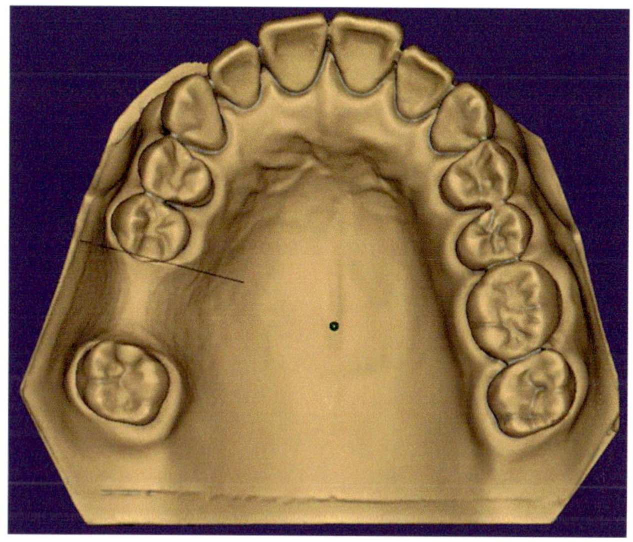

Fig. 5.19 Determining the insertion path

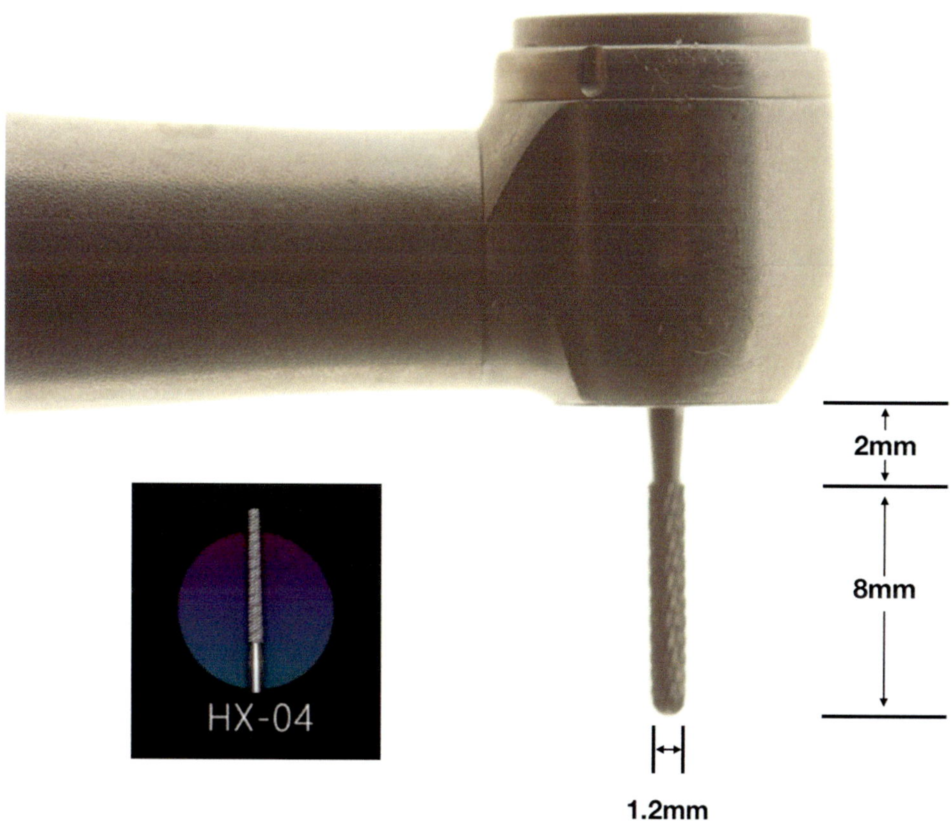

Fig. 5.18 HX-04. The geometric dimensions of HX-04 bur

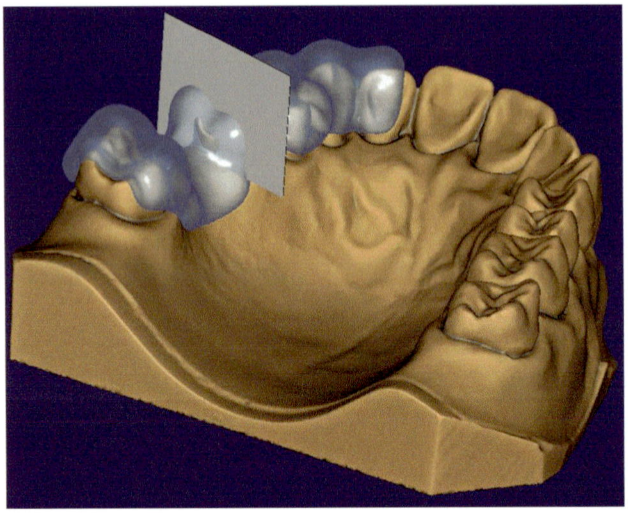

Fig. 5.20 Design of the major structure of the template

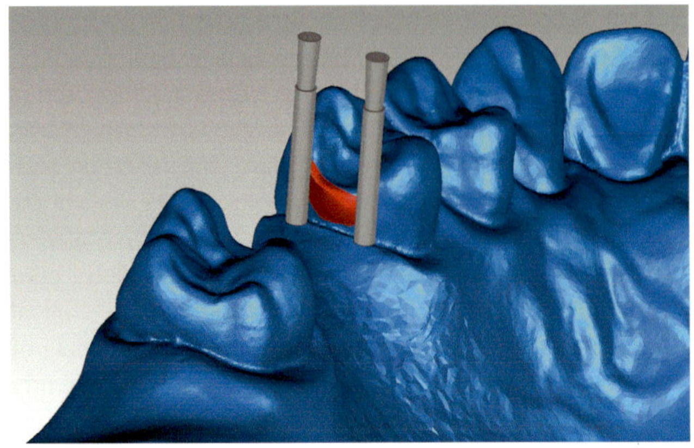

Fig. 5.21 Designing the starting point and the terminus of the bur

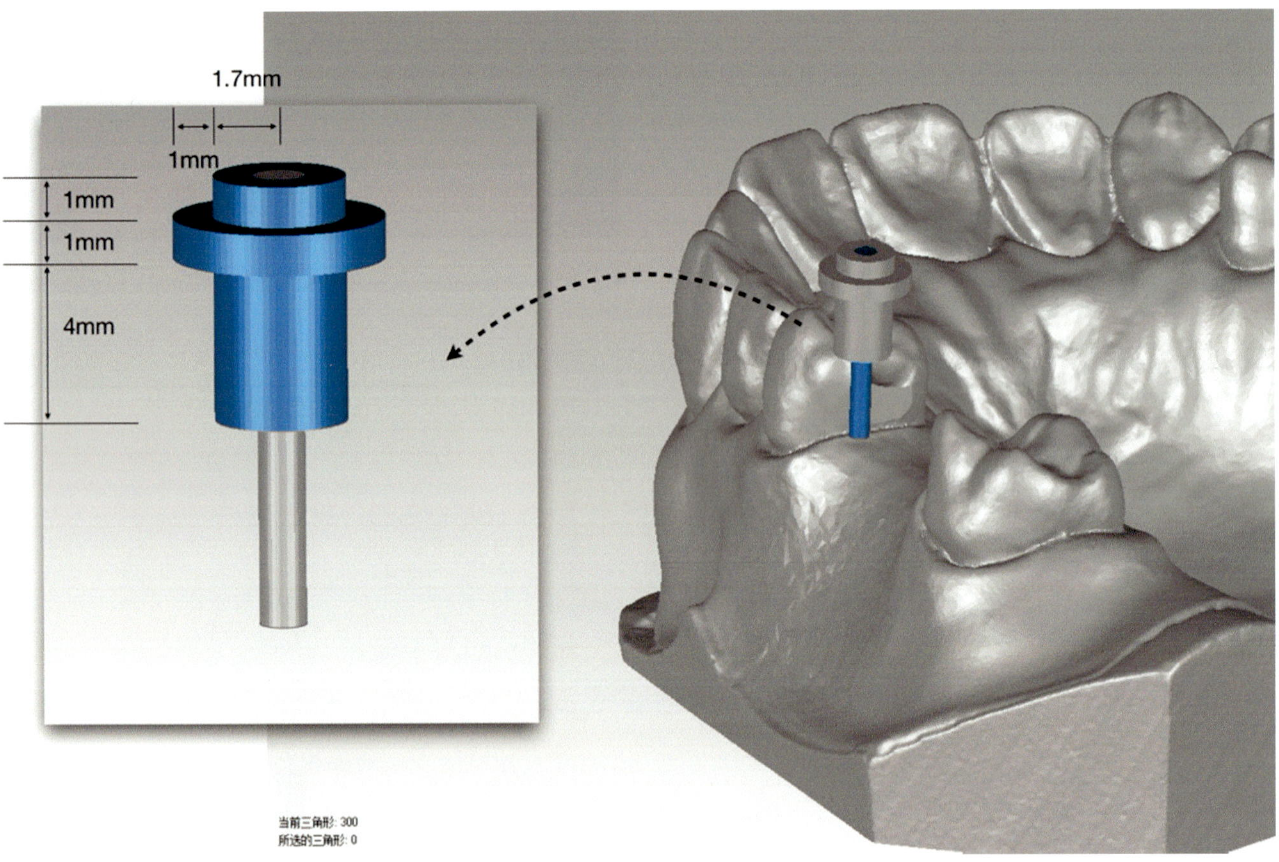

Fig. 5.22 Constructing the sleeve

4. Construct the sleeve.

   Construct a zirconia sleeve encircling the bur. Figure 5.22 shows the dimensions of the sleeve.

5. Simulate the preparation track of the bur.

   According to the starting point and the terminus of the bur, construct the preparation track of the bur by cutting the template (Figs. 5.23 and 5.24).

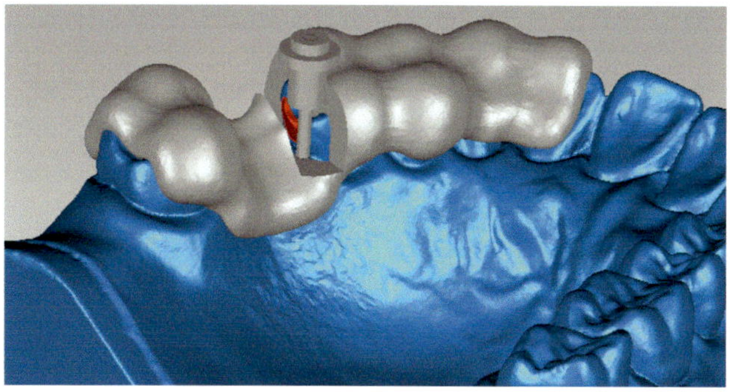

Fig. 5.23 The preparation track of the bur (starting point)

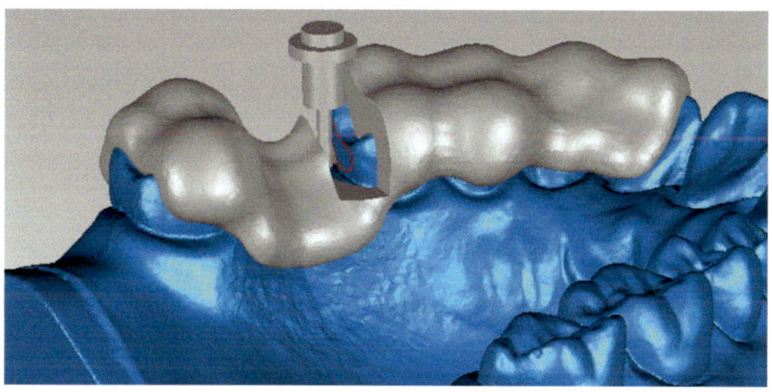

Fig. 5.24 The preparation track of the bur (terminus)

6. Design the retainer of the sleeve.

   Add the retainer of the zirconia sleeve to complete the design of the template (Fig. 5.25).

7. Prepare the guide plane under the guidance of the template.

   Place the template on the dentition, and check whether it is in place through the window opening on the template. Place the bur into the sleeve from the occlusal side, and place the sleeve with the bur into the track of the template laterally. Then the guide plane is prepared along the preparation track. Keep the handpiece in close contact with the template during the overall process (Fig. 5.26).

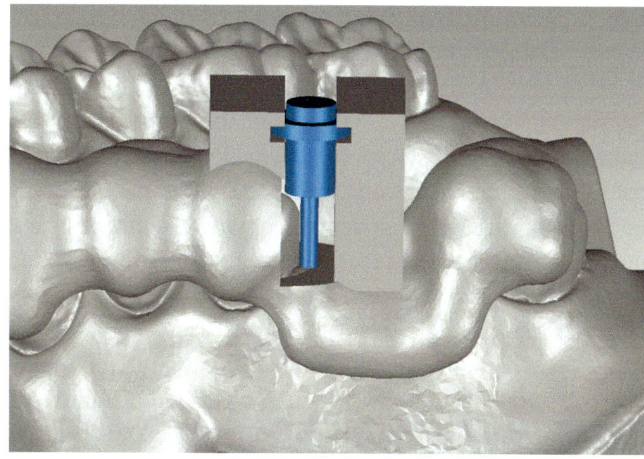

Fig. 5.25 The retainer of the sleeve

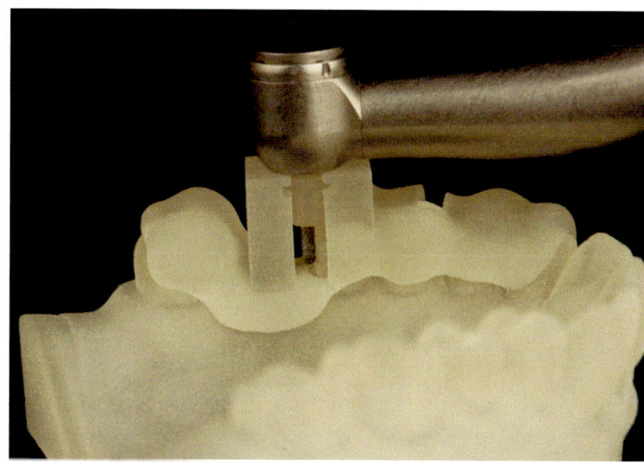

Fig. 5.26 Preparing the guide plane under the guidance of the template

5.4 The Digital Frameworks of RPD Design and Production

The digital frameworks of RPD design use CAD software to realize the virtual restoration step, which is very different from the manual framework wax made in the past. It omits the steps of filling the concave, copying the fire-resistant model, and making the bracket wax and saves the working procedure and manpower.

In the digital mode, using CAD software for computer operation, which not only does not have the dirty and messy environment of the mobile stent in the past but also reduces the human error in the production process, the stent design is more accurate, and the design process and design results can be easily used as medical-technical communication materials, which can effectively avoid the rework phenomenon caused by poor communication.

The digital framework of RPD's production process is detailed in Chap. 4 (Figs. 5.27, 5.28, 5.29, and 5.30).

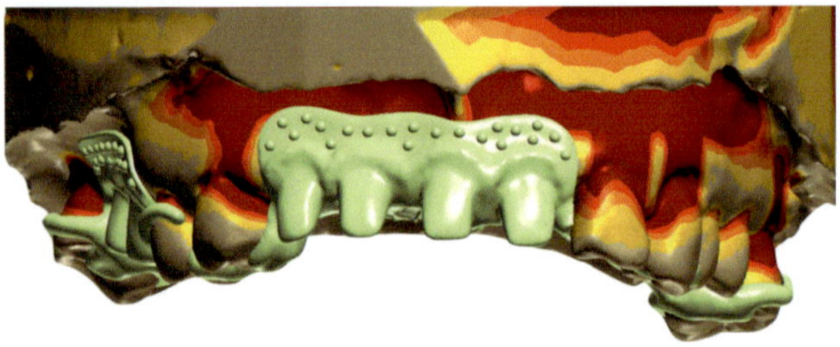

Fig. 5.27 The digital framework of RPD design

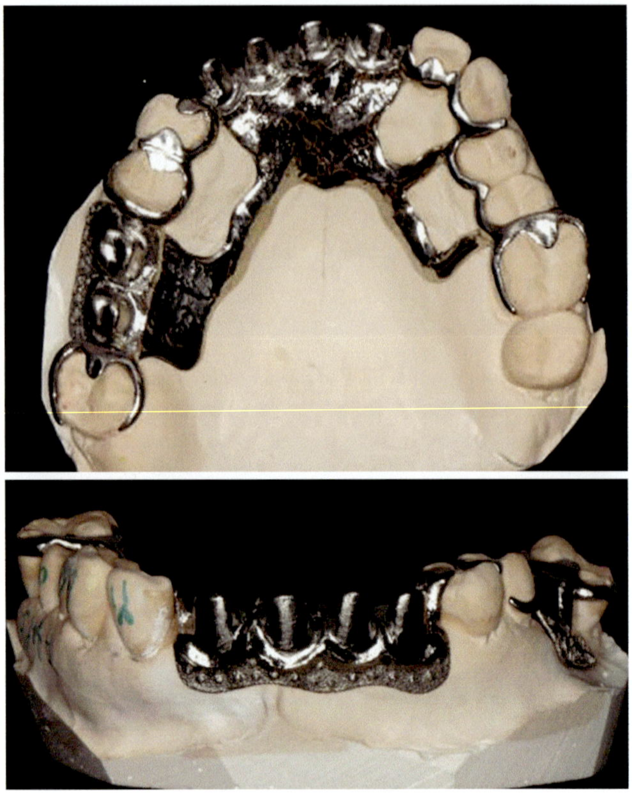

Fig. 5.28 Fabrication of the digital framework of RPD

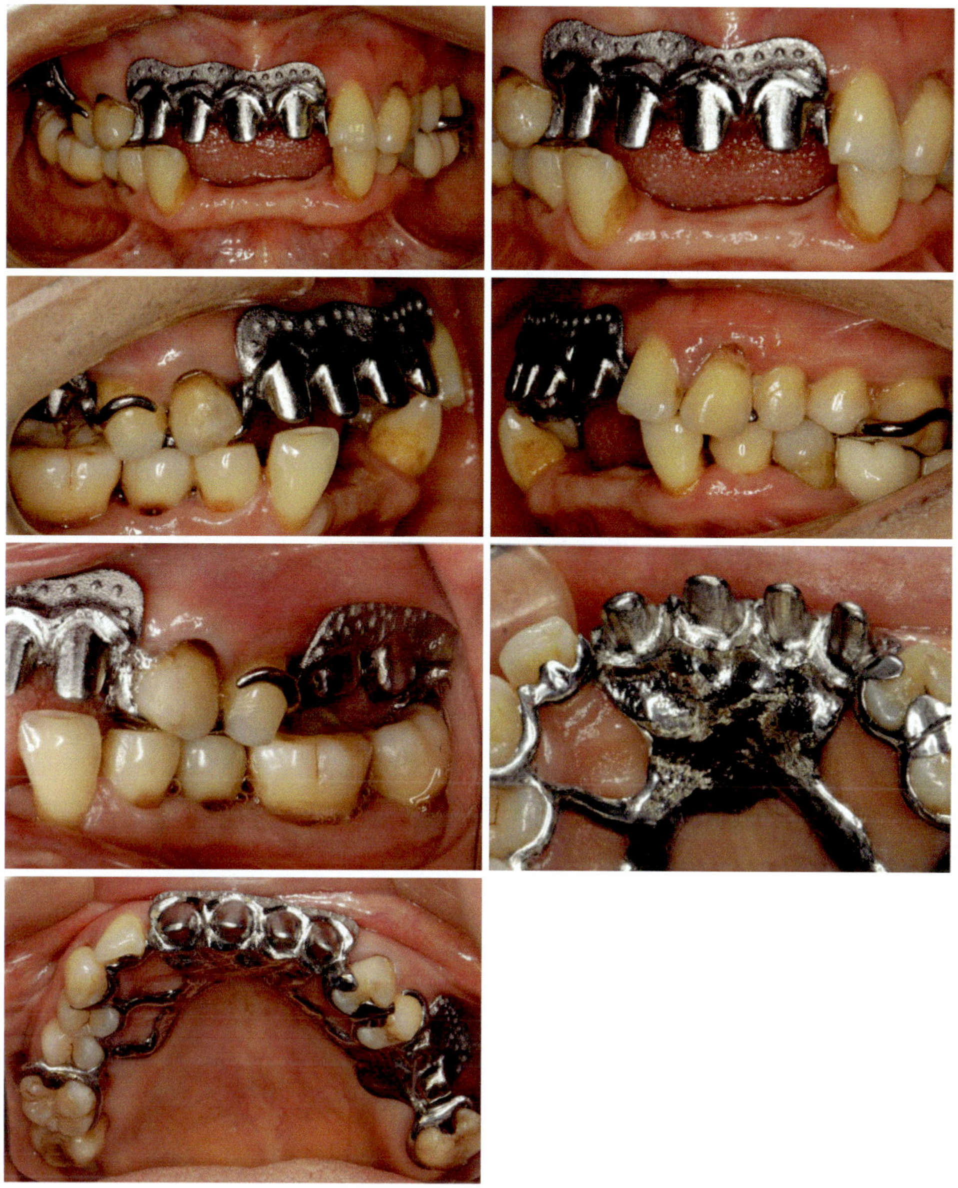

Fig. 5.29 Try-in of the framework

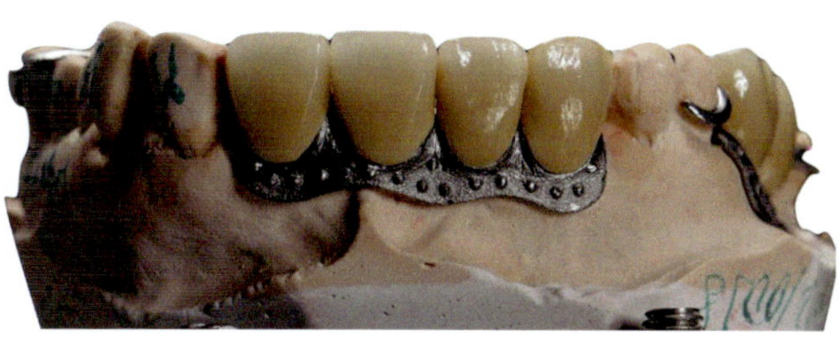

Fig. 5.30 Bonding porcelain teeth

5.5 Personalized Porcelain Teeth and Simulation Denture Base Production

1. *Opaque coating:*

   On the framework of the bonded porcelain teeth, the contact surface between metal and resin is treated, and the opaque porcelain is coated.

   The first layer, thin coating, plays a bonding role, and the second layer covers the metal color (Fig. 5.31).

   In order to achieve good simulation results, personalized gingival colorimetry is very important.

   You can use the existing gingival shade, or you can match the color on the spot. The gum resin is placed on the gingiva to compare the color on the spot, which shows

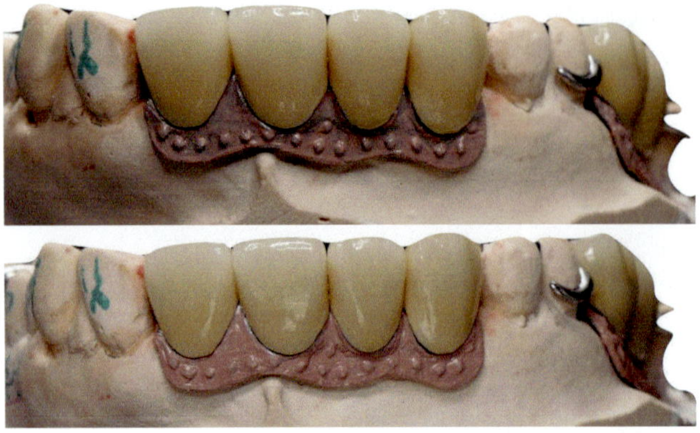

Fig. 5.31 Opaque coating

that the color is a little light. Add an appropriate amount of dye to the resin, then compare the color (this time the color is close to the gingival color of the patient), and determine the color matching scheme (Fig. 5.32).

2. *Coat the bonding layer on the opaque porcelain* (Fig. 5.33).
3. *In order to simulate the color of gingival blood vessels, deeper underlying stains such as crimson and blue are used at the membranous-gingival junction* (Fig. 5.34).
4. *Layered stacking of gingival resin:*

   Different colors of gingival resin are used in different positions of the gums to achieve a vivid simulation effect.

   The following is a brief introduction to the process of layering (Figs. 5.35, 5.36, 5.37, 5.38, and 5.39):

Fig. 5.32 Color matching for internal colorimetry

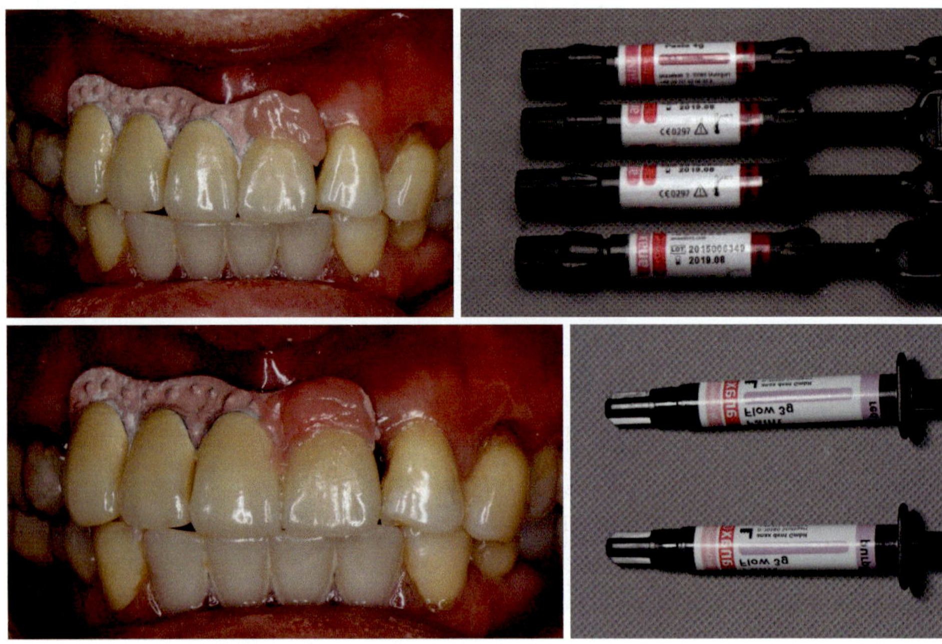

Fig. 5.33 Coating the bonding layer

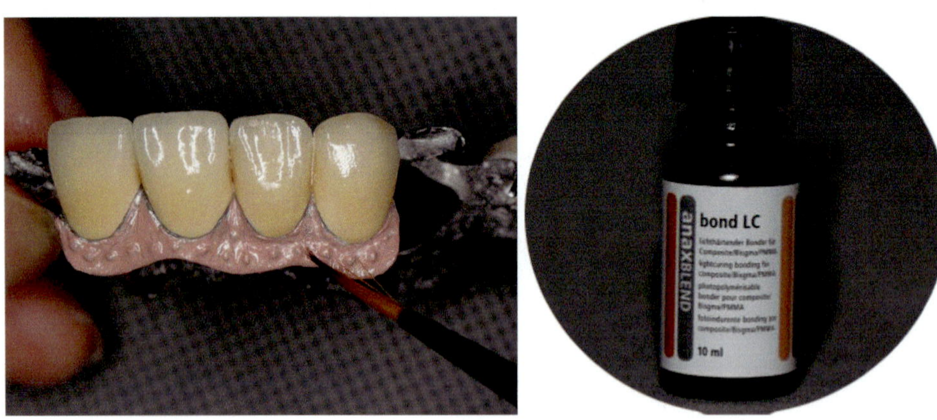

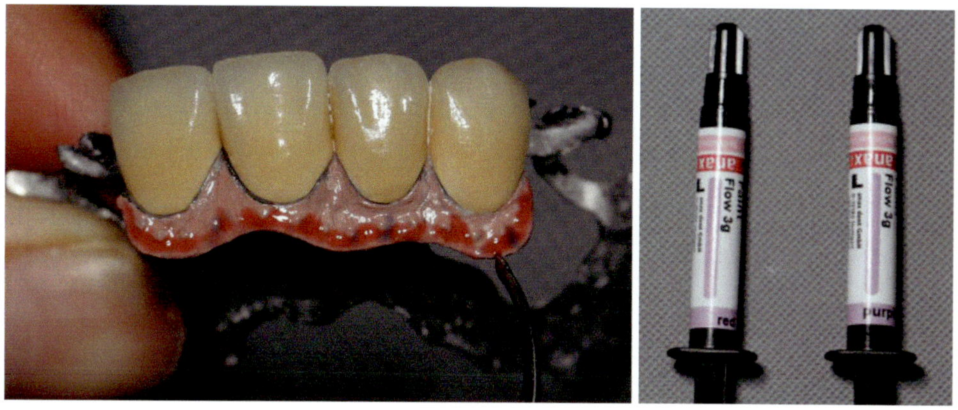

Fig. 5.34 The bottom staining

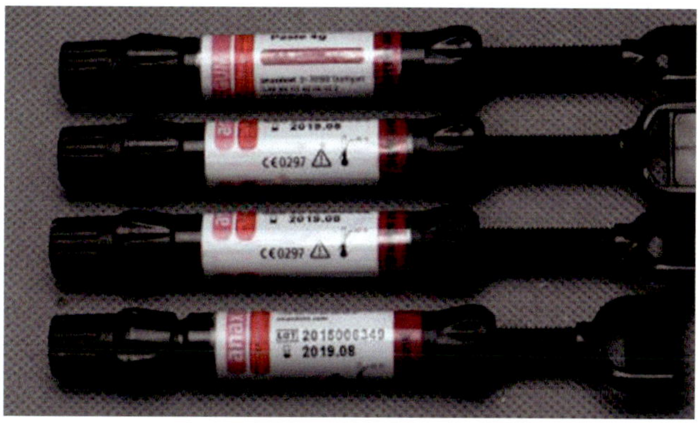

Fig. 5.35 Gingival resin

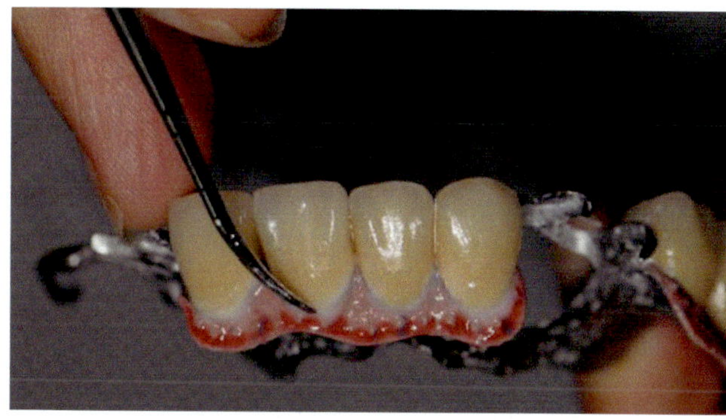

Fig. 5.36 Treatment of junctions

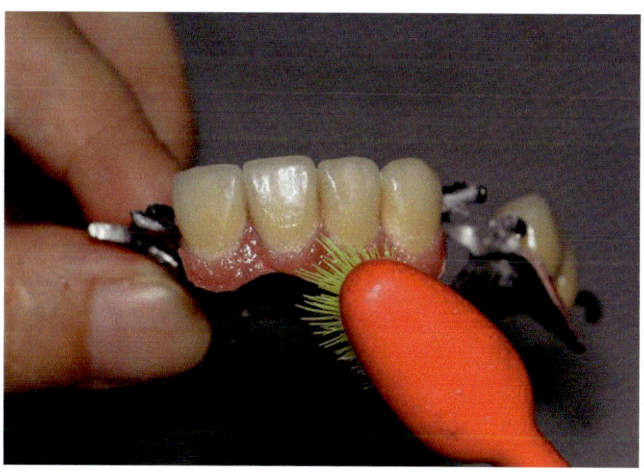

Fig. 5.37 Making gingival stippling stippling

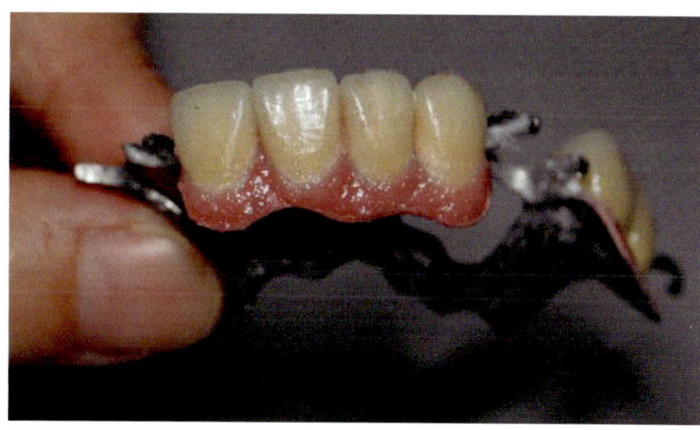

Fig. 5.38 Gingival stippling

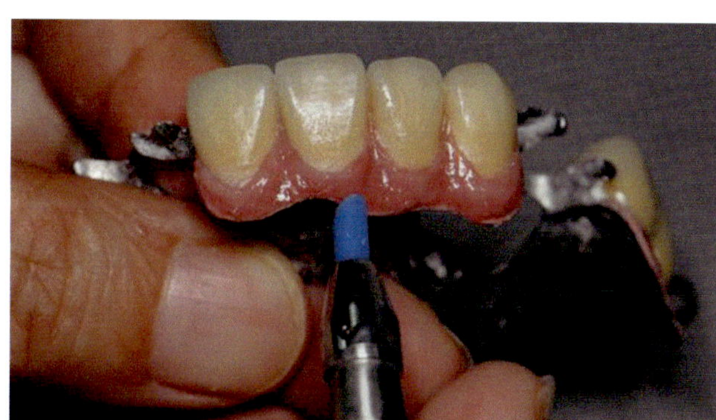

Fig. 5.39 Polish smooth surface

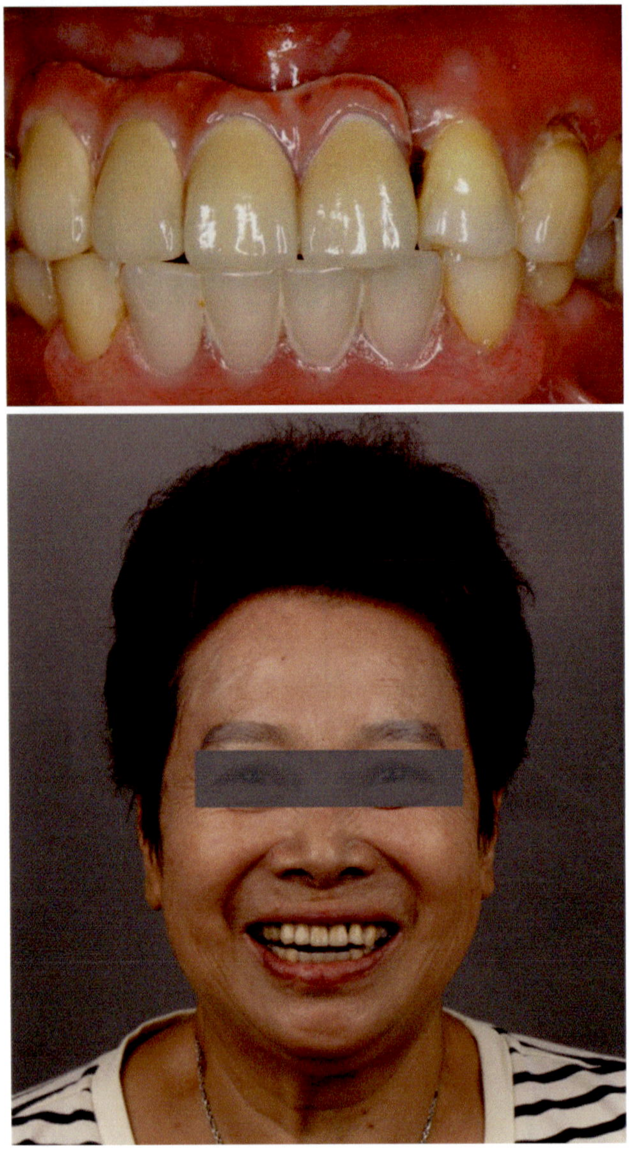

Fig. 5.40 Trying in the RPD

(a) The treatment of the connection between the framework and the neck of porcelain teeth can make the gingiva slightly cover the neck of the teeth. Use a lighter or root-colored gingival resin.
(b) Fill the main area of the gingiva with resin, using a predetermined color scheme.
(c) Make a stippling effect with a toothbrush.
(d) The free gingiva of the neck should be transparent, and the gingival resin with high transparency should be selected.
(e) Smooth the surface to ensure a good color mixture between the layers.
(f) The stacking of the simulation denture base is completed by light curing, and then polish it.

5. *Finished and ready to try in the RPD* (Fig. 5.40).

References

1. Beaumont AJ. An overview of esthetics with RPDs. J Quintessence Int. 2002;33(10):747–55.
2. Aras MA, Chitre V. Direct retains: esthetics solutions in the smile zone. J Indian Prosthod Soc. 2005;5(1):4–9.
3. Haiyang Y, Huang W. Classification design and clinical application of beautiful clasp. West China J Stomatol. 2012;43–49(5):30.

Case Analysis of Esthetic Clasp

6

Following the clinical pathway of esthetic clasp in this book, prosthodontist can design RPD with esthetic clasp for patients easily. Through 32 typical cases, this chapter explains the clinical steps and skills of the esthetic clasp. These real cases are certainly not the art performances, but real records of the current clinical situation in China. In our daily clinical work, we will encounter various problems. For example, the periodontal conditions of the elderly patients are generally not good, the patients' awareness of self-health care is not strong, it is difficult for patients to adhere to the correct brushing method, and the basic treatment of dental pulp and periodontal is not satisfactory. These problems deserve our attention.

Dentists should remember that although RPD is suitable for almost all the dentition defects, its efficacy is limited. According to the complaints and the actual situation of patients, the purpose is to improve the esthetics of RPD as much as possible on the basis of a reasonable design, rather than every case must pursue the ultimate metal-free exposure. And long term, stable, and effective are the highest clinical pursuit.

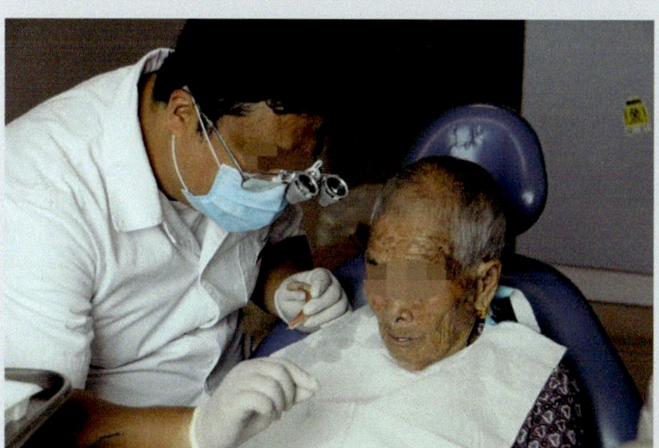

6.1 Case 1

When it comes to the restoration in esthetic area, prosthodontists should take into account the chewing, pronunciation, and other functions when designing. In RPD design, how to use adjacent surface to retain is often ignored. In the following case, we are going to introduce a proximal-retentive e-clasp that we designed for anterior tooth:

1. *Before restoration*

   He is a 48-year-old female patient, who is Kennedy III for the upper jaw and Kennedy I for the lower jaw (Figs. 6.1 and 6.2).
2. *RPD design and manufacturing*

   On A2 and A3, we designed adjacent surface hidden clasps for anterior tooth, both of which have plate-shaped retainer (Figs. 6.3 and 6.4). The difference is the lingual design—palate plate and lingual rest. Others are traditional design.

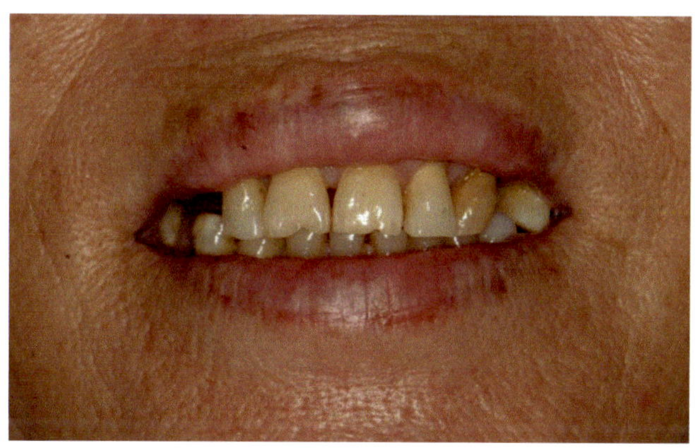

Fig. 6.1 Maxillary esthetic teeth: A1–A5, B1–B5

H. Yu, *Digital Removable Partial Denture Technology*, https://doi.org/10.1007/978-981-19-7923-1_6

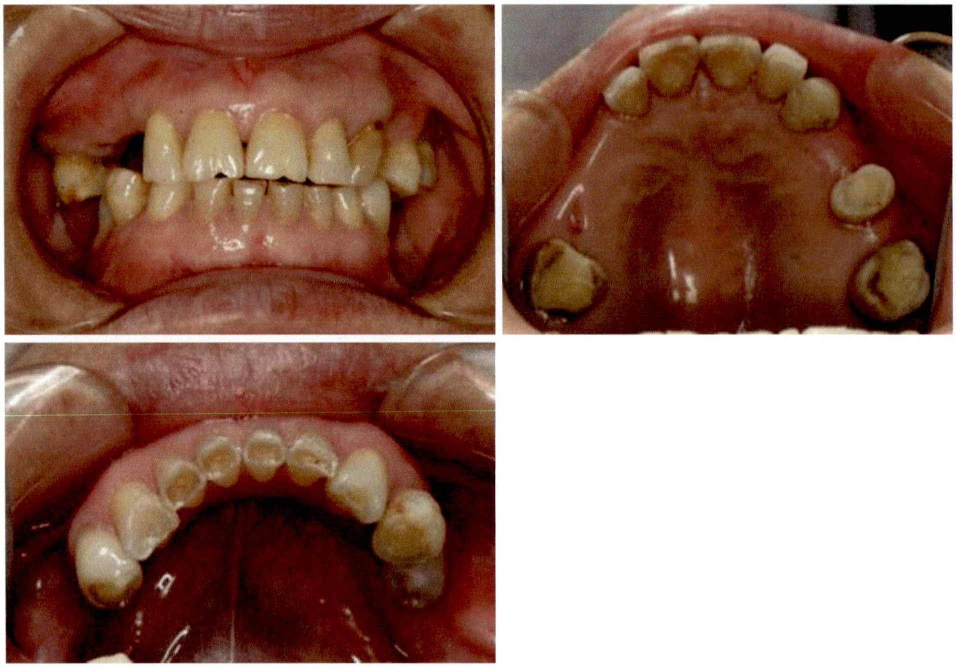

Fig. 6.2 Missing teeth: A3–A5; B4, B6; C6–7; D5–7

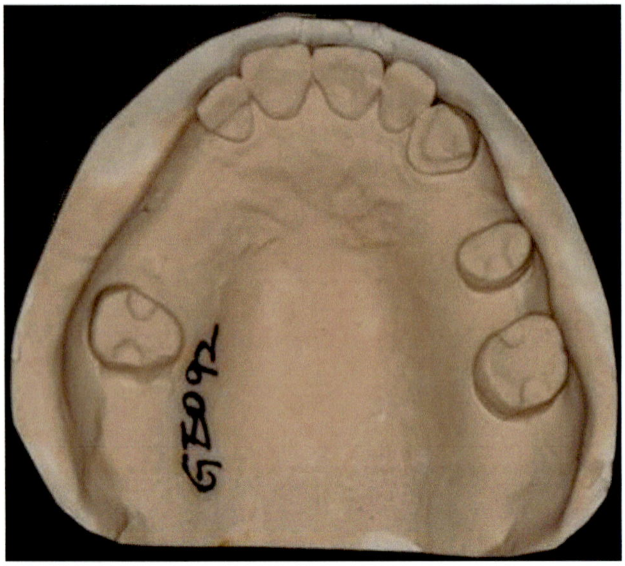

Fig. 6.3 A2, B3—adjacent surface hidden clasp for anterior tooth

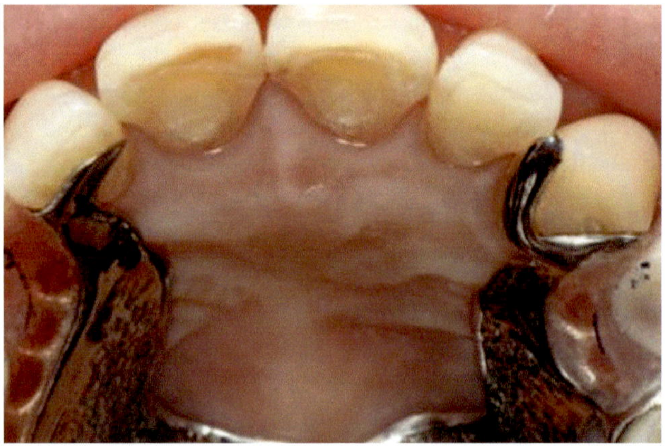

Fig. 6.4 Intraoral effect of A2, B3—adjacent surface hidden clasp for anterior tooth

For the lower jaw, the patient's smile line is low, so there is minimal tooth exposure. Thus, we placed low T clasps with mesial rest on D4 and C5 (Fig. 6.5). We also designed sublingual bar for major connector.

3. *After restoration*

   The final result is shown in Figs. 6.6 and 6.7.

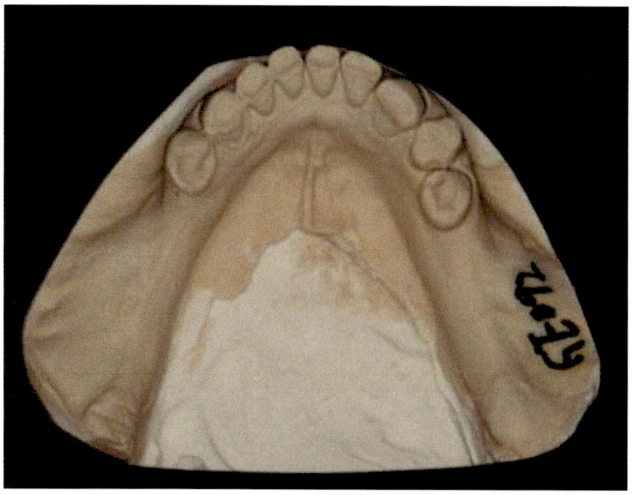

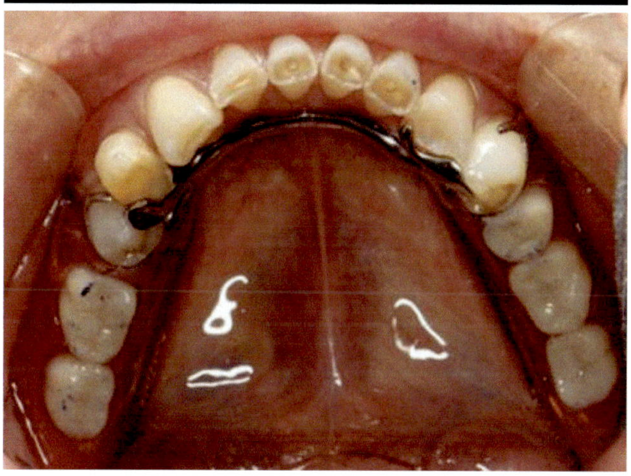

Fig. 6.5 C5, D4-T clasp

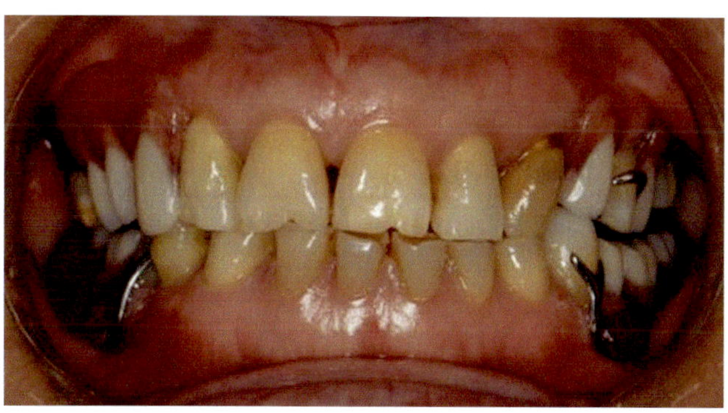

Fig. 6.6 Intraoral effect

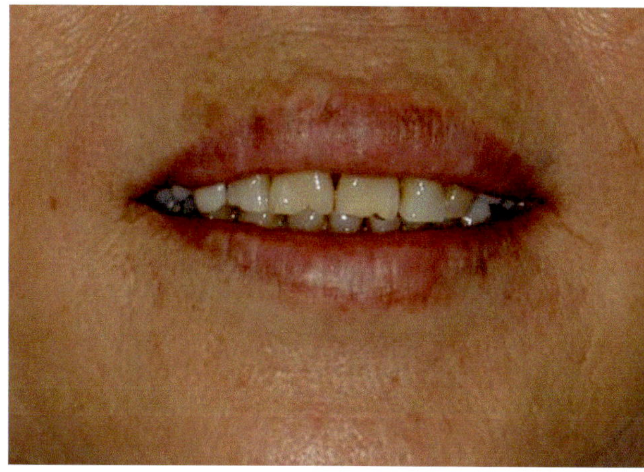

Fig. 6.7 Final effect

6.2 Case 2

1. *Before restoration*

   Mrs. Zhou, 66 years old. Both her maxillary and mandibular teeth are Kennedy I type—bilateral free-end edentia. The esthetic area teeth of this patient are A4–B4 and C3–D3, and C4 was I°loose. The point of this case is the esthetic design of clasp put on the A4 and B4.

   Conditions are shown in Figs. 6.8, 6.9, and 6.10.

2. *RPD design and manufacturing*

   On maxillary, A area and B area lost the same teeth. To improve retention, we let first premolar to be an abutment besides the second premolar near the gap. We put a double T clasp on the two adjacent teeth (Figs. 6.11, 6.12, and 6.13).

   C4 and C5 could have been designed according to the maxillary, but considering that C4 was I°loose, we just put a T clasp on C5 (Fig. 6.14). On the opposite side, the buccal space of the mesial abutment D6 was not enough to put a T clasp, so we designed a traditional three-arm clasp (Fig. 6.15).

3. *After restoration*

   The final effect with denture is shown in Figs. 6.16, 6.17, and 6.18. The patient was very satisfied.

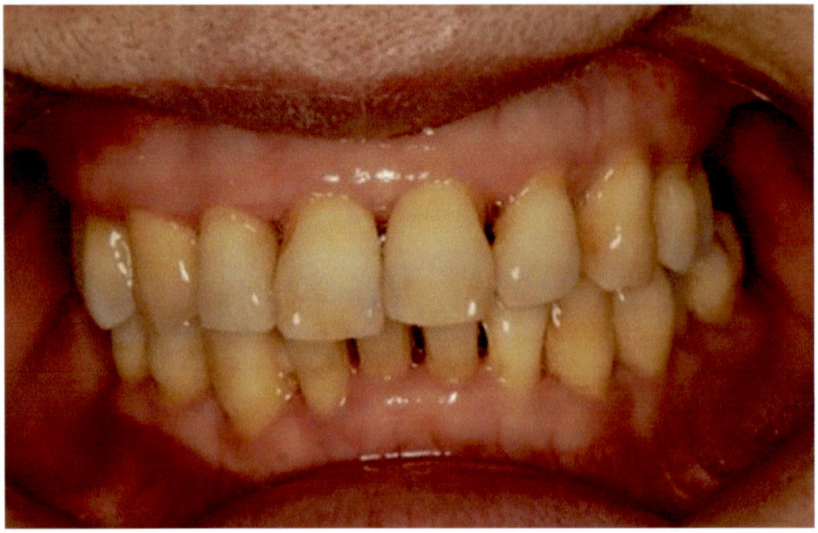

Fig. 6.8 Free-end loss of posterior teeth

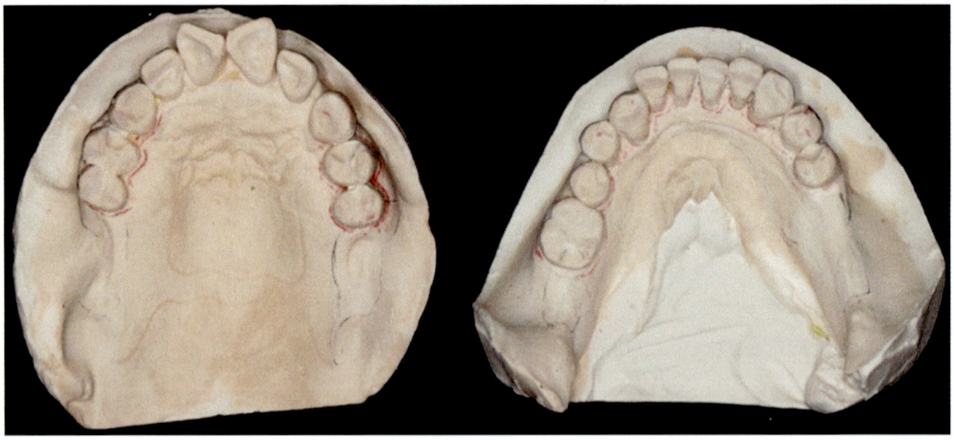

Fig. 6.9 Dentition defect: A6, A7, B6, B7, C6, C7, D7

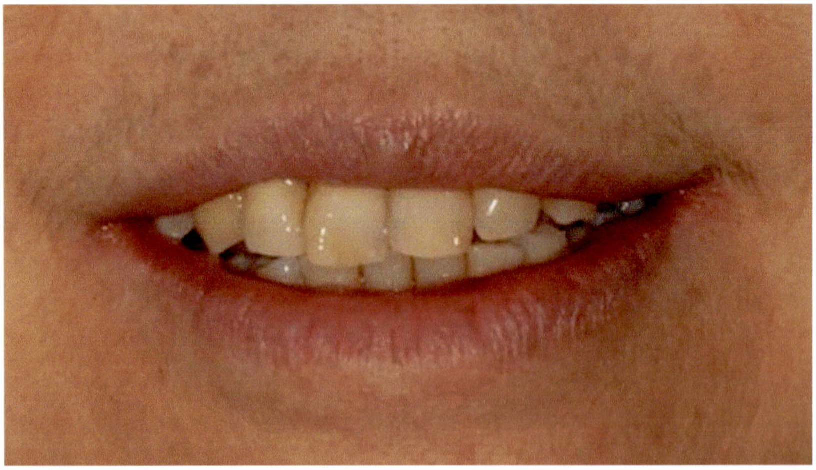

Fig. 6.10 Esthetic teeth: A4–B4, C3–D3

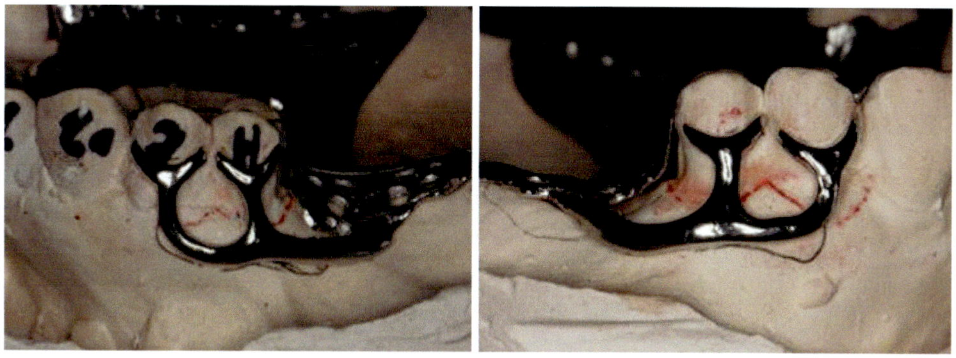

Fig. 6.11 A45, B45—double T clasp

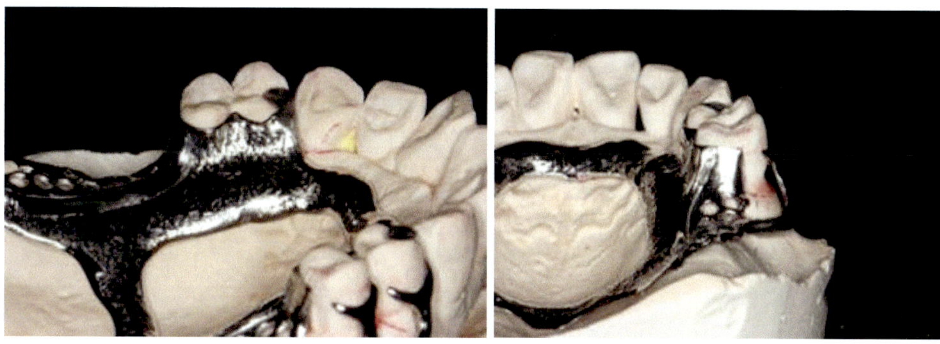

Fig. 6.12 Lingual surface and one side of the double T clasp

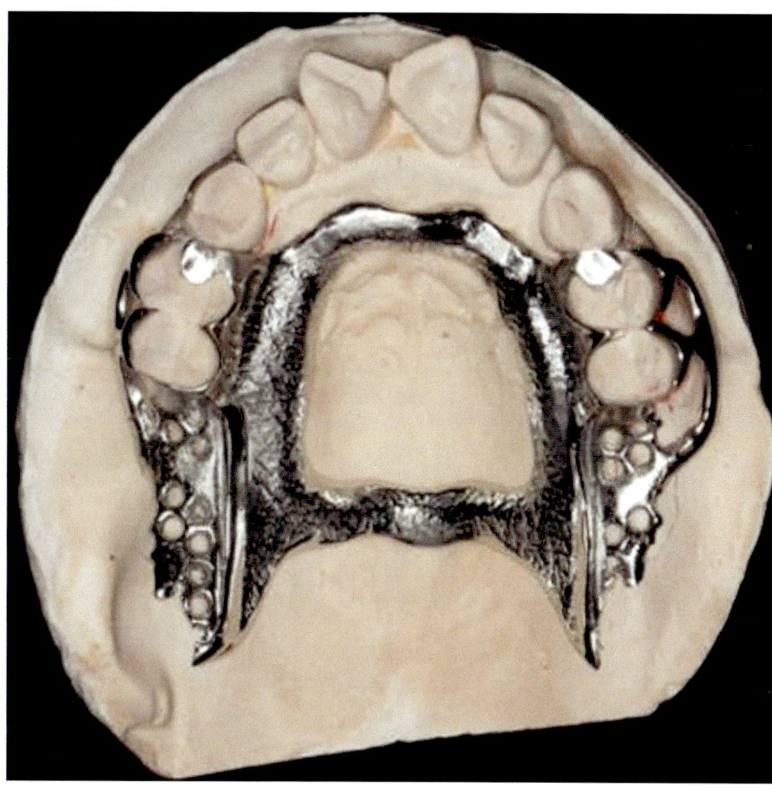

Fig. 6.13 Free end combined with two teeth as abutment

Fig. 6.14 C5, T-type clasp; D6, three-arm clasp

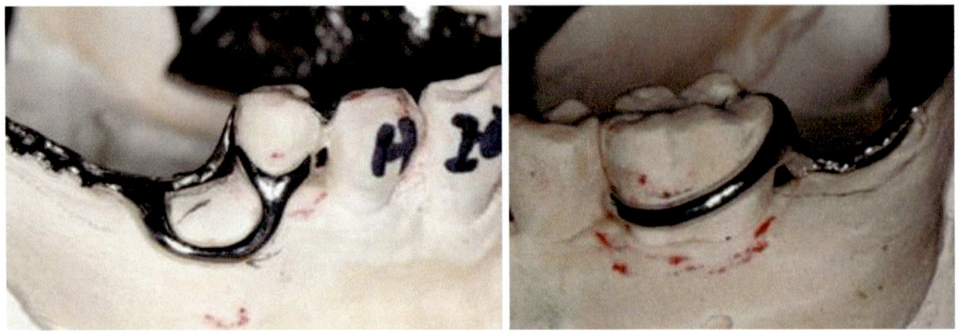

Fig. 6.15 Design of mandible framework

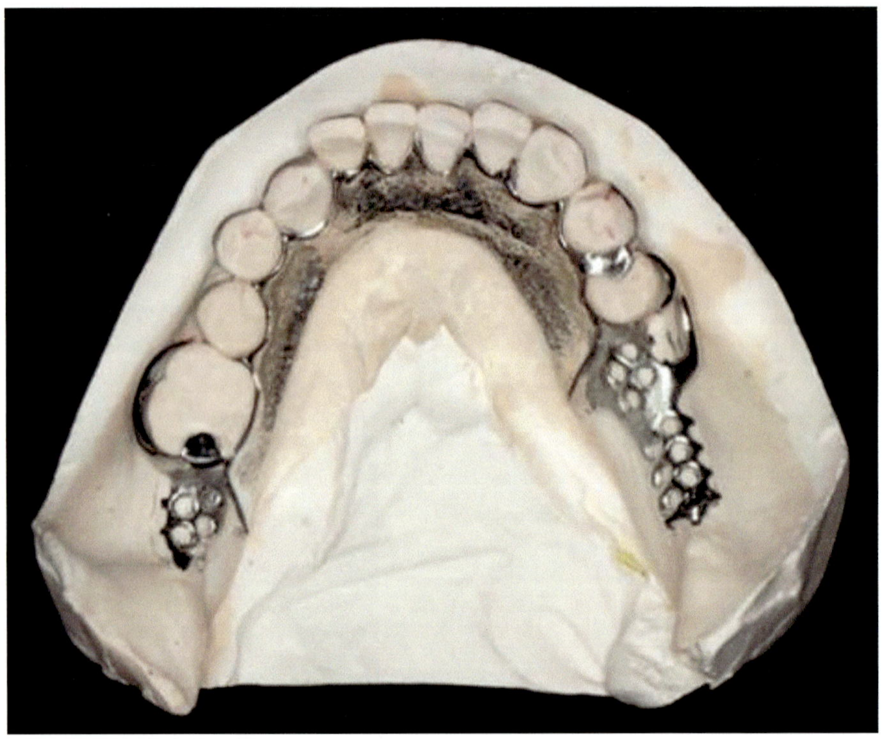

Fig. 6.16 Intraoral renderings of T-type clasps

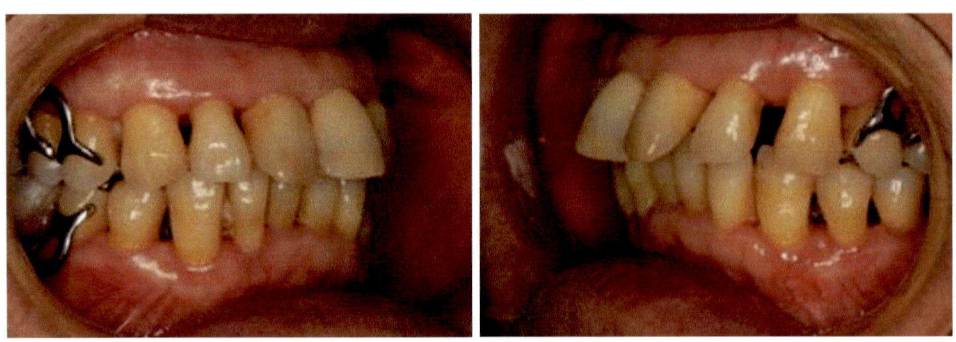

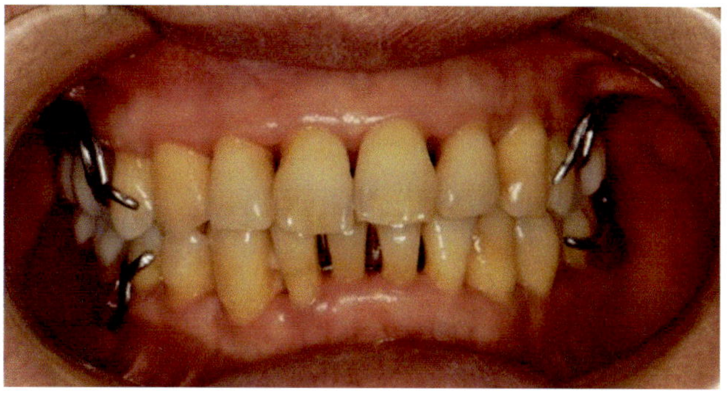

Fig. 6.17 The intraoral renderings

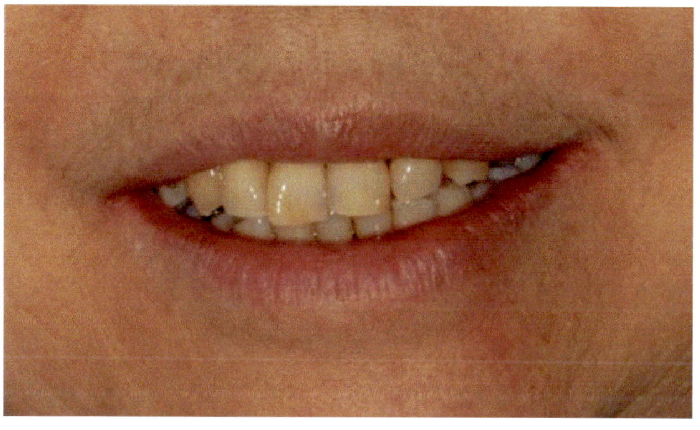

Fig. 6.18 The final effect with denture

6.3 Case 3

1. *Before restoration*

   Mrs. Zhang, 76 years old. Her maxillary edentia have lost A6, A7, B6, and B7 teeth. And similar to previous patient, she has free-end edentia as well.

2. *RPD design and manufacturing*

   In this case, we used the modification of T clasp. But considering she is little old, to make it easy to take off, we designed the clasp to be another shape (Fig. 6.19). A part of clasp arm is extended from the mesial end of the T clasp and then got into the undercut in the distal surface of the mesial adjacent tooth's buccal axial ridge. It finally ended on the buccal axial ridge, hidden by adjacent teeth and lips (Fig. 6.20). This flexible design is called extended T clasp.

3. *After restoration*

   The final effect with denture is shown in Figs. 6.21 and 6.22.

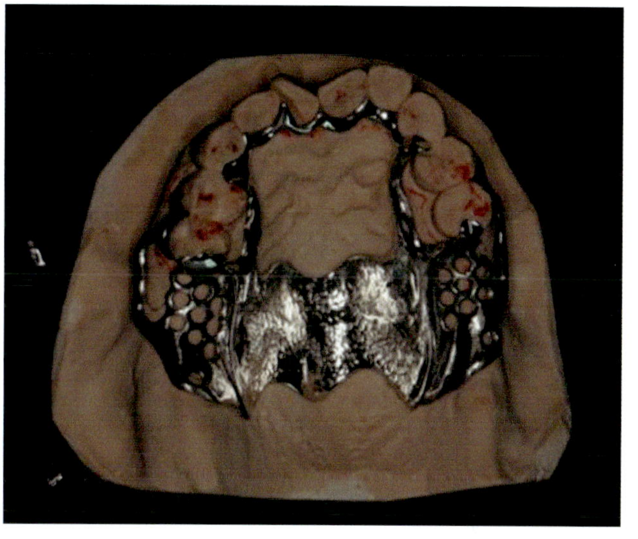

Fig. 6.19 Dentition defect A67, B67

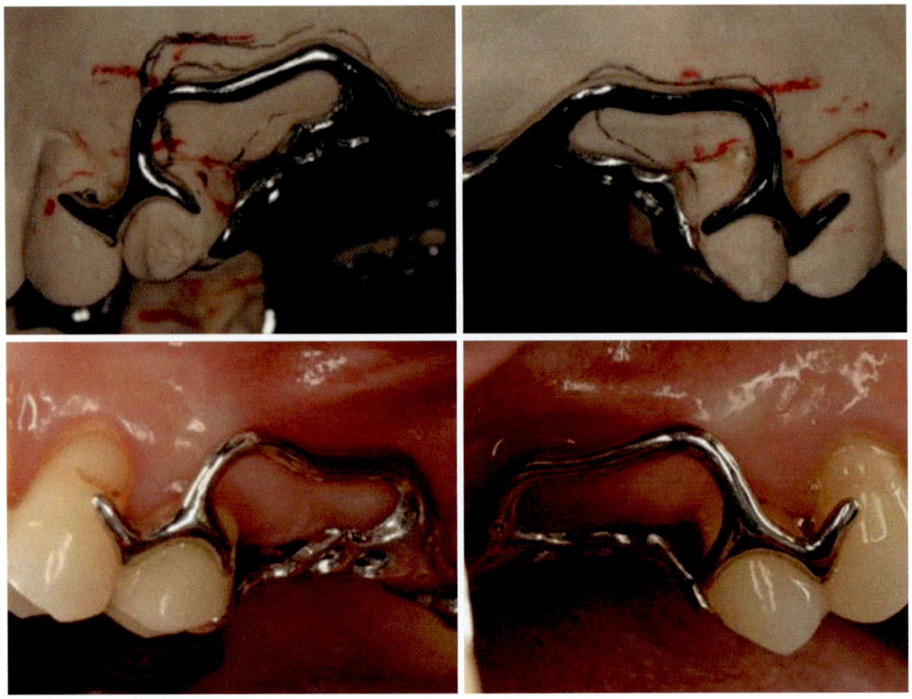

Fig. 6.20 Extended T-type clasp on A45 and B45

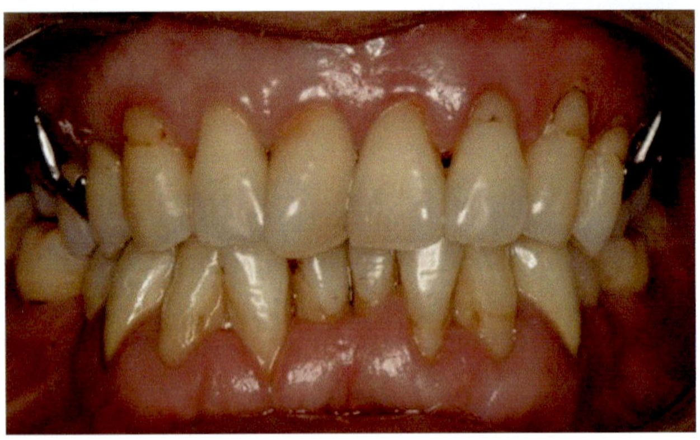

Fig. 6.21 The intraoral rendering

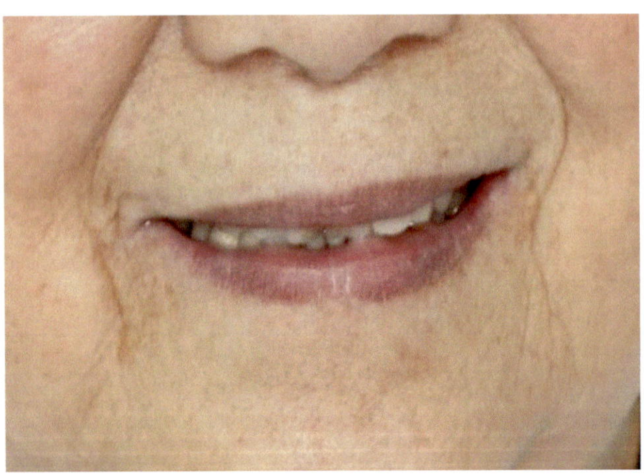

Fig. 6.22 The final effect with denture

6.4 Case 4

1. *Before restoration*

   A woman, 65 years old. In this case, we used buccal short-arm clasp combined with T-type clasp to repair bilateral free-end dentition defect.

   Smile analysis: Median smile line, deep overbite, and all the remaining teeth can be seen when smiling, while mandibular anterior teeth are exposed only 1/3 of the neck (Fig. 6.23). Esthetic area teeth are A3–B3 and C5–D4 (Fig. 6.24). Abutment teeth are in good health and have proper undercuts (Fig. 6.25).

2. *RPD design and manufacturing*

   Maxillary framework design: Because the abutment teeth on both sides of the gap are in good health, there is a suitable undercut. Buccal short-arm clasps were designed for both maxillary canine teeth (Fig. 6.26).

   Mandible framework design: The mandible teeth are not exposed too much, so we used the original undercut of the teeth and designed the T clasps on C5 and D4 (Fig. 6.27).

3. *After restoration*

   The final effect with denture is shown in Figs. 6.28 and 6.29.

   In previous cases, we have presented patients with Kennedy I single-ended free-end edentia and Kennedy II double-ended free-end edentia. So in this case, we will present Kennedy III non-free-end edentia. If only patients keep their oral condition well, the retention and stability of tooth-borne type RPD will be satisfying. The choice of esthetic clasps is wise.

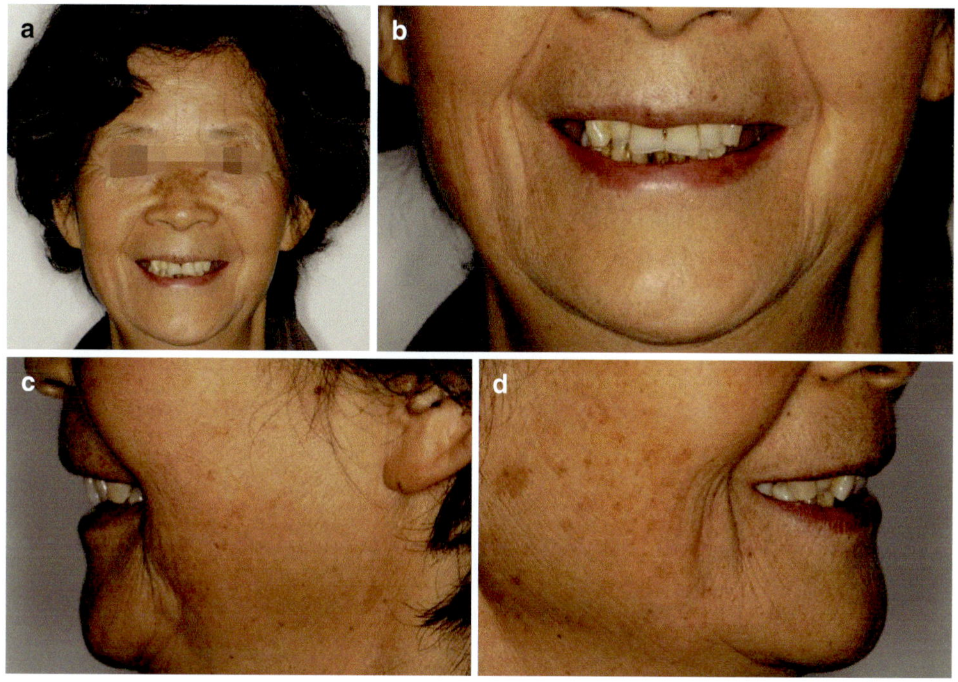

Fig. 6.23 Patient's facial analysis. (**a**) Full-face photo (**b**) Front photo of the lower third of the face (**c**) Left side photo of the lower third of the face. (**d**) Right side photo of the lower third of the face

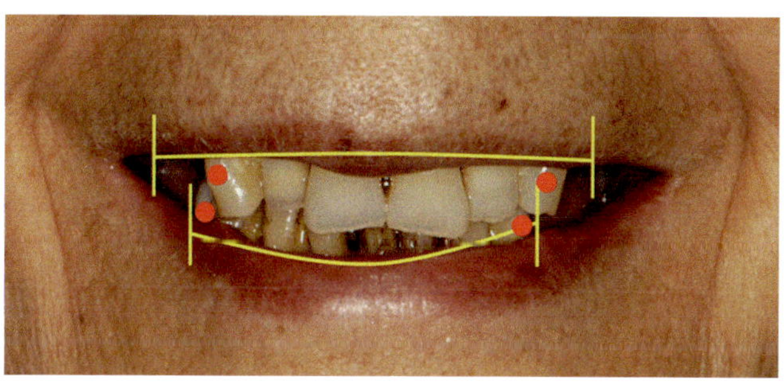

Fig. 6.24 Smile analysis: tooth position in esthetic area—A3–B3, C5–D4

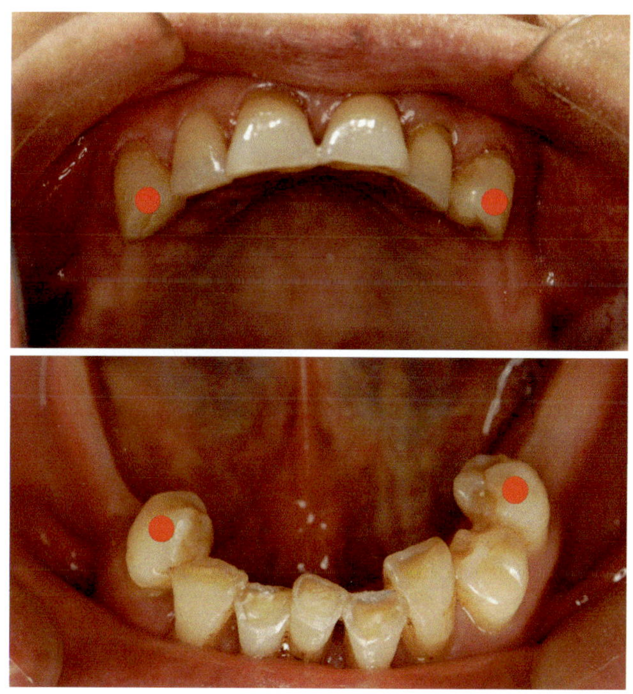

Fig. 6.25 Dentition analysis: design esthetic clasps on A3, B3, C5, and D4

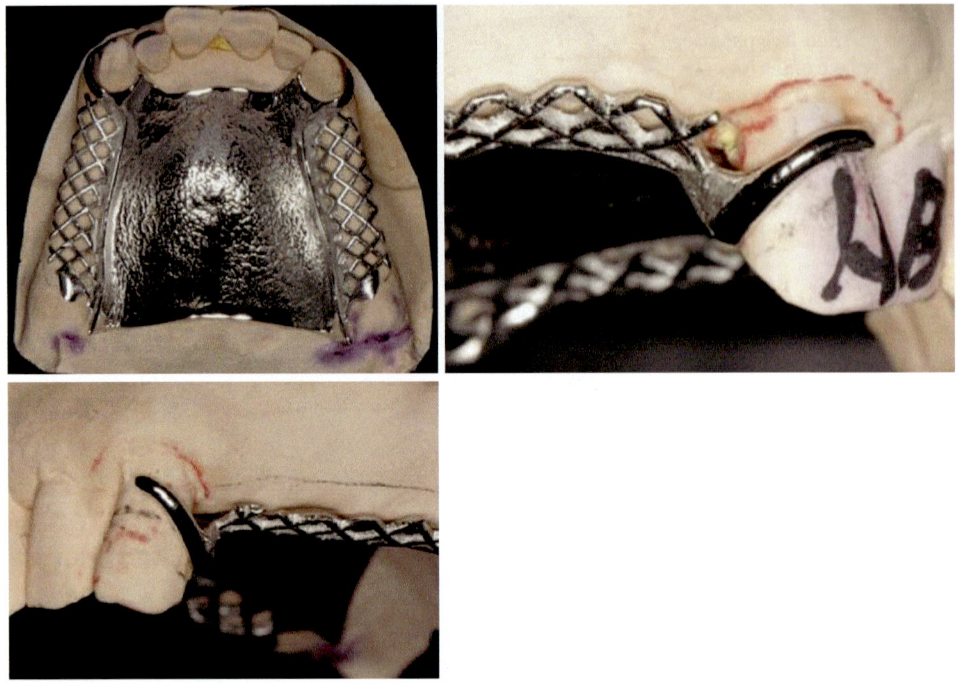

Fig. 6.26 Maxillary framework design: buccal short-arm clasps were designed for both maxillary canine teeth

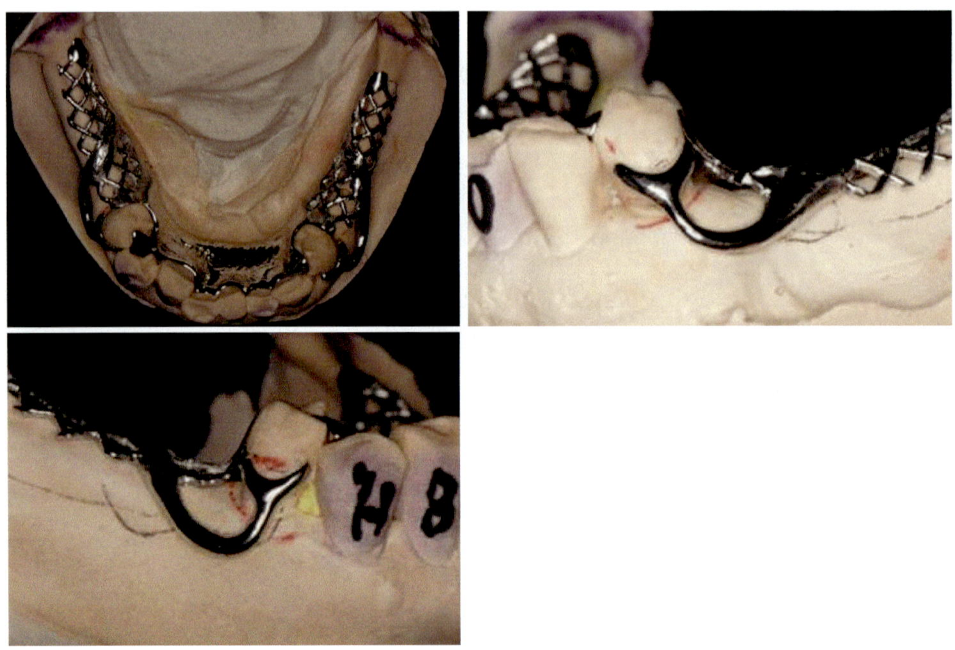

Fig. 6.27 Mandible framework design: T clasps were designed for C5 and D4

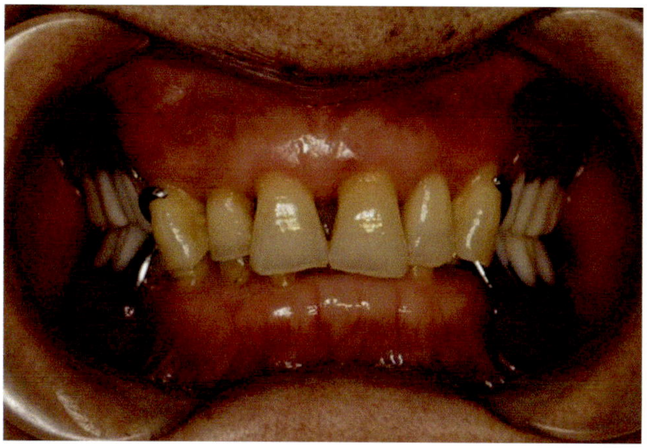

Fig. 6.28 The intraoral rendering

6.5 Case 5

1. *Before restoration*

   A female patient is 61 years old. She lost A6 and B6 on maxillary (Fig. 6.30), and both ends had the second molar left. The abutments were fine. Teeth in esthetic area are A5–B5 and C4–D4.

2. *RPD design and manufacturing*

   In this case, we put short buccally retained clasps on the A5 and B5, and the clasp arms ended at buccal axial ridge. We put traditional three-arm clasps on A7 and B7 the distal abutments of the gap. The back palate plate connected two sides of the RPD, making it symmetrical, esthetic, small, and exquisite (Fig. 6.31).

3. *After restoration* (Fig. 6.32)

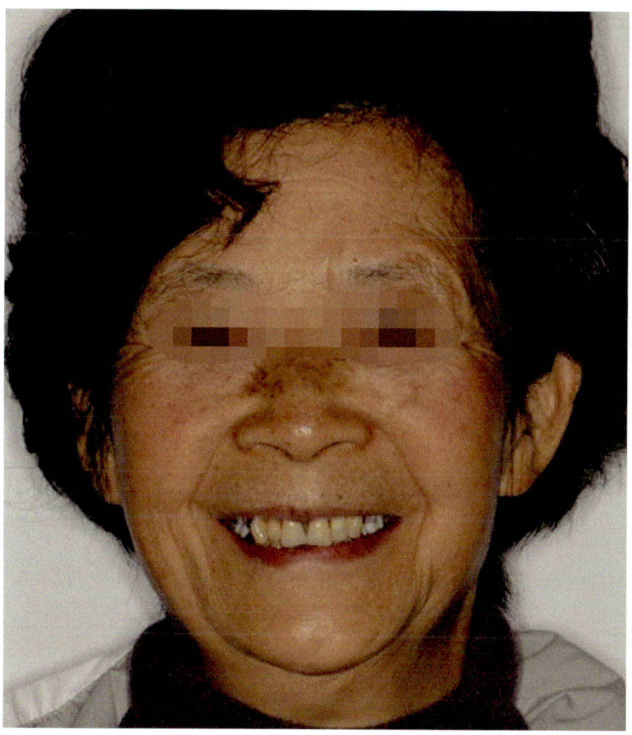

Fig. 6.29 The final effect with denture

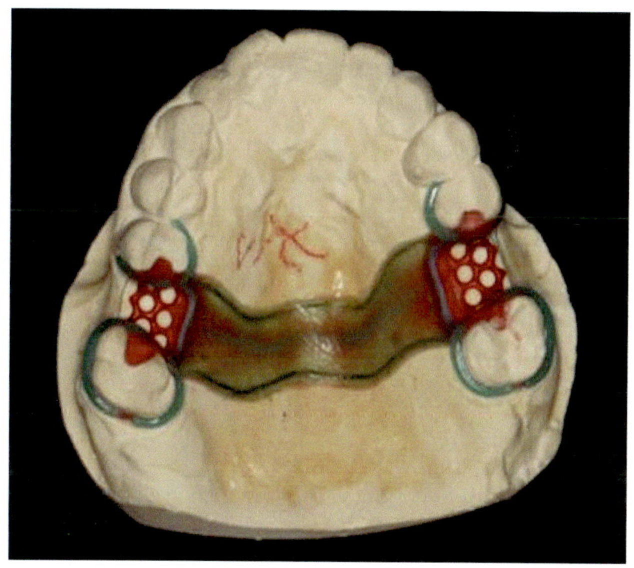

Fig. 6.30 Dentition defect:A6, B6

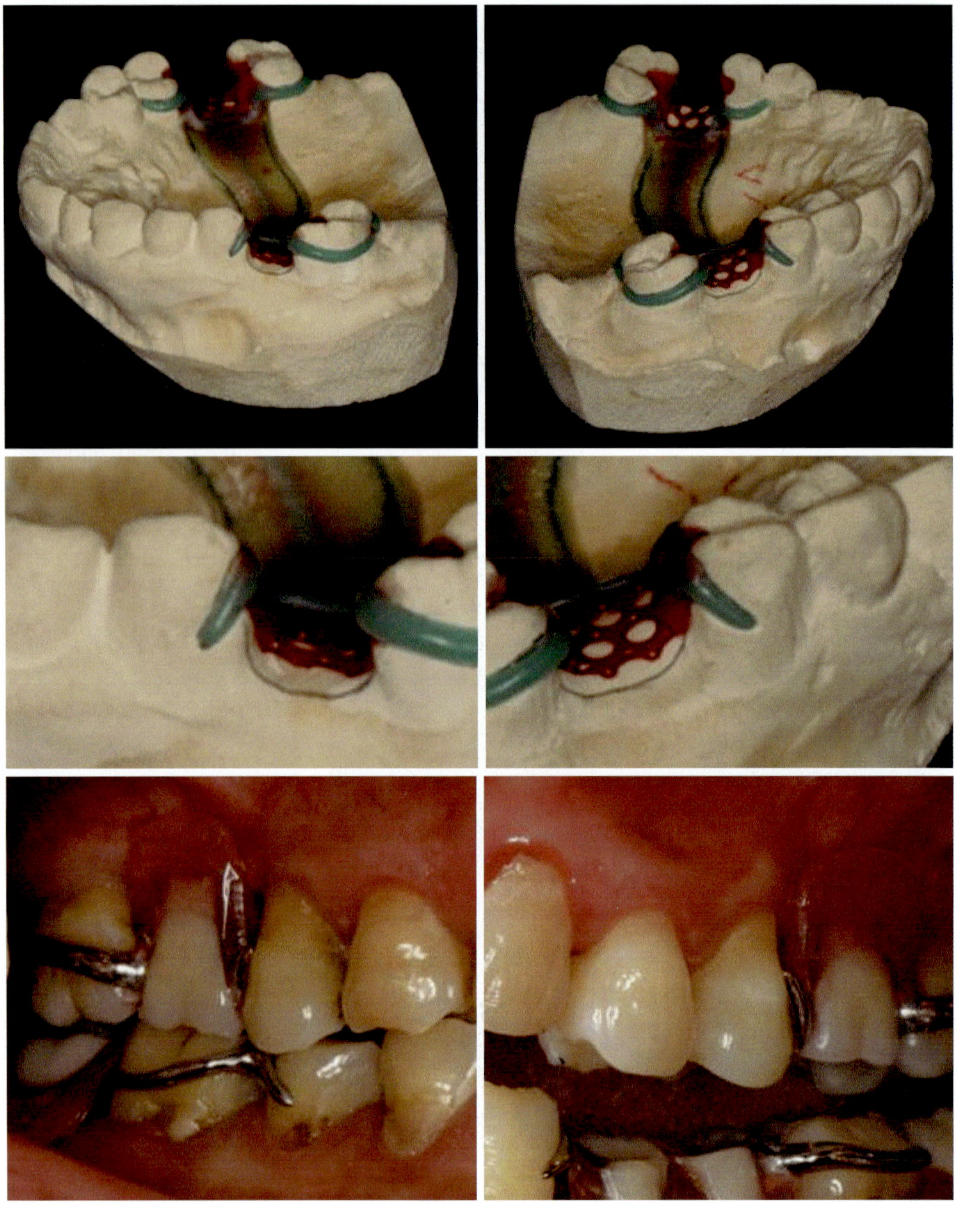

Fig. 6.31 The intraoral renderings: A5, B5—short buccally retained arm

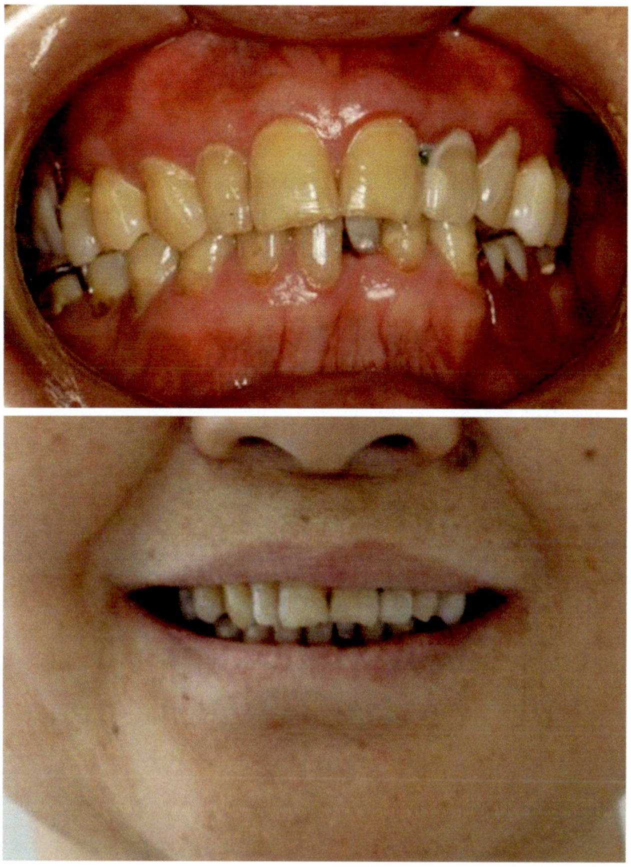

Fig. 6.32 Final effect with denture

6.6 Case 6

Short Buccally Retained Clasp Design for Patient with High Smile Line

1. *Before restoration*

   Mrs. Wang, 59 years old.

   Smile analysis: The patient's smile line is high. When she smiles, the gum exposure is seriously large (Fig. 6.33). B1 is a residual root, which has been finished with root canal therapy. A2 is a residual crown and the patient refuses to remove the tooth for repair. The overbite and overjet of anterior teeth are deep. The esthetic teeth of the patient is A5–B4 and C3–D3, and the overdenture is made after grinding the B1. The remaining abutments have suitable undercuts.

   Dentition analysis: The patient has Kennedy III dentition defect in the upper jaw and Kennedy II dentition defect in the lower jaw. Missing tooth are 7 which will not be repaired in A area; 1, 2, and 4 in B area; 5–7 in C area; and 5–7 in D area, and there is also a gap between 1 and 2 in A area. With regard to the selection of abutments, due to the serious caries of A2, the retention form is not good, so the clasp is not designed on A2. We design e-clasps on A4, B3, B5, C4, and D4 (Fig. 6.34).

2. *RPD analysis design and manufacturing*

   With regard to the selection of abutments, due to the serious caries of A2, the retention form is not good, so the

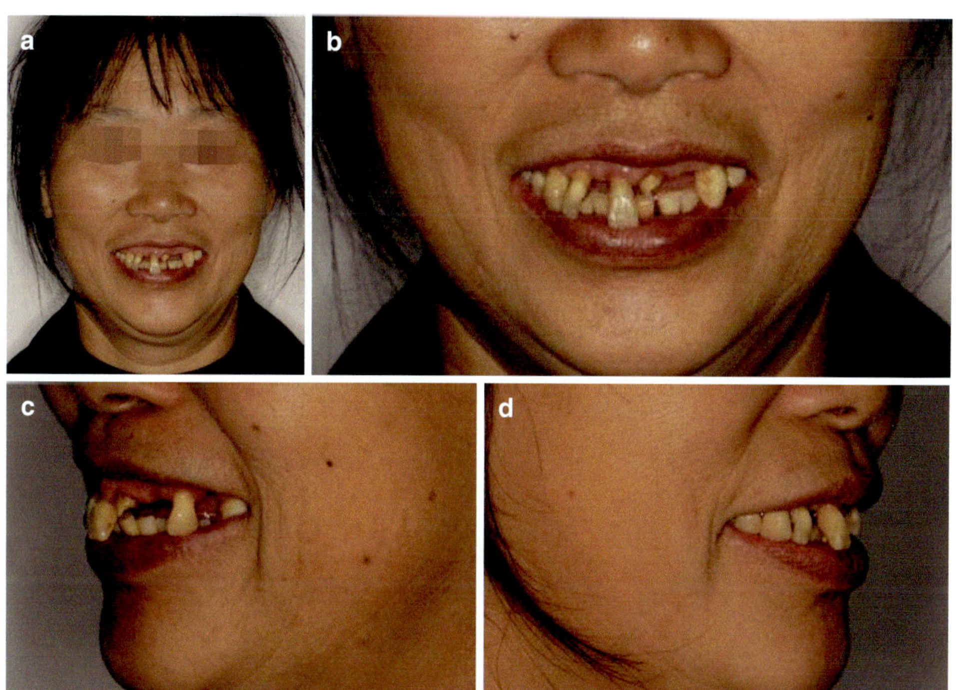

Fig. 6.33 Facial analysis. (**a**) Facial frontal view. (**b**) Lower facial 1/3 frontal view. (**c**) Lower facial 1/3 left lateral view. (**d**) Lower facial 1/3 right lateral view

clasp is not designed on A2. We design e-clasps on A4, B3, B5, C4, and D4 (Fig. 6.34).

Maxillary framework design: An embrasure clasp is designed on A4, and a short buccally retained clasp is designed on B3, which has good concealment effect. A three-arm clasp is put on B5 to provide sufficient retention (Fig. 6.35). Mandibular framework design: Two bar clasps are, respectively, set on C4 and D4 to utilize the labial undercut for retention (Fig. 6.36).

3. *After restoration*

The final effect with denture is shown in Figs. 6.37, 6.38, 6.39, and 6.40. The patient is satisfied.

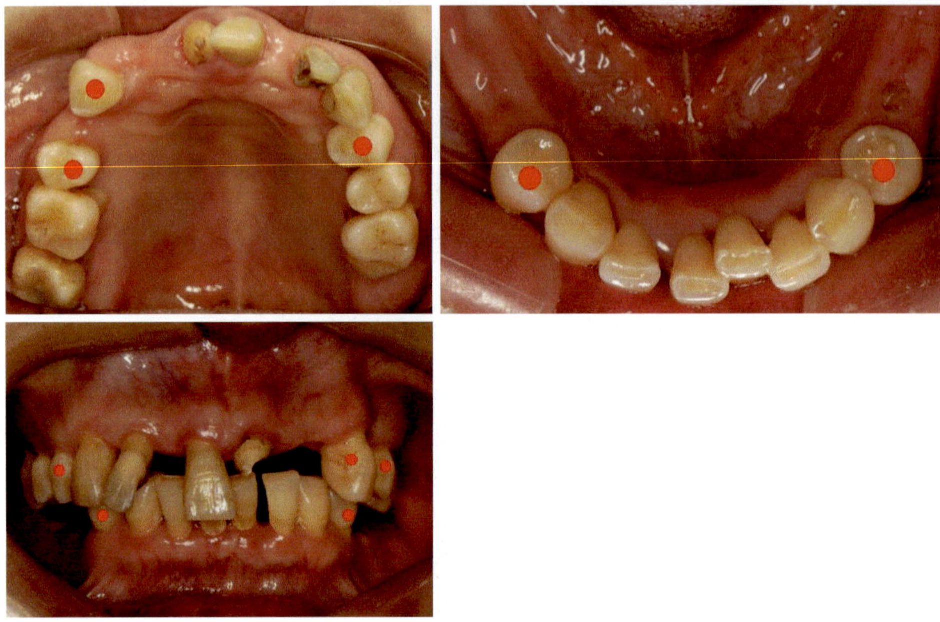

Fig. 6.34 Dentition analysis: the e-clasps are put on A4, B3, B5, C4, and D4. (It can be seen that the oral hygiene of the patient is poor, so it is recommended to restore after periodontal treatment. However, the patient refuses periodontal treatment due to cost problems)

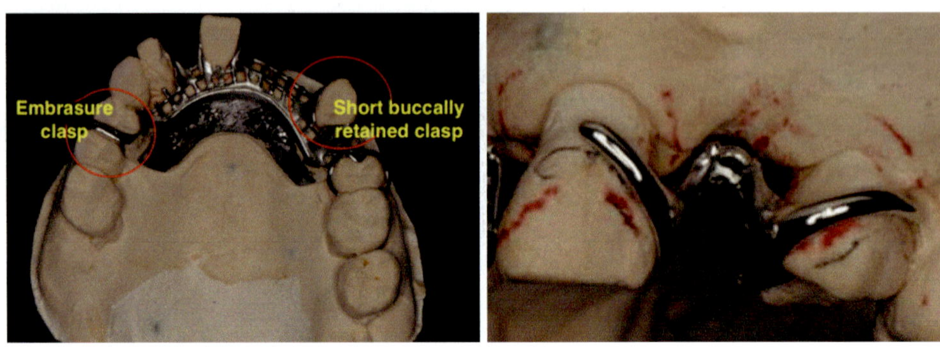

Fig. 6.35 Maxillary framework design: set an embrasure clasp on A4, a short buccally retained clasp on B3, and a three-arm clasp on B5 to provide sufficient retention

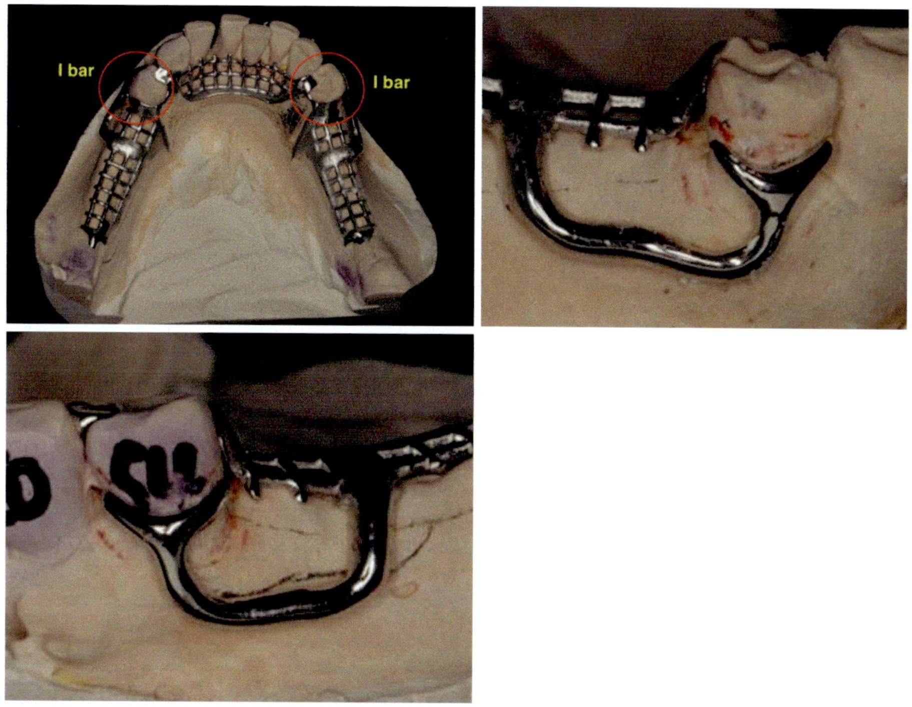

Fig. 6.36 Mandibular framework design: set bar clasps on C4 and D4 to utilize the labial undercut for retention

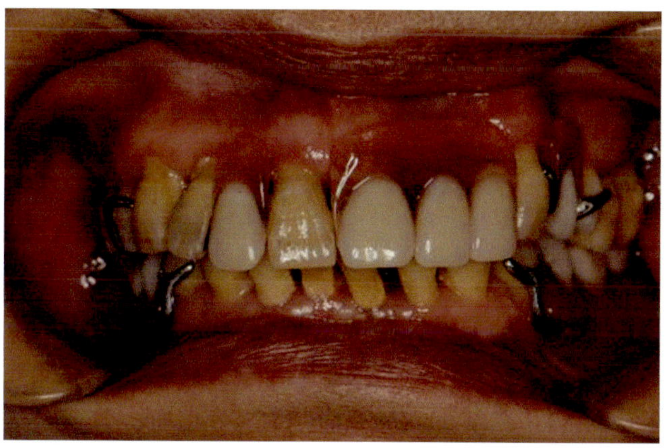

Fig. 6.37 Intraoral frontal view with denture

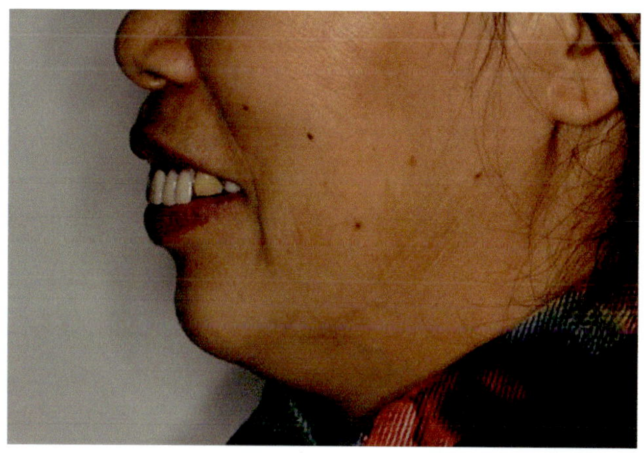

Fig. 6.39 Lower facial 1/3 lateral view with denture

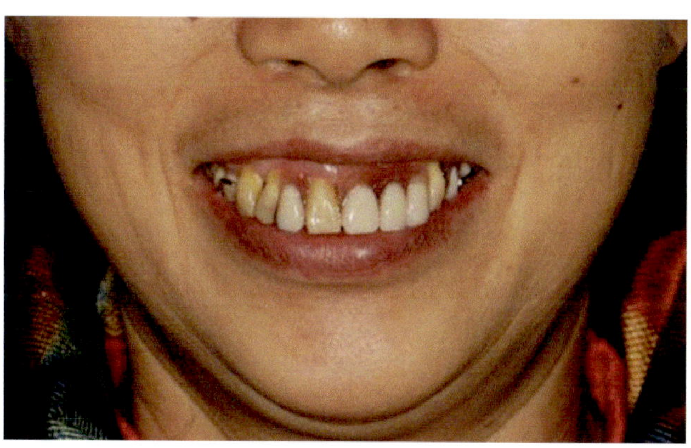

Fig. 6.38 Lower facial 1/3 frontal view with denture

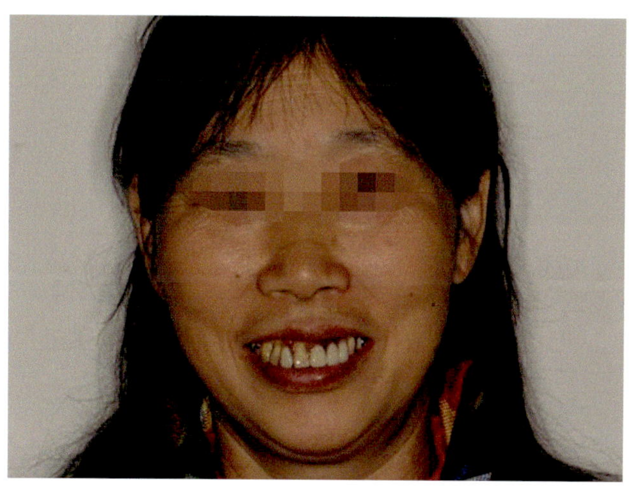

Fig. 6.40 Facial frontal view with denture

6.7 Case 7

E-Clasps Design for Patient with Tooth Defects and Gingival Atrophy

1. *Before restoration*

A man, 89 years old. He came to see the doctor because his old denture was not suitable after the tooth was lost. The patient reported that he had burning mouth syndrome, skewed tongue, advanced age, and low esthetic requirements.

Smile analysis: The smile line of Mr. Hu is low, and the lower teeth area is exposed more when talking. Most of lower anterior teeth is missing. The patient's esthetic teeth are A3–B3 and C3–D3 (Fig. 6.41).

Dentition analysis: The patient has Kennedy III dentition defect in the upper jaw. On the lingual side of A6, A7, and B7 on the maxilla, there are much gingival atrophy and root exposure. To protect the remaining teeth, they are not suitable for abutments. Furthermore, the patient has Kennedy I unilateral free-end edentia on the mandible. Most of the teeth have cervical wedge-shaped defects, and the abutments are in poor condition. Missing teeth are A3, B5, and B6, 1–2 and 5–7 in C area, and 1–2 and 6 in D area (Fig. 6.42). Besides, B7 is a residual crown. So we design e-clasps on A4, A5, B4, C3, C4, and D3, D4, D5 (Fig. 6.43).

2. *RPD analysis design and manufacturing*

Most of the teeth have cervical wedge-shaped defects, and the abutments are in poor condition. In summary, the e-clasps are designed on A4, A5, B4, C3, C4, and D3, D4, D5 (Figs. 6.44 and 6.45).

3. *After restoration*

The final effect is shown in Figs. 6.46, 6.47, and 6.48. The patient is much satisfied.

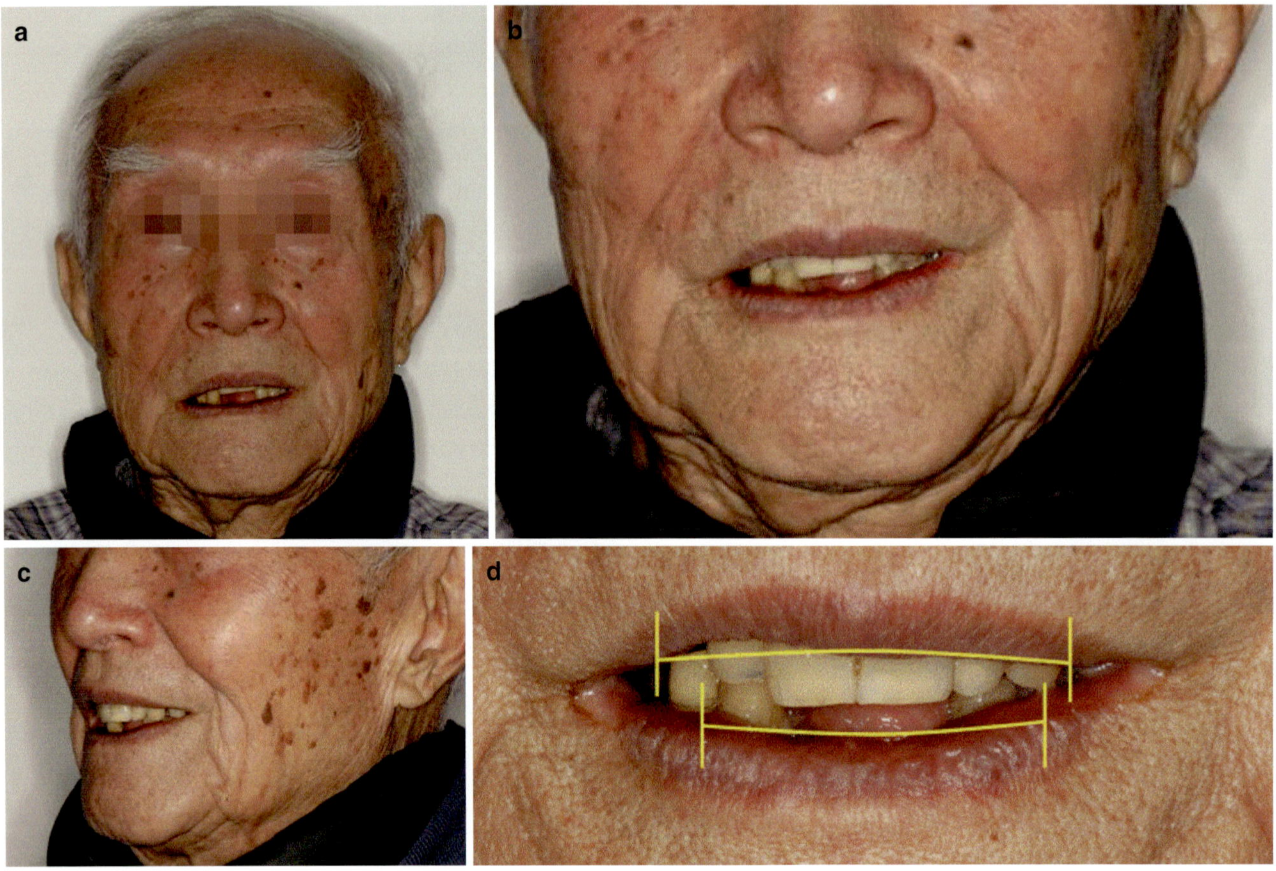

Fig. 6.41 Facial analysis. (**a**) Facial frontal view. (**b**) Lower facial 1/3 frontal view. (**c**) Lower facial 1/3 lateral view. (**d**) Smile analysis: The patient has a low smile line, and the esthetic teeth are A3–B3, C3–D3

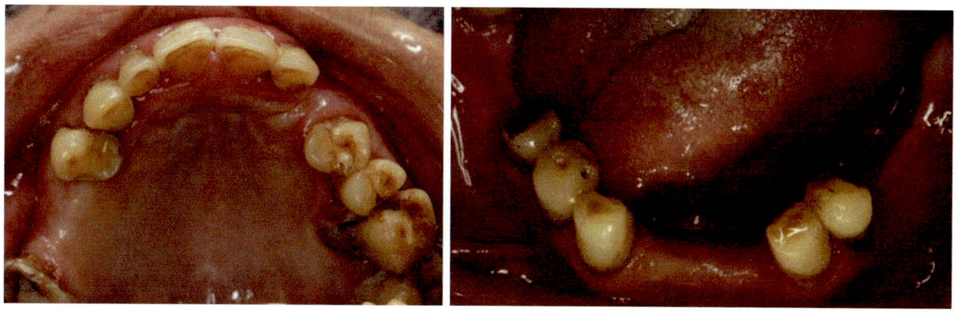

Fig. 6.42 Missing teeth: A3, B5, B6; 1–2, 5–7 in C area; 1–2, 6 in D area, and B7 is the residual crown

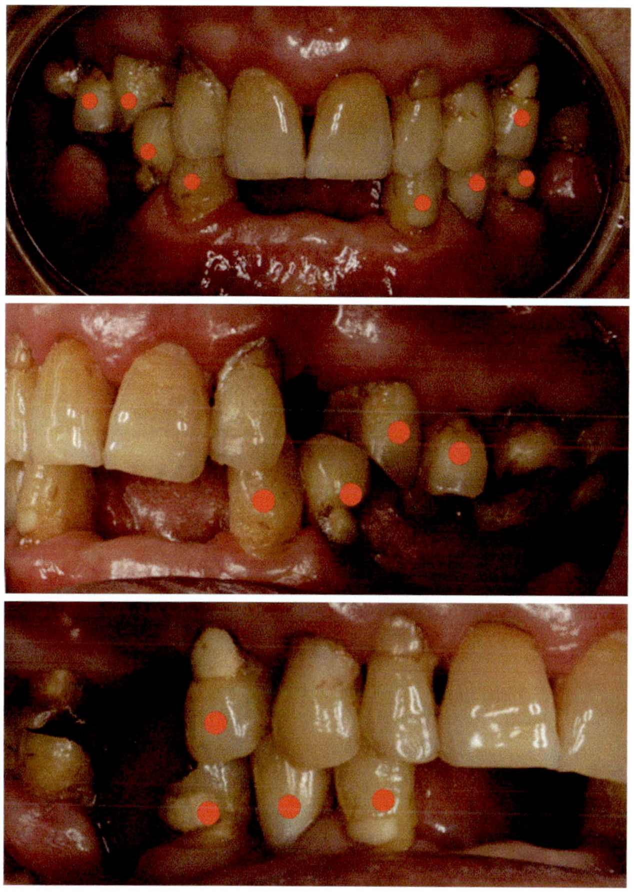

Fig. 6.43 Dentition analysis: set e-clasps on A4, A5, B4, C3, C4, and D3, D4, D5

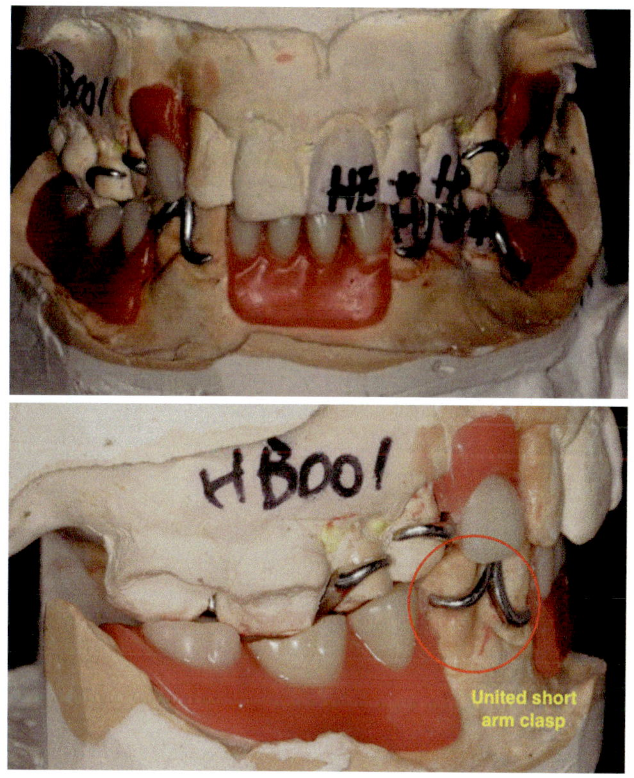

Fig. 6.44 Framework design: a one-arm clasp is set on A4, and an embrasure clasp is set on A5. Due to insufficient retention of the abutment in C area and cervical wedge-shaped defect, we design the united short-arm clasp and extend the clasp tip appropriately to improve the retention and support

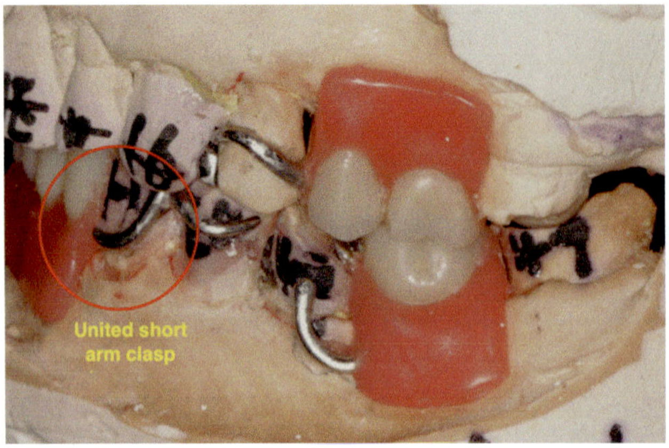

Fig. 6.45 Framework design: one-arm clasp is placed on B4; a united short-arm clasp is placed on D3 and D4; a I-bar is placed on D5

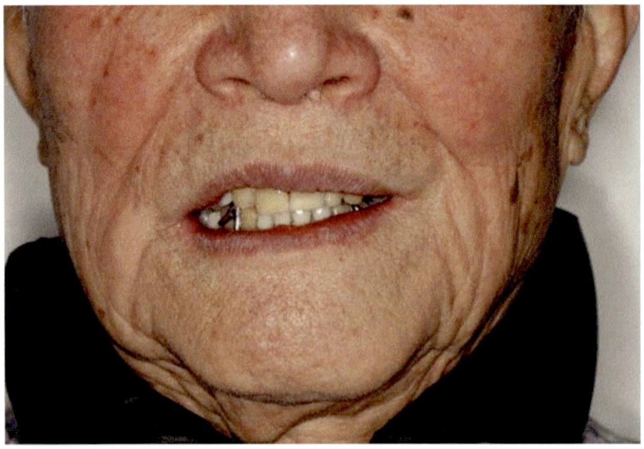

Fig. 6.46 Lower facial 1/3 frontal view with denture

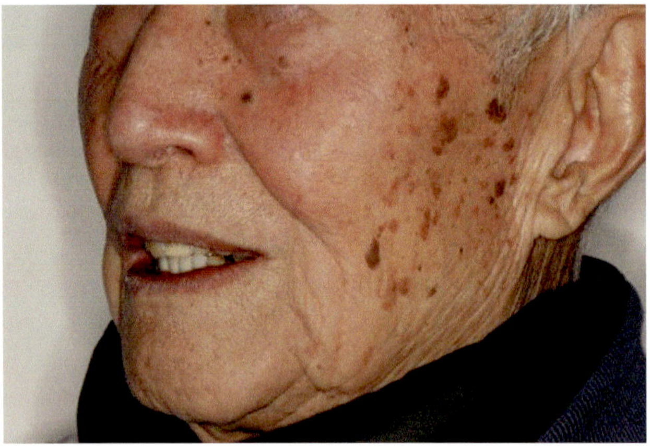

Fig. 6.47 Lower facial 1/3 lateral view with denture

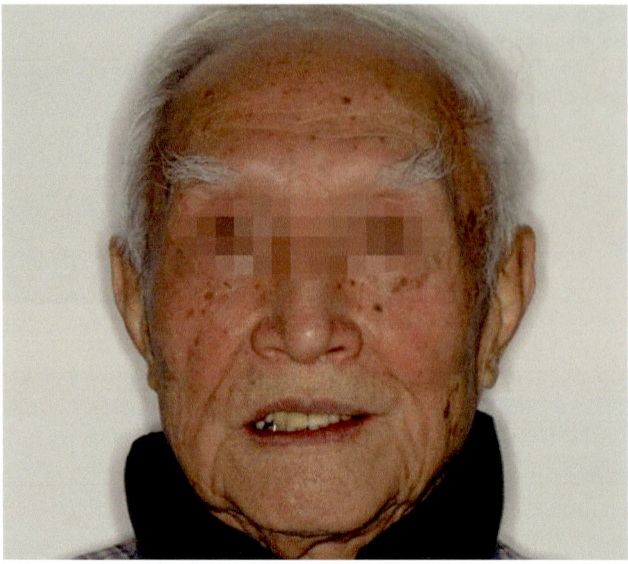

Fig. 6.48 Facial frontal view with denture

6.8 Case 8

E-Clasps Design for Patient with Dentition Defect in Long-Term Unrestored Condition

1. *Before restoration*

   A female, 67 years old. The patient reported that she had never made dentures before and chewed only with the first molars on the right for a long time.

   Smile analysis: The patient has a middle smile line. When she smiles, we can see the upper canines are torqued and the missing teeth area on mandible is exposed. The vertical distance of lower 1/3 face is insufficient, and there is an apparent aging face. The patient's esthetic teeth are A3–B3 and C3–D3 (Fig. 6.49).

   Dentition analysis: There are a large number of missing teeth. The patient has Kennedy III dentition defect in the upper jaw, and two canines have a large torsion (Fig. 6.50) with an undercut on the mesial. There is defect in the mesial buccal wall of 6. The maxillary alveolar ridge is full and the roots of 8 are exposed. Missing teeth are 1–2, 4–5, and 7 in A area and 1–2 and 4–7 in B area (Fig. 6.51). The patient has Kennedy III dentition defect without 8 in the lower jaw, and alveolar ridge is sharp (Fig. 6.52). Missing teeth are 1–5 and 7 in C area and 1 and 7 in D area (Fig. 6.53). There are third molars in the upper jaw and no third molar in the lower jaw.

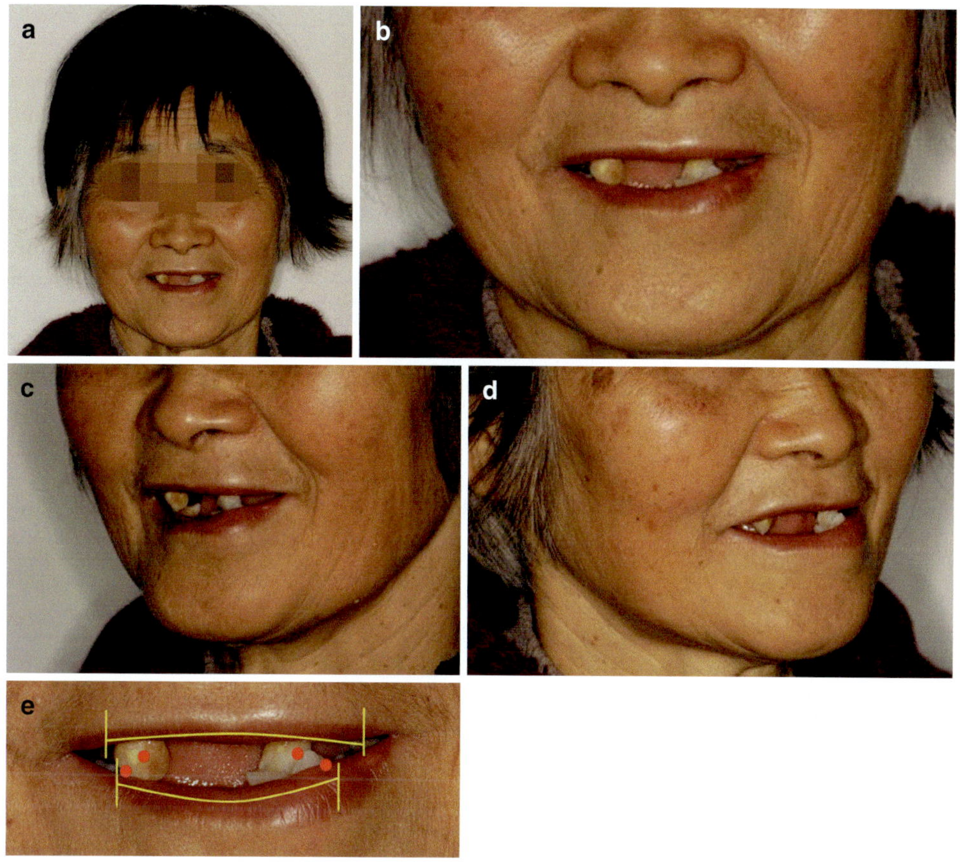

Fig. 6.49 Facial analysis. (**a**) Facial frontal view. (**b**) Lower Facial 1/3 frontal view. (**c**) Lower Facial 1/3 left lateral view in 45°. (**d**) Lower Facial 1/3 right lateral view in 45°. (**e**) Smile analysis: The patient has a middle smile line, and the esthetic teeth are A3–B3, C3–D3

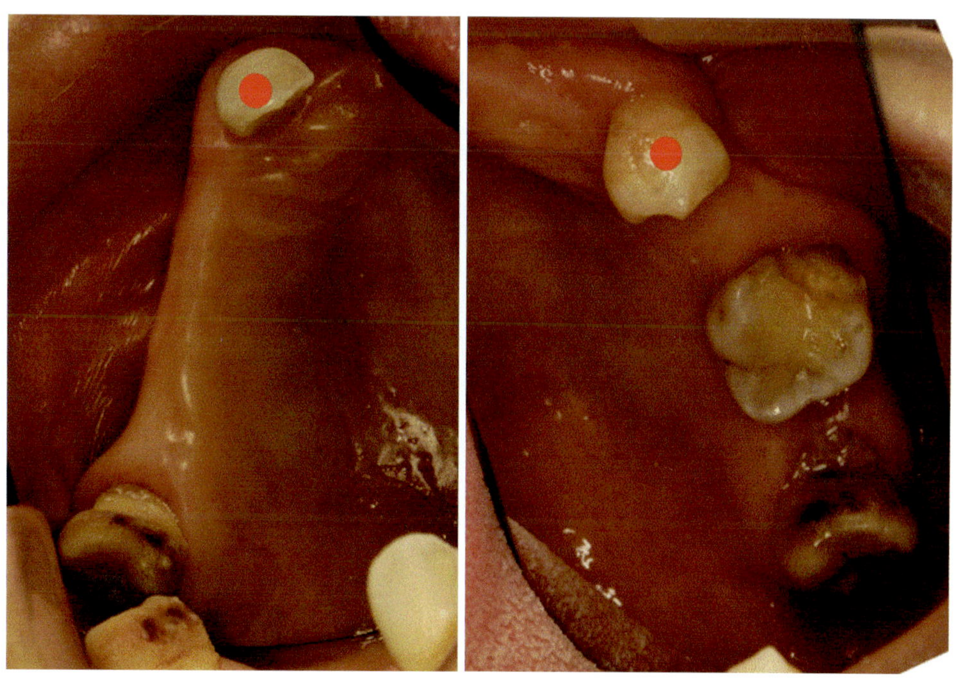

Fig. 6.50 Dentition analysis: Kennedy III dentition defect in the upper jaw and torqued canines

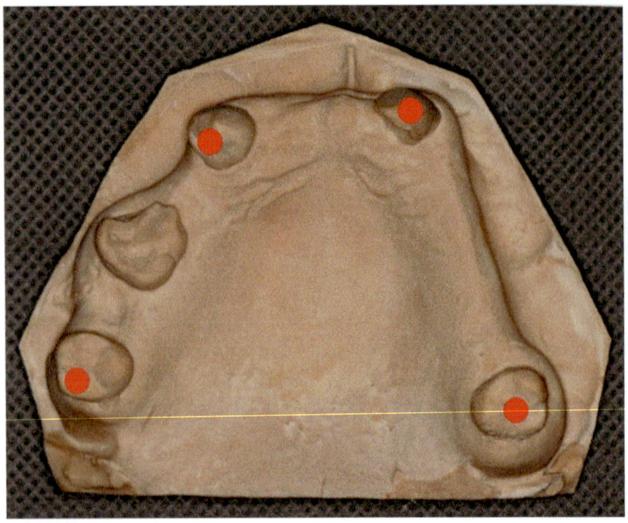

Fig. 6.51 Missing teeth: 1–2, 4–5, 7 in A area; 1–2, 4–7 in B area

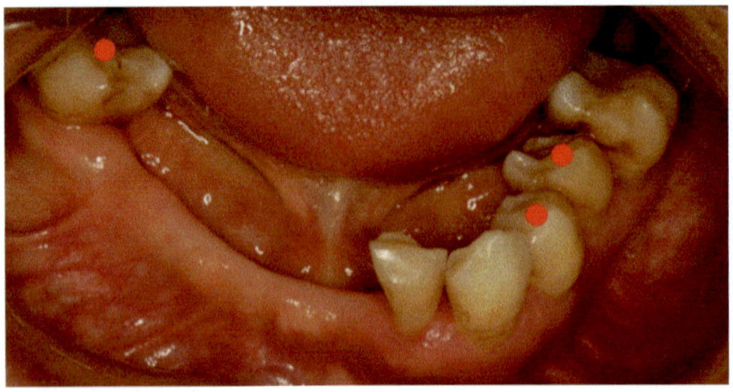

Fig. 6.52 Dentition analysis: Kennedy III dentition defect in the lower jaw and sharp alveolar ridge

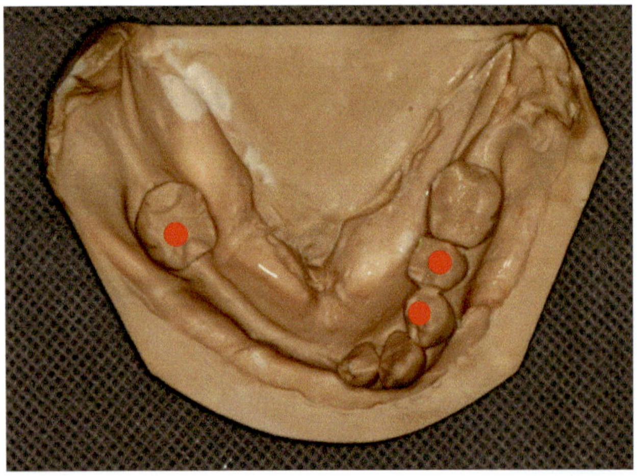

Fig. 6.53 Missing teeth: 1–5, 7 in C area; 1, 7 in D area

It can be seen from the occlusion situation that the anterior crossbite is very serious (Fig. 6.54). Therefore, it is recommended to increase the occlusal height during restoration to restore the height and occlusal relationship of the paired jaw teeth with the self-curing resin on the occlusal surface of 6 in A area.

2. *RPD analysis design and manufacturing*

Maxillary framework design: Two adjacent surface hidden clasps are designed on A3 and B3, respectively, and are retained by the undercut of teeth's adjacent surface. Because of the mesial defect of A6, the occlusal surface of A6 is raised. and then three-arm clasps are put on A8 and B8, respectively (Fig. 6.55).

Mandibular framework design: D7 in mandible is not repaired, a ring clasp is placed on C6, and a united short-arm clasp is set on the gap between D4 and D5 (Fig. 6.56).

3. *After restoration*

The final result is shown on Figs. 6.57 and 6.58. The patient is contented.

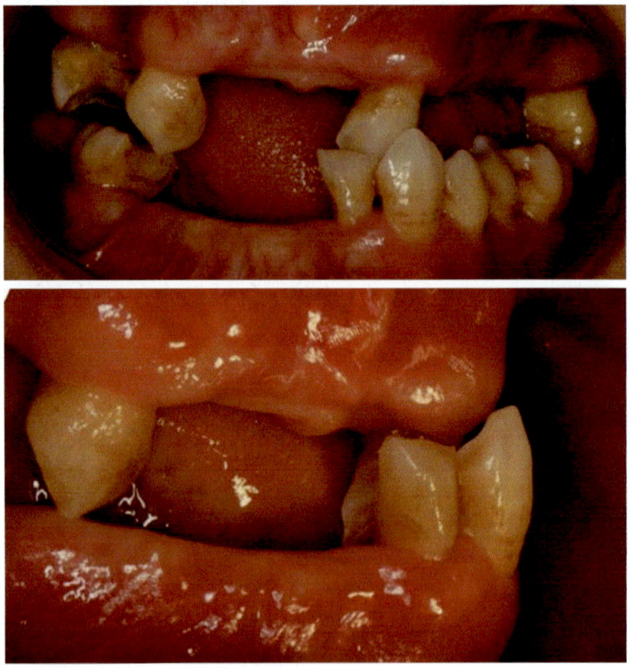

Fig. 6.54 Serious anterior crossbite

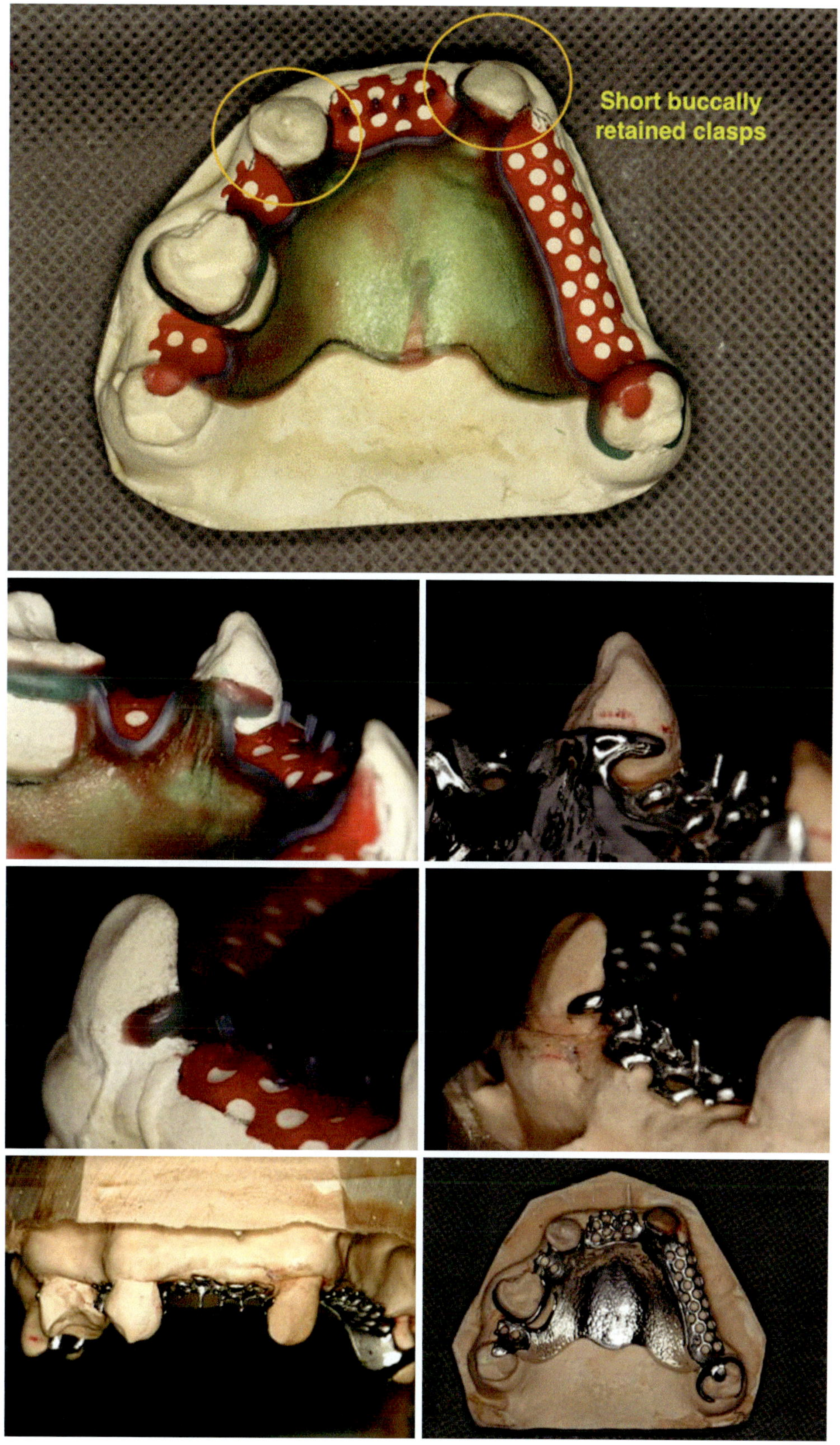

Fig. 6.55 Maxillary framework design: two adjacent surface hidden clasps are designed on A3 and B3, respectively, and are retained by the undercut of teeth's adjacent surface. Because of the mesial defect of A6, the occlusal surface of A6 is raised, and then two three-arm clasps are put on A8 and B8, respectively

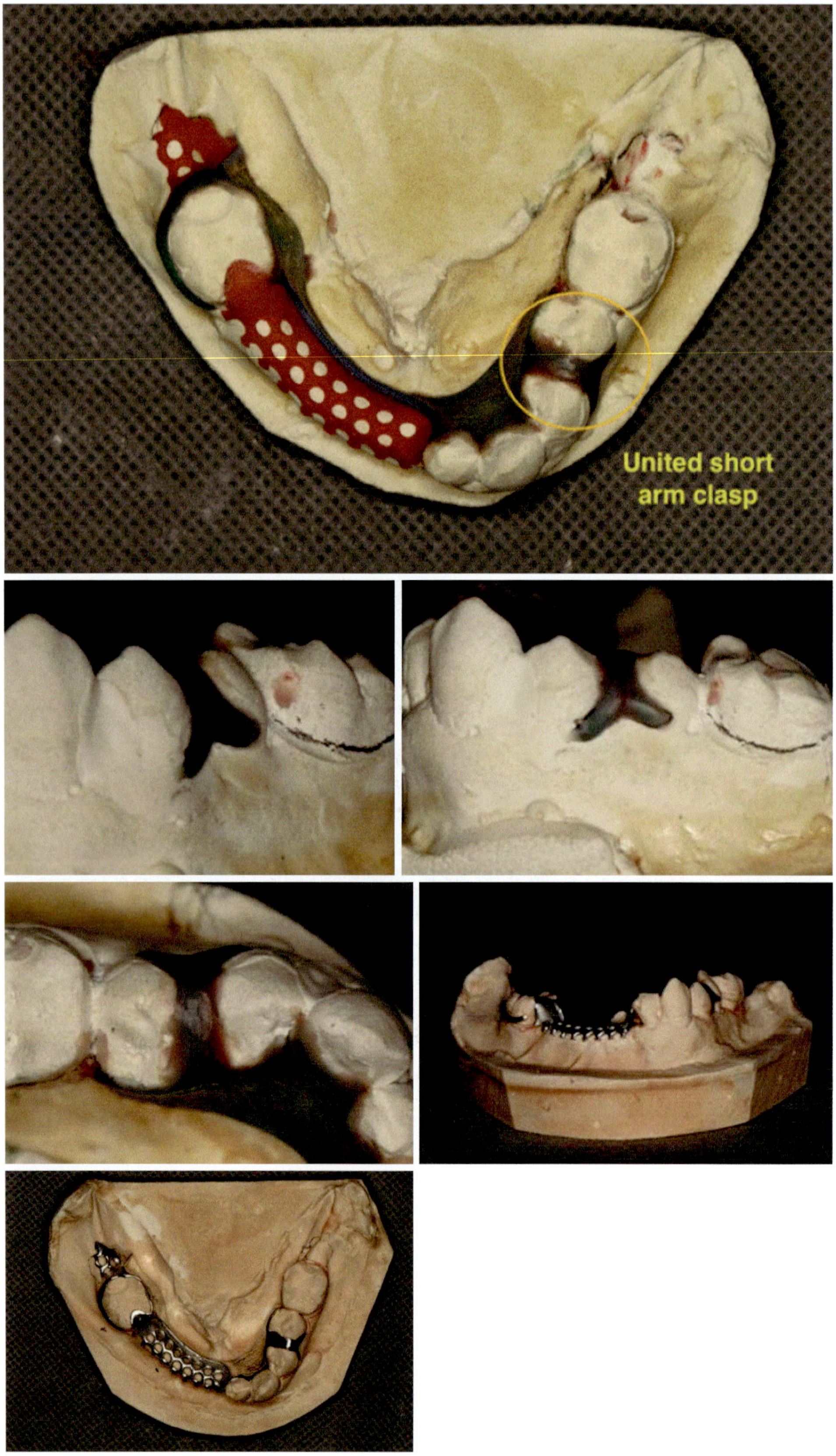

Fig. 6.56 Mandibular framework design: D7 in mandible is not repaired, a ring clasp is placed on C6, and a united short-arm clasp are set on the gap between D4 and D5

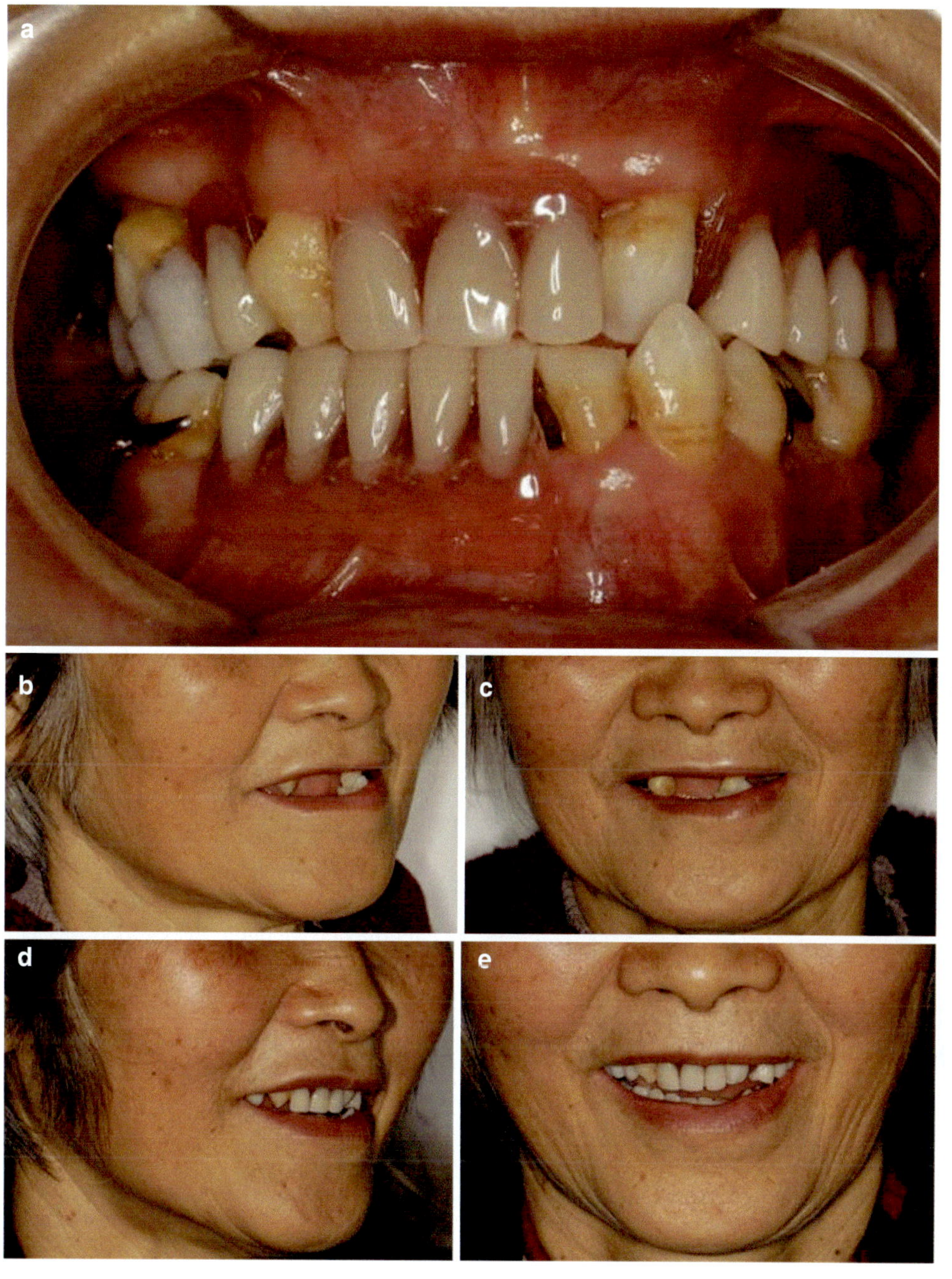

Fig. 6.57 Comparison before and after restoration. (**a**) Intraoral frontal view with denture. (**b**) Facial lateral view before restoration. (**c**) Facial frontal view before restoration. (**d**) Facial lateral view after restoration. (**e**) Facial frontal view after restoration. (**f**) Before restoration. (**g**) After restoration

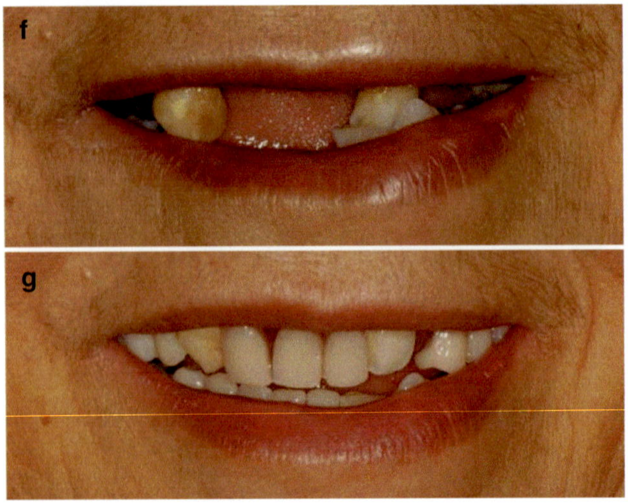

Fig. 6.57 (continued)

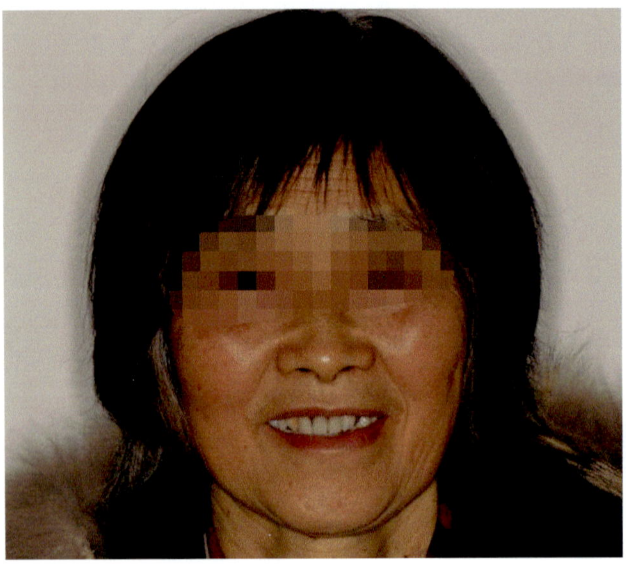

Fig. 6.58 Facial frontal view with denture

6.9 Case 9

Combined C Clasps Design for Patient with Bilateral Maxillary Free-End Edentia

1. *Before restoration*

   A man, 46 years old.

   Smile analysis: The patient has a median smile line, whose overbite and overjet are normal. His upper lip covers the cervix of teeth, and the lower lip covers 1/3 of the incision. The mandibular missing area of teeth can be seen when smiling. The esthetic teeth are A4–B3 and C5–D5 (Fig. 6.59). Four in the right upper jaw is I°loose. The remaining abutments are relatively stable and have suitable undercuts.

   Dentition analysis: The patient has Kennedy I dentition defect in the upper jaw and Kennedy III dentition defect in the lower jaw. Missing teeth are A5–A7; B4–B7; C1, C2, and C4; and D1 and D7. Due to the severe torsion, the clasp cannot be designed on C3. On A4, B3, C6, C7, and D6, e-clasps are designed. (Fig. 6.60).
2. *RPD analysis design and manufacturing*

   Maxillary framework design: Two split C clasps are designed on A4 and B3, respectively, which protects the II°loose abutment in A area to extend the remaining time of the abutment. Besides, the clasps enter the cervical undercut, which is good for concealment (Fig. 6.61).

   Mandibular framework design: We design combined clasps on C6 and C7. Due to the large gap between two abutments, we put a special food-resistant impactor to fill in the gap and a three-arm clasp on D6 (Fig. 6.62).
3. *After restoration*

   The final repair effect is shown in Figs. 6.63, 6.64, and 6.65 The patient was contented.

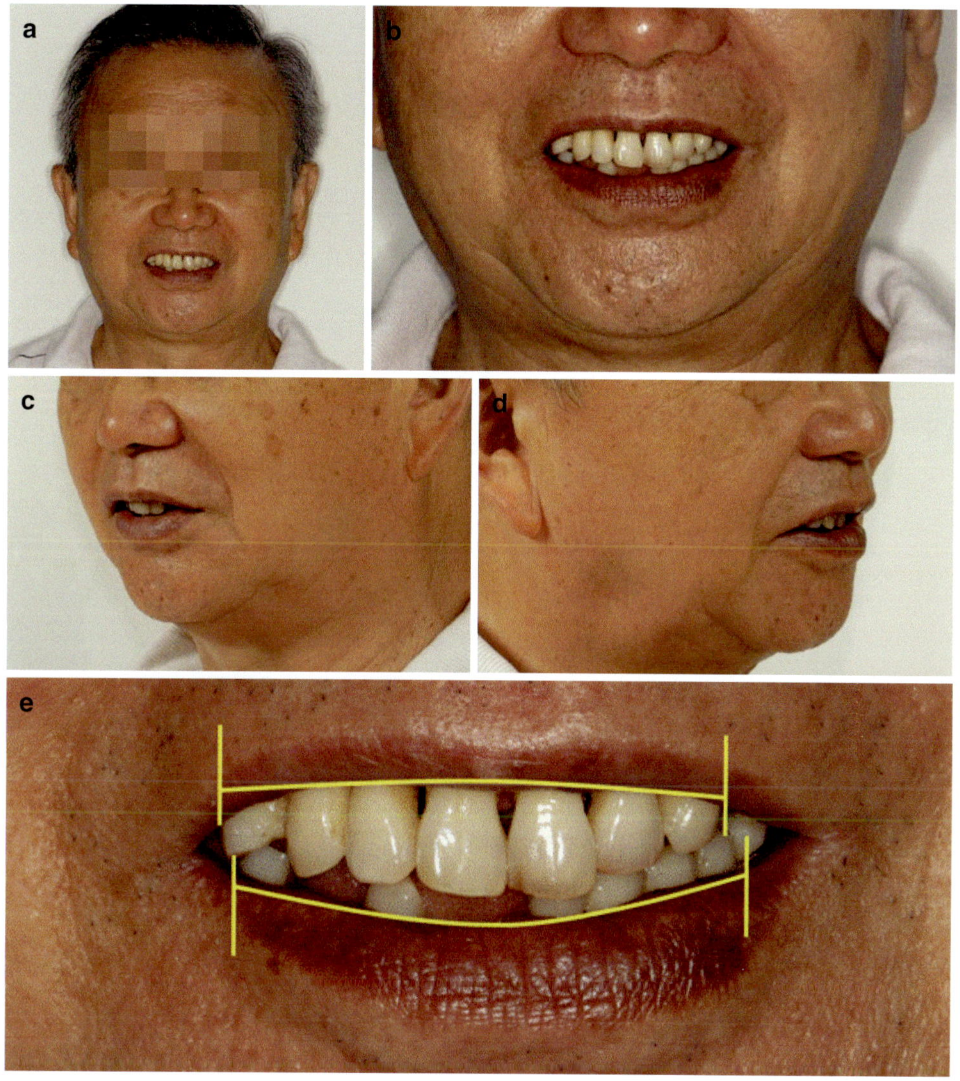

Fig. 6.59 Facial analysis. (**a**) Facial frontal view. (**b**) Lower facial 1/3 frontal view. (**c**) Lower facial 1/3 left lateral view in 45° (**d**) Lower facial 1/3 right lateral view in 45°. (**e**) Esthetic teeth are A4–B3 and C5–D5

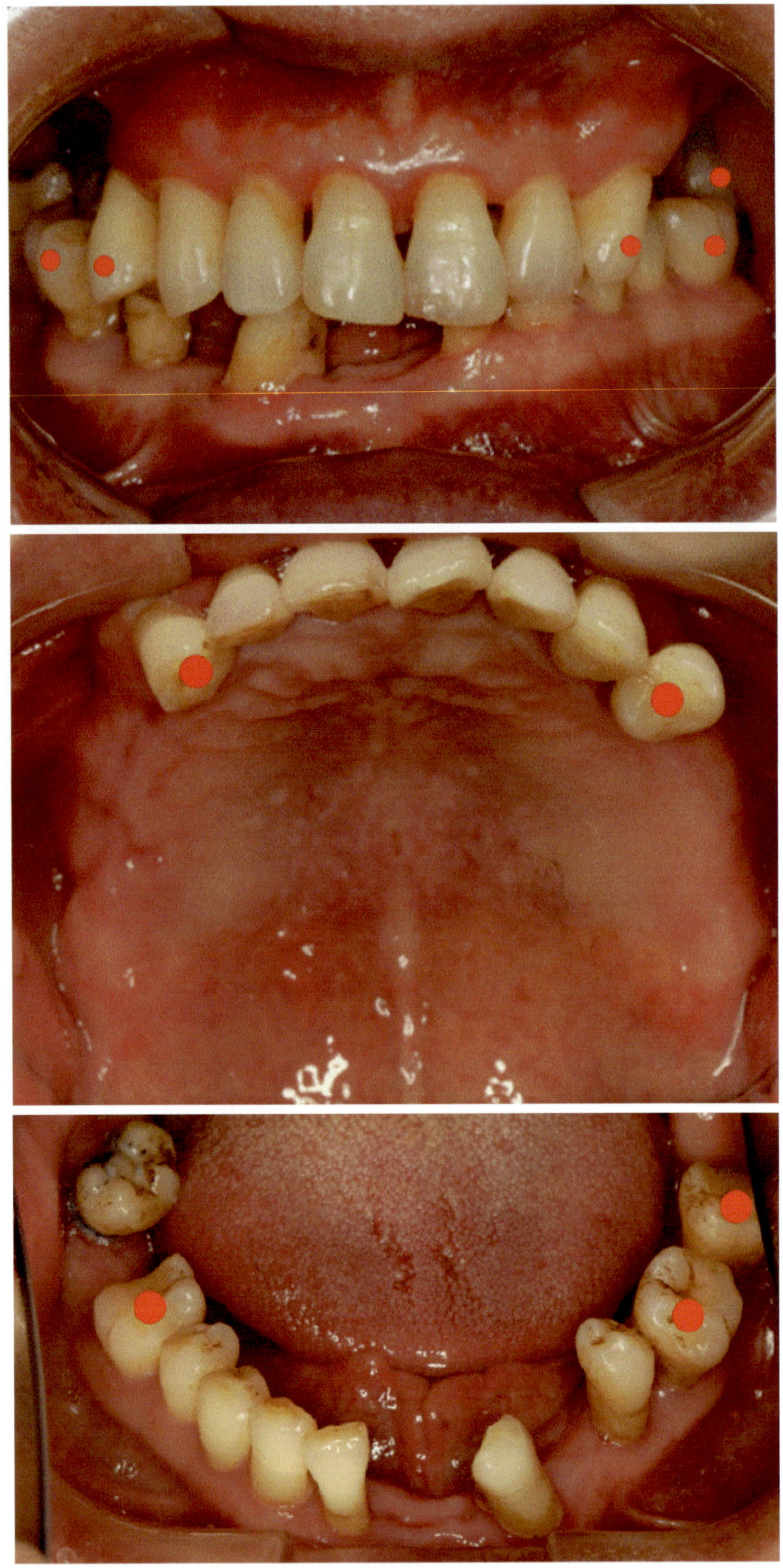

Fig. 6.60 Missing teeth: A5–A7; B4–B7; C1, C2, C4; D1, D7. Due to the severe torsion, clasp cannot be designed on C3. On A4, B3, C6, C7, and D6, e-clasps are designed

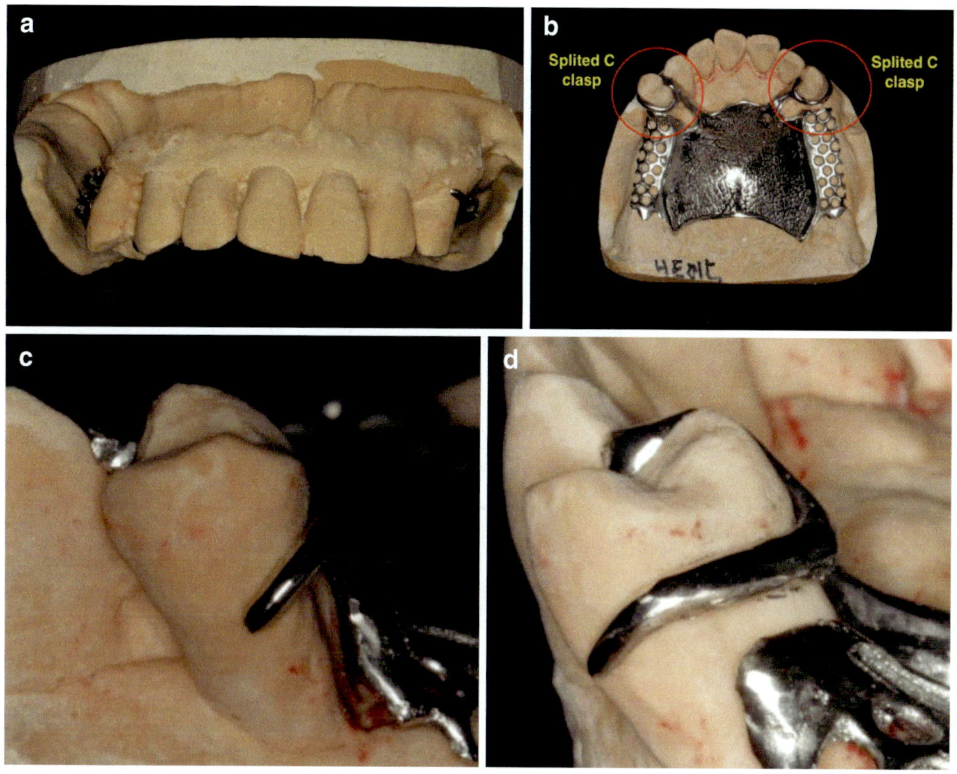

Fig. 6.61 Maxillary framework design. (**a**) The clasps enter cervical undercut, which is good for concealment. (**b**) Two split C clasps are designed on A4 and B3, respectively. (**c**) Buccal view of clasp on A4. (**d**) Proximal view of clasp on A4

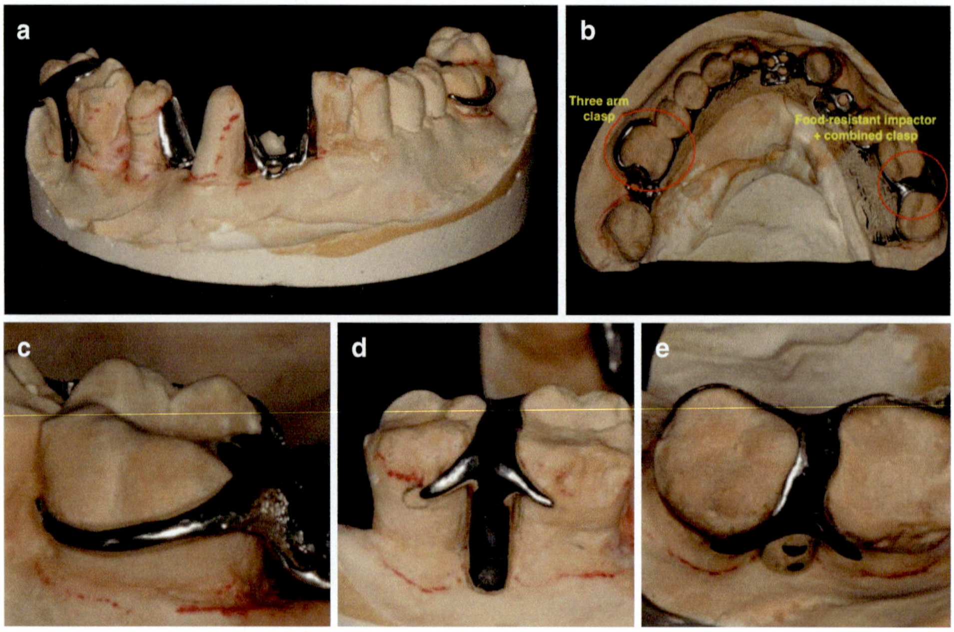

Fig. 6.62 Detail view of mandible framework: combined clasp is designed on C6 and C7. Three-arm clasp is designed on D6. (**a**) Labial view of mandibular framework. (**b**) Occlusal view of mandibular framework. (**c**) Three-arm clasp. (**d**) Food-resistant impactor. (**e**) Combined clasp

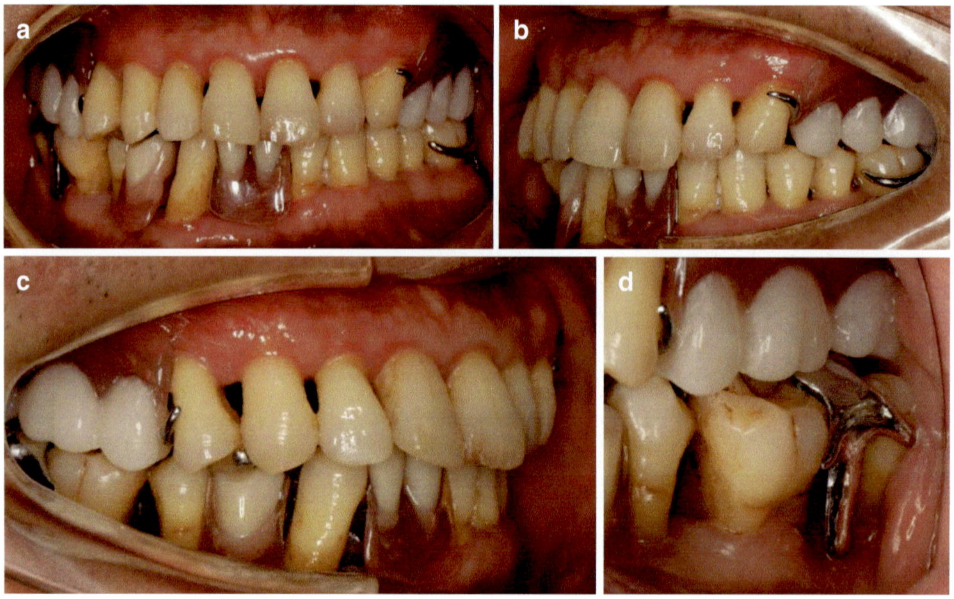

Fig. 6.63 Intraoral view with denture. (**a**) Intraoral frontal view with denture. (**b**) Intraoral left lateral view with denture. (**c**) Intraoral right lateral view with denture. (**d**) Intraoral view of food-resistant impactor

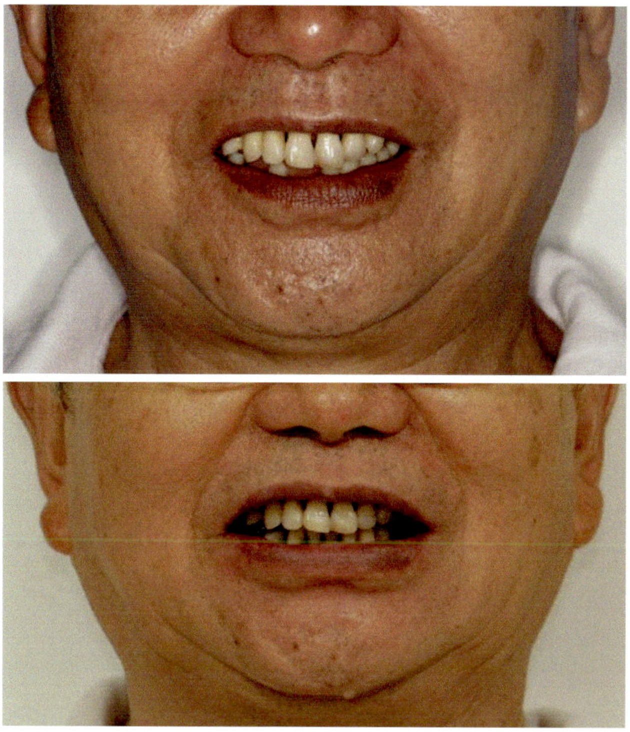

Fig. 6.64 Comparison before and after restoration

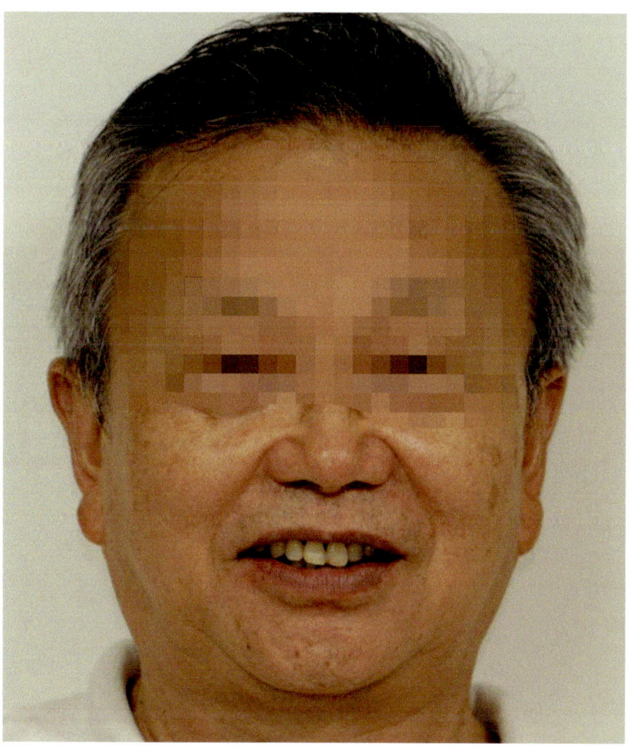

Fig. 6.65 Facial frontal view with denture

6.10 Case 10

C Clasps Combined with Ring Clasp Design for Patient with Unilateral Free-End Edentia

1. *Before restoration*

   A man, 87 years old.

   Smile analysis: The patient has a low smile line with asymmetrical face and average overbite and overjet (Fig. 6.66). The esthetic teeth are A5–B4 and C4–D4 (Fig. 6.67). Missing teeth are maxillary dentition, C5–C6, and D5–D7.

2. *RPD analysis design and manufacturing*

   Maxillary design: Restoration of complete denture.

   Mandibular framework design: For adequate space of lingual side and mouth floor, we design double lingual bar as major connector. Two C clasps are put on C4 and D4, respectively, to protect the remaining abutment, and the buccal side of the clasps enters the distal cervical undercut of the abutments which is good for concealment (Fig. 6.68). C8 has an obvious mesial incline, and a ring clasp is designed on it (Fig. 6.69).

3. *After restoration*

   The final effect is shown in Figs. 6.70 and 6.71. The patient is satisfied.

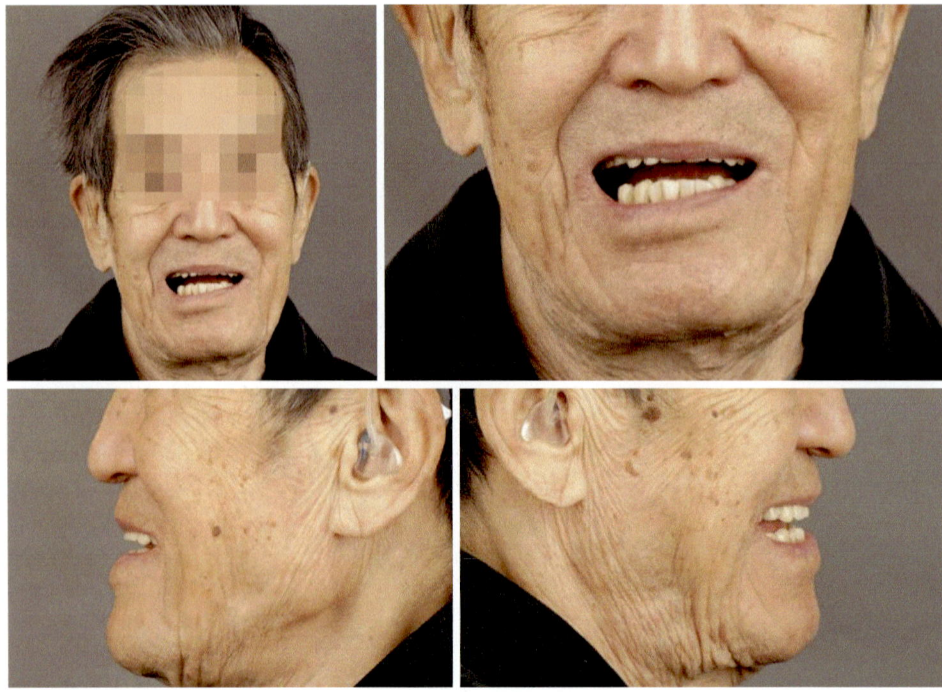

Fig. 6.66 Facial analysis

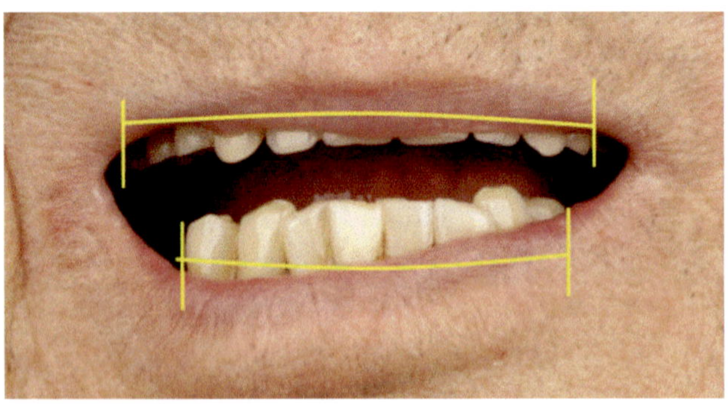

Fig. 6.67 Esthetic teeth: A5–B4, C4–D4

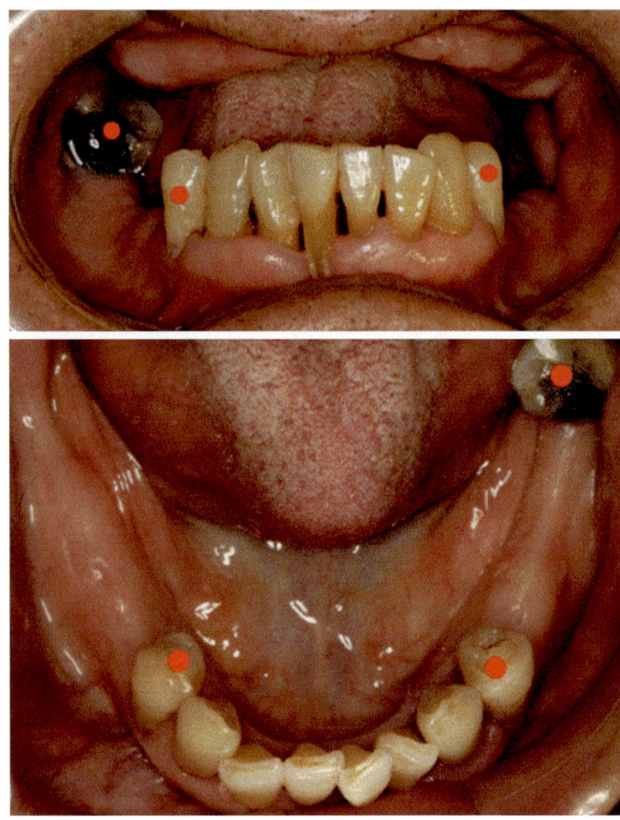

Fig. 6.68 Dentition analysis: design e-clasps on C4, C8, and sD4

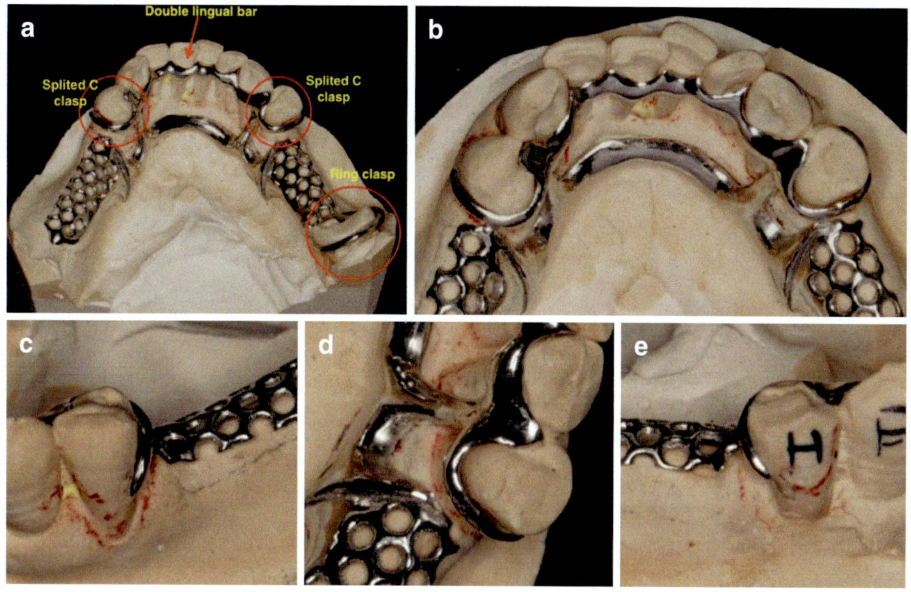

Fig. 6.69 Mandibular framework design: design double lingual bar, put C clasps on C4 and D4, and put a ring clasp on C8, which has an obvious mesial incline. (**a**) Occlusal view of mandibular framework. (**b**) Double lingual bar and clasps fit on the model in the lingual view. (**c**) Splited C clasp on D4. (**d**) Occlusal view of splited C clasp on C4. (**e**) Buccal view of splited C clasp on C4

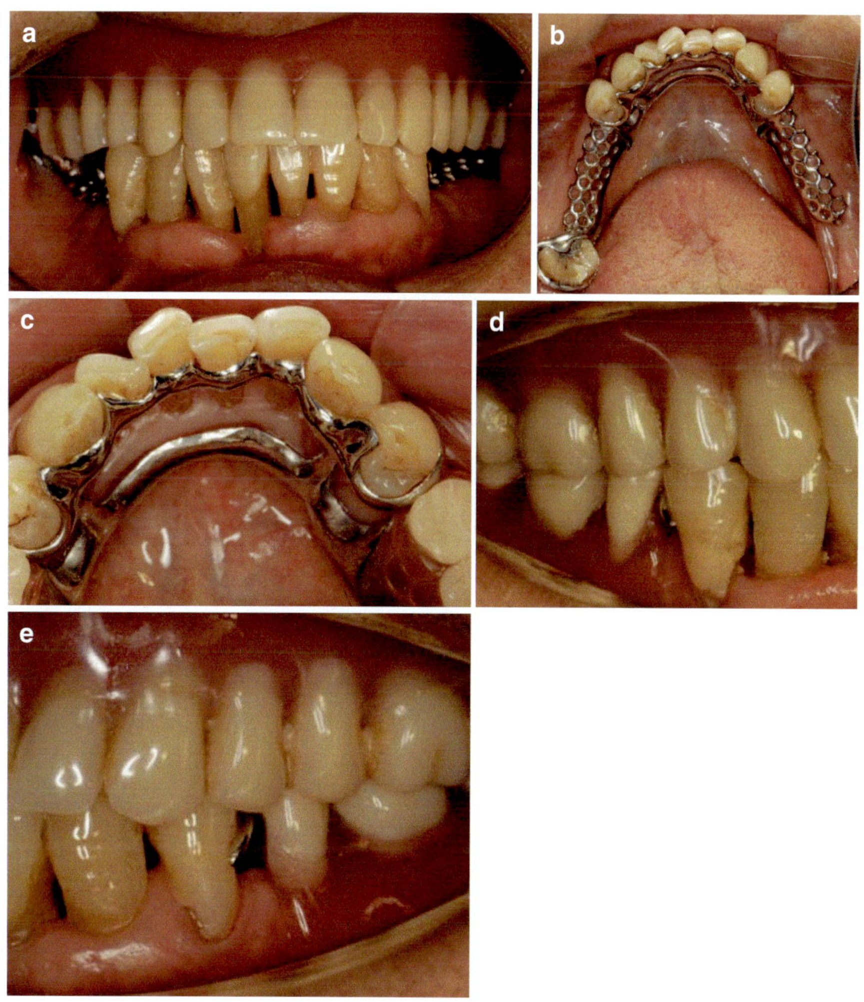

Fig. 6.70 Intraoral view with denture. (**a**) Frontal view. (**b**) Occlusal view. (**c**) Double lingual bar and clasps fit in the lingual view. (**d**) Right lateral view. (**e**) Left lateral view

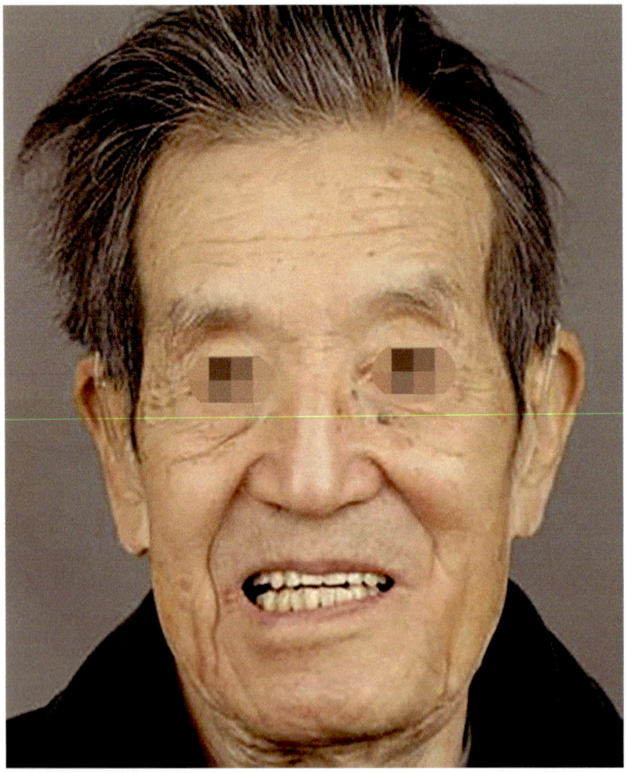

Fig. 6.71 Facial frontal view

6.11 Case 11

Modified Extension Clasps Design for Patient with Unilateral Free-End Edentia on Mandibular

1. *Before restoration*

   A man, 58 years old

   Smile analysis: The patient has a middle smile line with average overbite and overjet (Fig. 6.72). Esthetic teeth are A4–B4 and C5–D5 (Fig. 6.73).

   Dentition analysis: The patient has Kennedy II dentition defect in the lower jaw. Missing teeth are 1, 2, 6, and 7 in C area; 1, 2, and 5–7 in D area; and 3 and 4 in D area. Due to the small gap in the anterior mandible, only three anterior teeth are restored. As a result, e-clasps are designed on C4, C6, D3, and D4 (Fig. 6.74).

2. *RPD analysis design and manufacturing*

   Framework design: An extension clasp is designed on D3 and D4 to protect the abutments in D area which are II° loose and extend the remaining time of the abutment. A C clasp is designed on C4, and a three-arm clasp is designed on C6. (Fig. 6.75)

3. *After restoration*

   The final repair effect is shown in Figs. 6.76 and 6.77. The patient is satisfied.

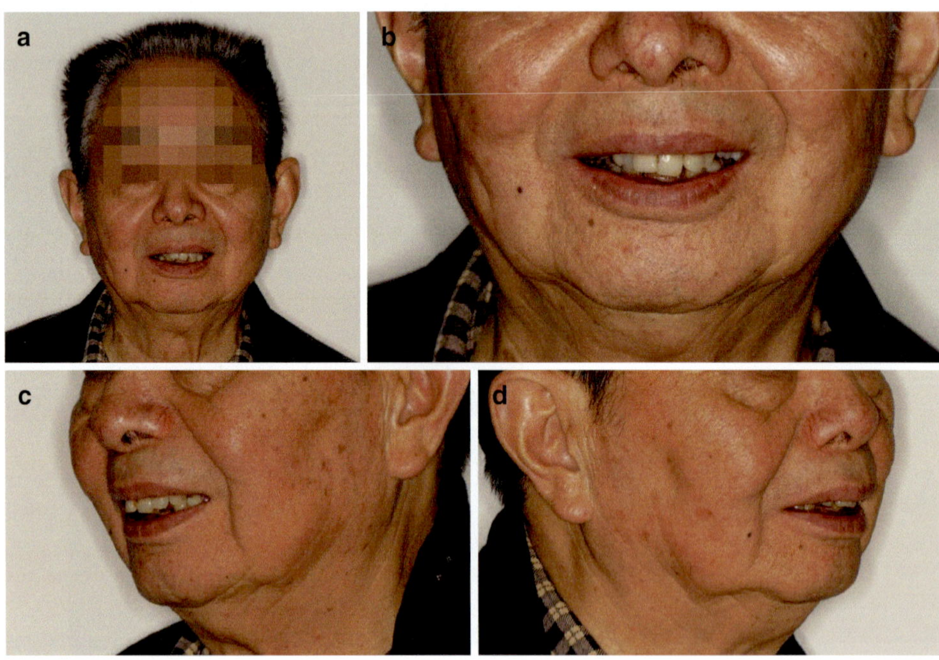

Fig. 6.72 Facial analysis. (**a**) Facial frontal view. (**b**) Lower facial 1/3 frontal view. (**c**) Lower facial 1/3 left lateral view in 45°. (**d**) Lower facial 1/3 right lateral view in 45°

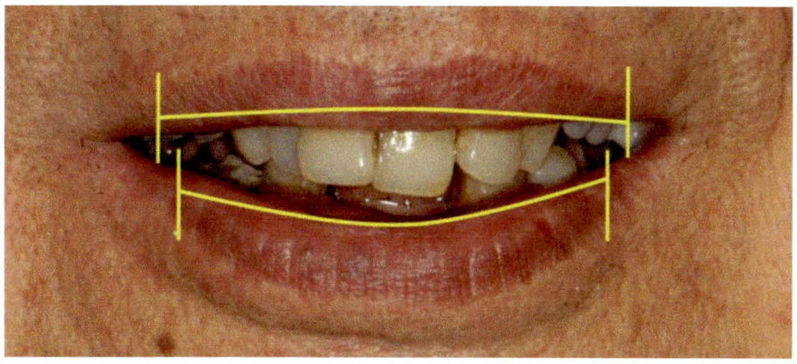

Fig. 6.73 Esthetic teeth: A4–B4, C5–D5

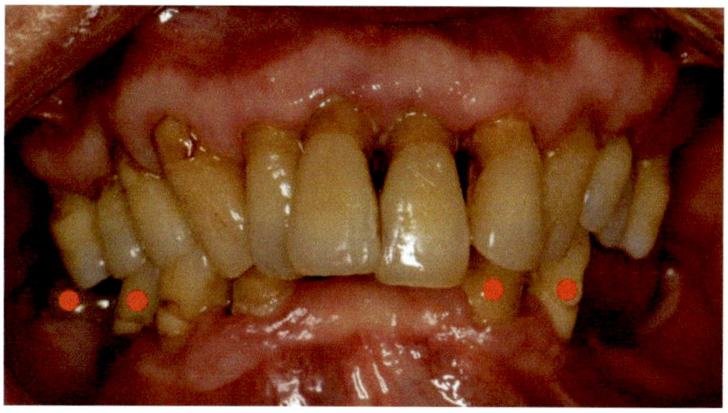

Fig. 6.74 Dentition analysis: e-clasps are put on C4, C6, D3, and D4

Fig. 6.75 Mandibular framework design

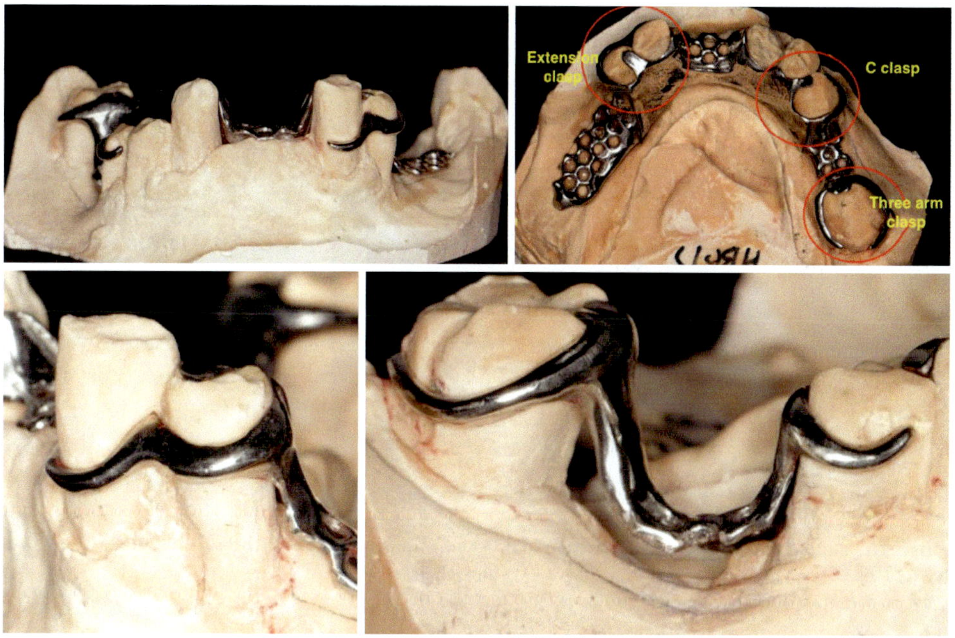

Through the analysis design, manufacturing, and clinical application of the abovementioned cases, we find it not difficult to apply e-clasps, and the patient's esthetic effect is also significantly improved. In clinical application, we should take attention that the oral health consciousness of patients in China is generally poor and the necessary preparations such as scaling and pulling residual roots and loose teeth before restoration are also difficult to achieve. Some patients first time to run prosthetics even think it is the accepted simplest requirement that "Can eat with prosthesis." Moreover, they think their requirement of chief complaint is very low and make little of the difficulty of dental prosthetists. Therefore, around the long-term, stable, and effective goals of clinical treatment, we must strengthen the doctor-patient communication, actively participate in design, and think it over clinically. Only in this way we can know their shortcomings, take full use of their strengths, and finally obtain the clinical effect patients satisfy with. Furthermore, there are also many secondary repair patients who replace dentures are very satisfied with the esthetic clasps, which proves the importance of fine design in another way.

In the aforementioned cases, all the e-clasp frameworks are manufactured with traditional casting techniques. With the rapid popularization and application of various digital technologies in dentistry, 3D printing technology has become the latest technology for denture framework fabrication. It combines traditional prosthetic manufacturing technology with computer-aided design and computer-aided manufacturing (CAD-CAM) technologies, taking incremental manufacturing as its core feature. So it can use 3D printing to realize the wax mold fabrication of denture framework, which can reduce the labor cost and digital equipment investment of traditional

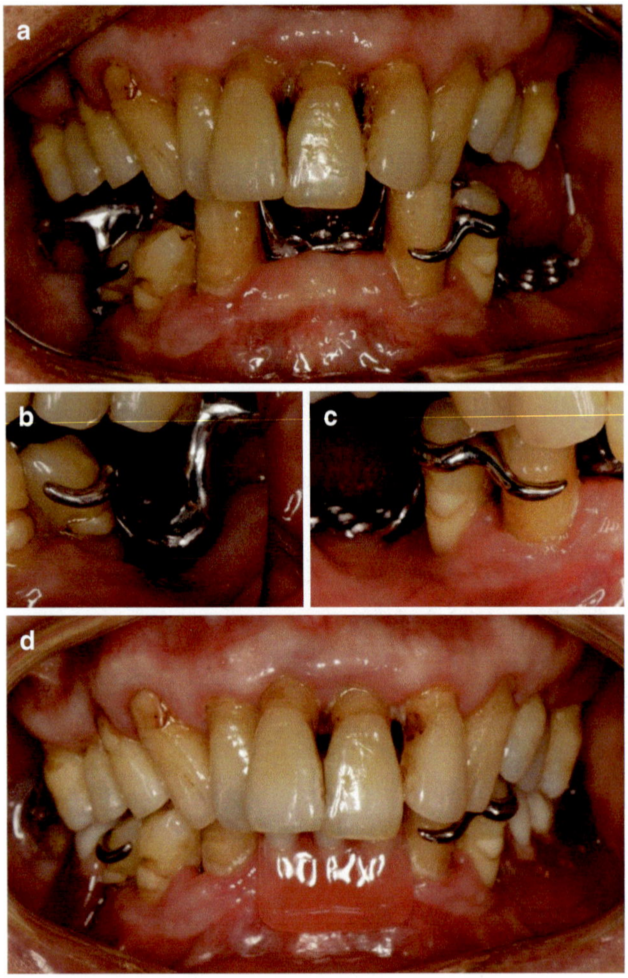

Fig. 6.76 Intraoral view with denture. (**a**) Frontal view of framework try-in. (**b**) C Clasp on C4. (**c**) Extension clasp on D3 and D4. (**d**) Frontal view of denture

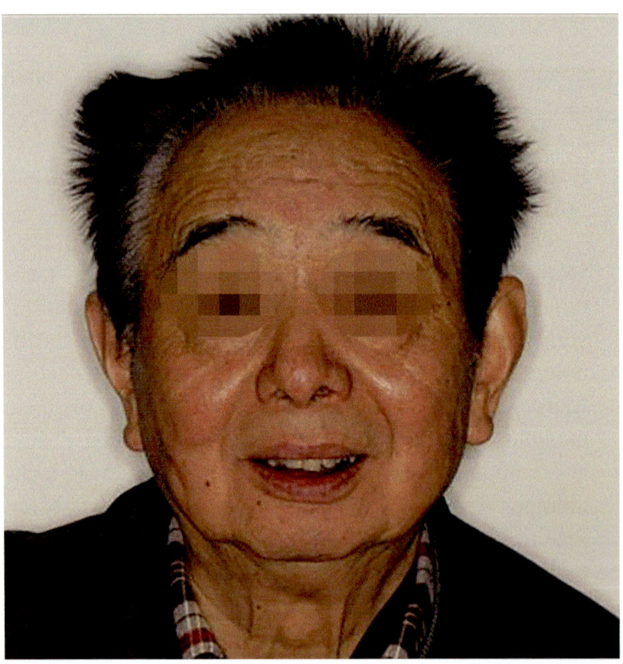

Fig. 6.77 Facial frontal view with denture

wax making, etc. and then use the traditional dental casting technology to complete the framework fabrication. Moreover, it can also directly print metal framework by direct selective laser melting (SLM) technology, etc. Through framework design in the CAD software and 3D printing, finally a high-density, highly precise, and highly personalized prosthesis is finished.

Digital technology also can make up for insufficient information in work authorization form on processing. As an effective tool for information exchange, digital technology is conducive to communication among dentist, technician, and patient, determination of the treatment plan, as well as fabrication of the prosthesis.

In the following cases, we are going to complete the design and printing processes of e-clasp frameworks with digital technology.

6.12 Case 12

Plate Clasp on Isolated Abutment in Digital Framework RPD Design for Patient with Unilateral Free-End Edentia

1. *Before restoration*

   A woman, 78 years old.

   Smile analysis: The patient has a low smile line. When smiling, the lower anterior teeth are exposed, and the lower lip covers the cervix of the lower anterior teeth. At the same time, we can see the patient has the mandibular defection of anterior teeth and maxillary edentia. What's more, she shows collapsed upper lip, deep nasolabial groove, as well as upward corner of the mouth in the frontal view (Fig. 6.78).

   Dentition analysis: The upper jaw is edentulous, while the lower jaw has the Kennedy II dentition defect, and the gap of missing C7 is not repaired. Missing teeth are C5, D1–D3, and D5–D7. Besides, D4 is II°loose. So e-clasps are designed on C4, C6, and D4. C6 inclinate mesially, in which undercut is in the mesiolingual; the remaining abutments have moderate undercut (Fig. 6.79).
2. *RPD analysis design and manufacturing*

   Mandibular framework design: A C clasp is designed on C4, and a ring clasp is designed on C6, whose tip enters the mesiolingual undercut and then a mesio-occlusal rest recovers the occlusal height. A plate clasp is put on D4 to protect II°loose abutment (Fig. 6.80).
3. *After restoration*

   The final repair effect is shown in Figs. 6.81, 6.82, and 6.83.

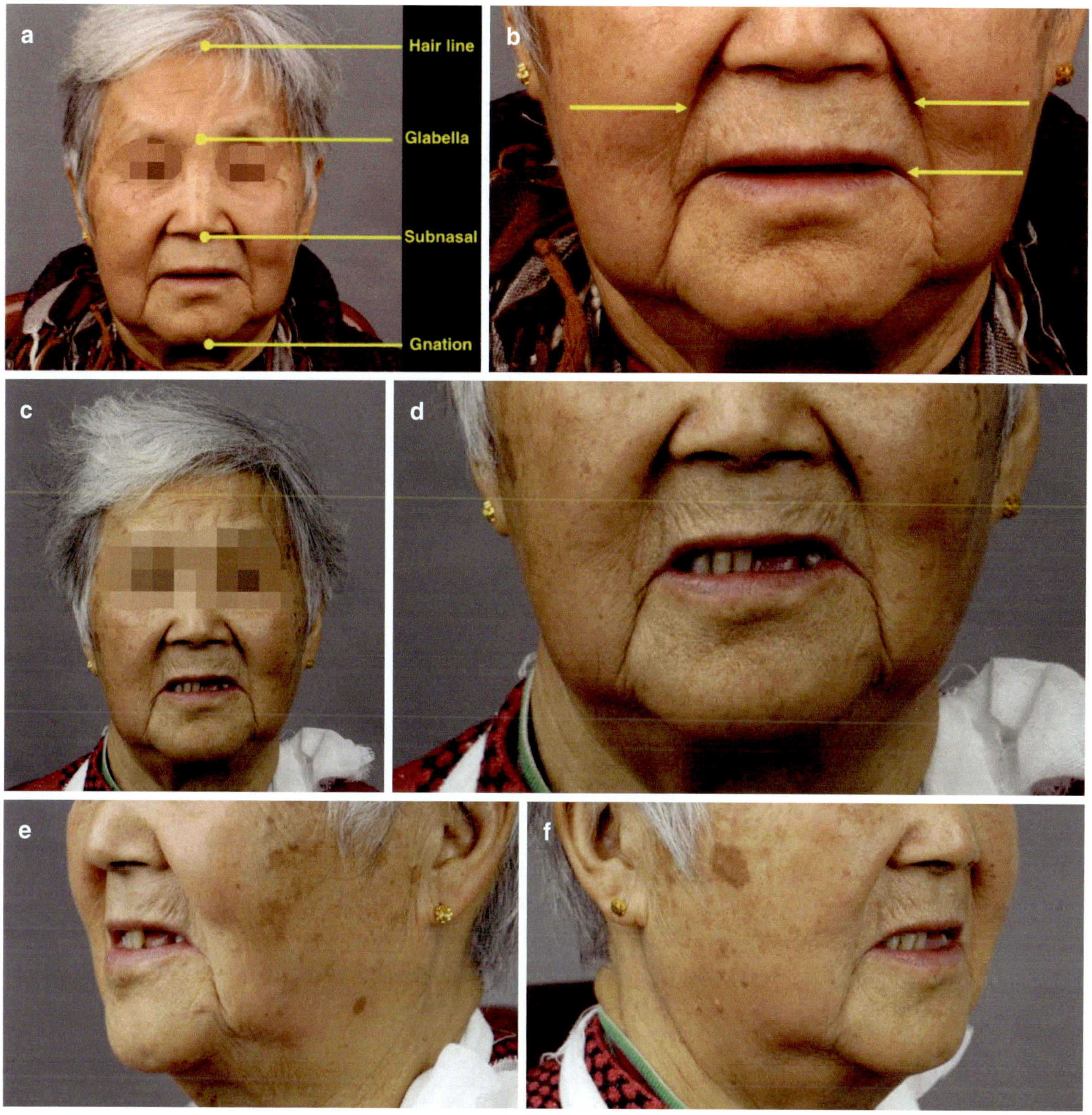

Fig. 6.78 Facial analysis. (**a**) Facial frontal view. (**b**) Lower facial 1/3 frontal view. (**c**) Facial frontal view when smiling. (**d**) Lower facial 1/3 frontal view when smiling. (**e**) Lower facial 1/3 left lateral view in 45°. (**f**) Lower facial 1/3 right lateral view in 45°

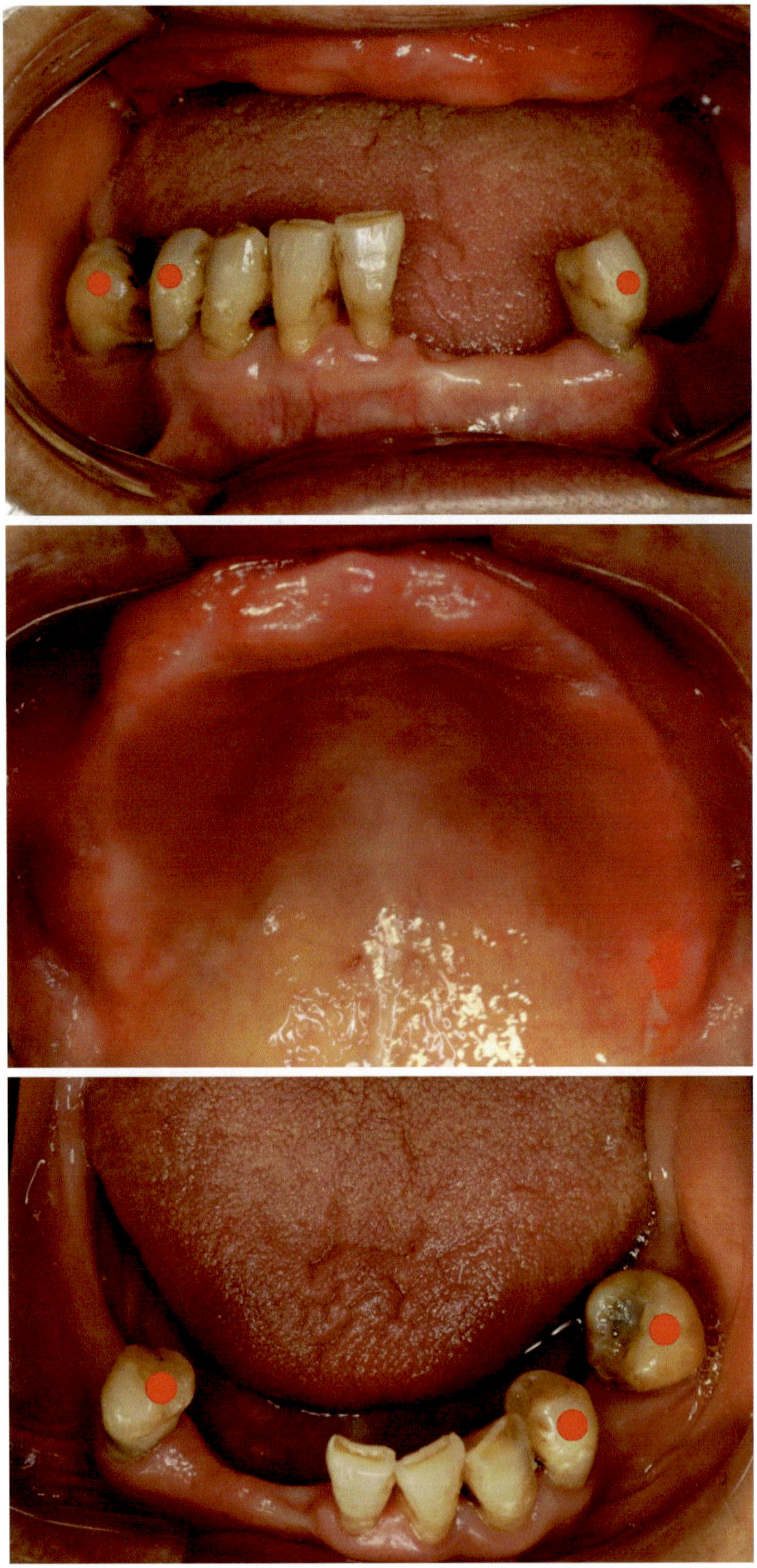

Fig. 6.79 Dentition analysis: e-clasps are designed on C4, C6, and D4

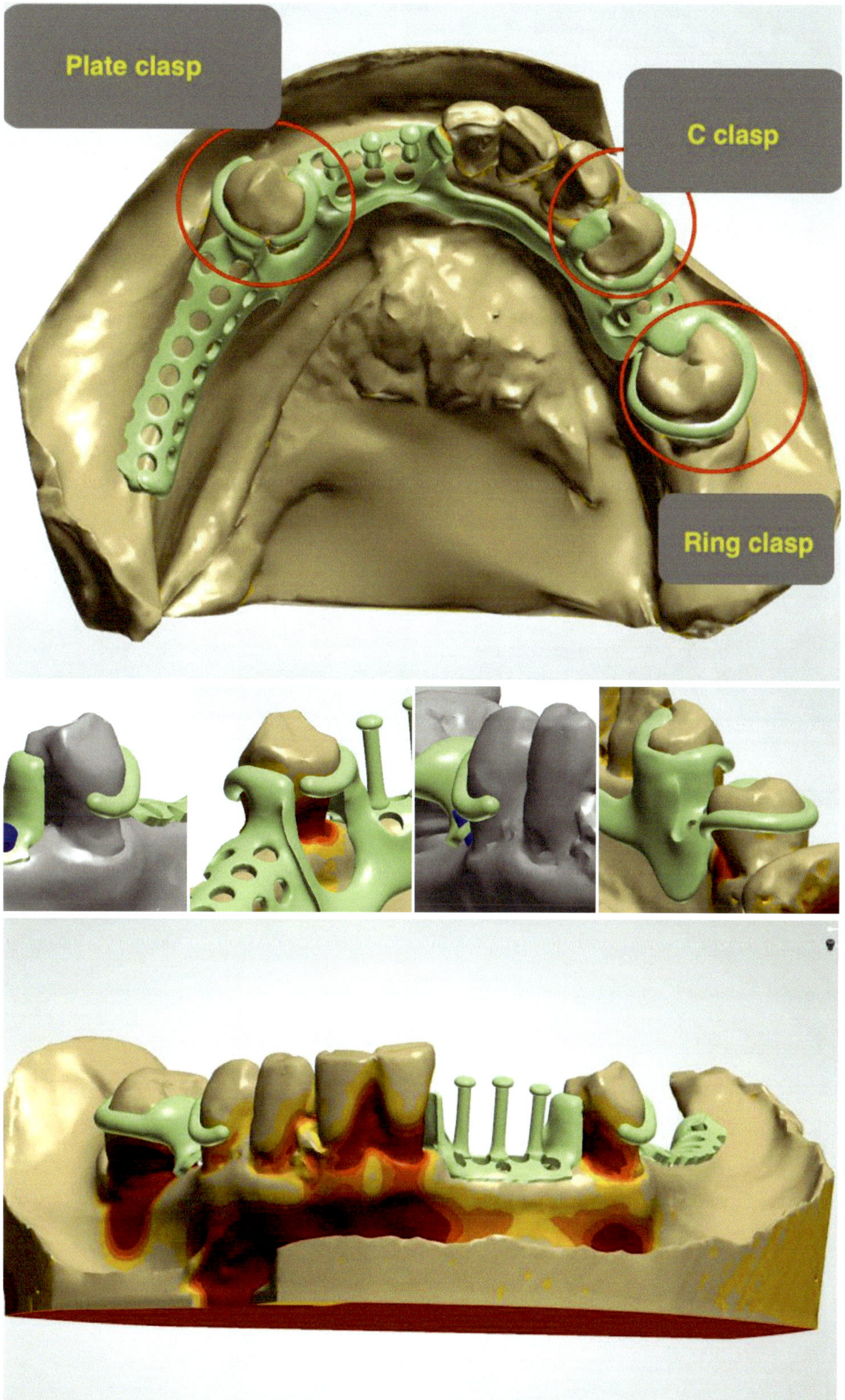

Fig. 6.80 Mandibular framework design

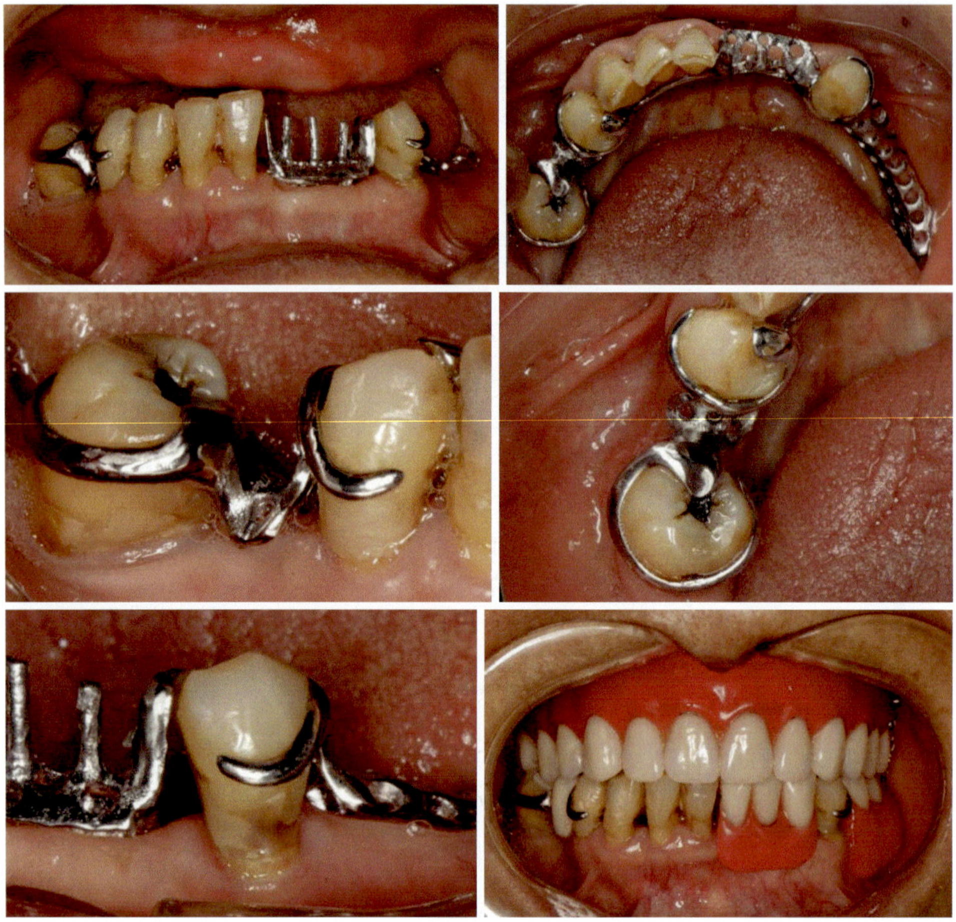

Fig. 6.80 (continued)

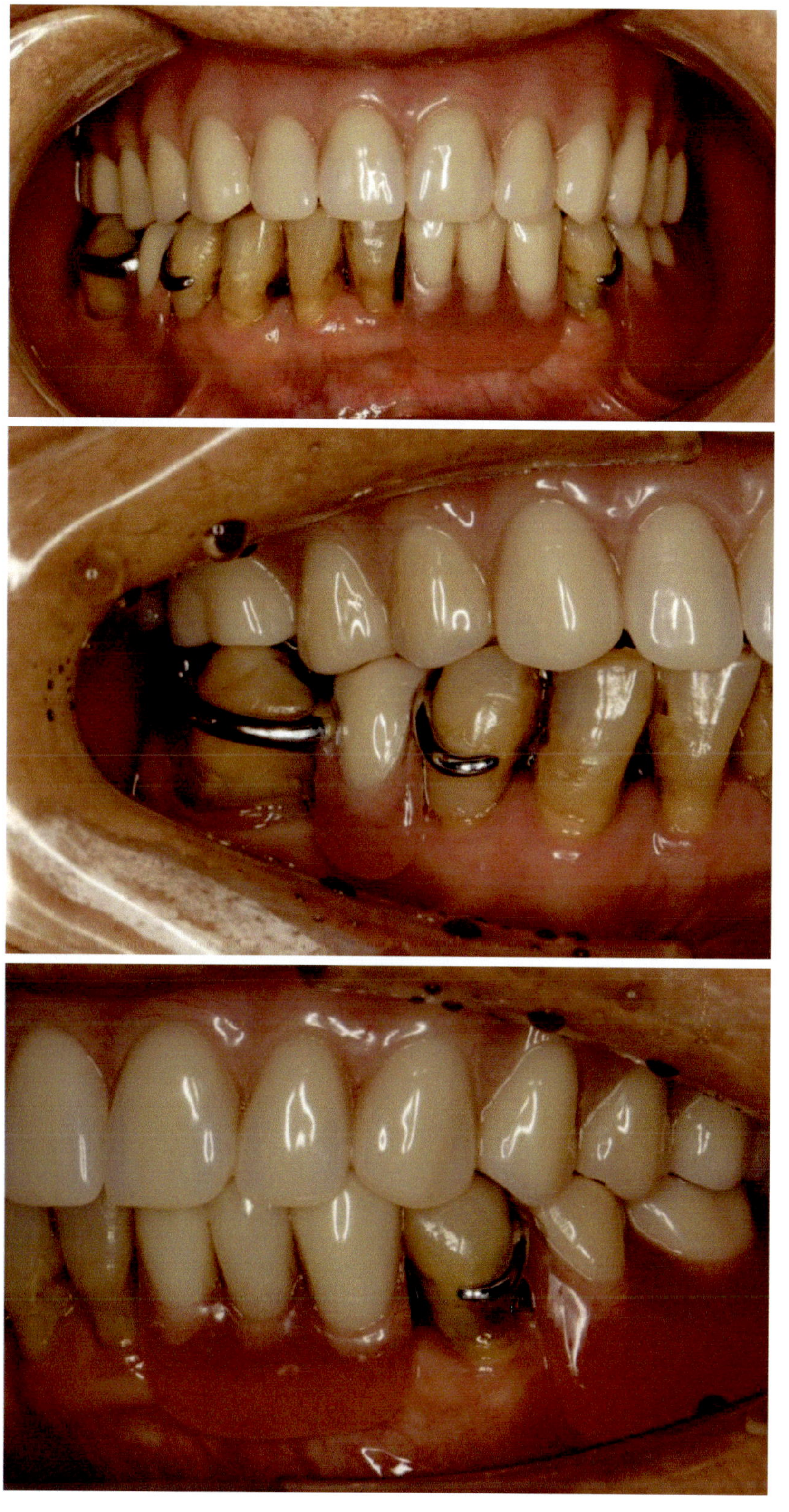

Fig. 6.81 Intraoral view with denture

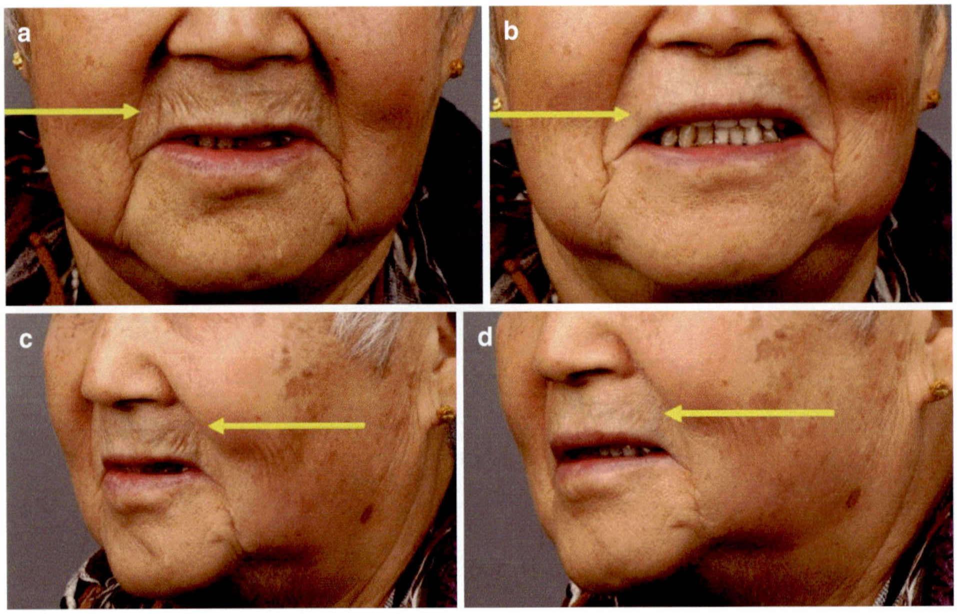

Fig. 6.82 Comparison before and after restoration. (**a**) Lower facial 1/3 frontal view before restoration. (**b**) Lower facial 1/3 frontal view after restoration. (**c**) Lower facial 1/3 lateral view before restoration. (**d**) Lower facial 1/3 lateral view after restoration

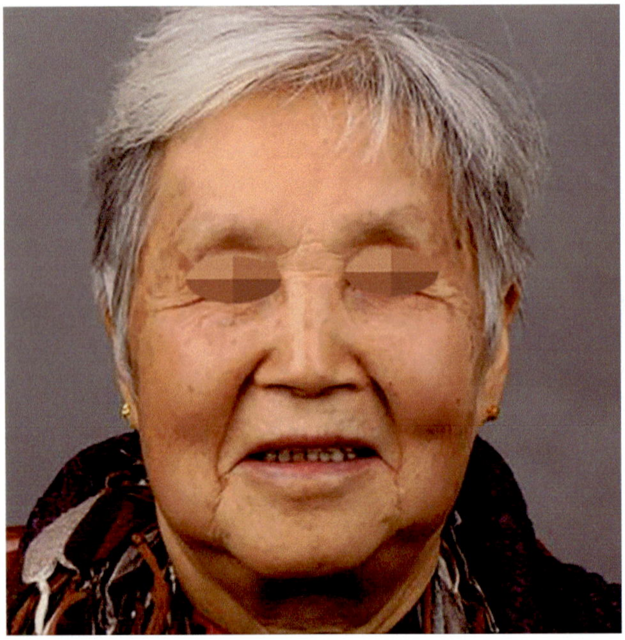

Fig. 6.83 Facial frontal view with denture

6.13 Case 13

Buccally Short-Arm Clasp Combined with C Clasp in Digital Framework RPD Design for the Patient with Non-free-End Deletion

1. *Before restoration*

   A woman, 76 years old.

   Face analysis: The nasolabial groove is deep and the corner of the mouth is upward.

   Smile analysis: The patient has a middle smile line as well as deep overbite (Fig. 6.84), and the esthetic teeth are A4–B4 (Fig. 6.85).

   Dentition analysis: The cervical gingivae of the entire mouth recede and the roots are exposed. Furthermore, the overbite and overjet of anterior teeth are deep. C6, D6, and D7 in the mandibular are dental implants. Missing teeth are A4, A5, B6, and B7. Besides, A6 is I°loose, and the remaining teeth all have appropriate undercuts (Fig. 6.86). We put e-clasps on A3, A6, B5, and B8 (Fig. 6.87).

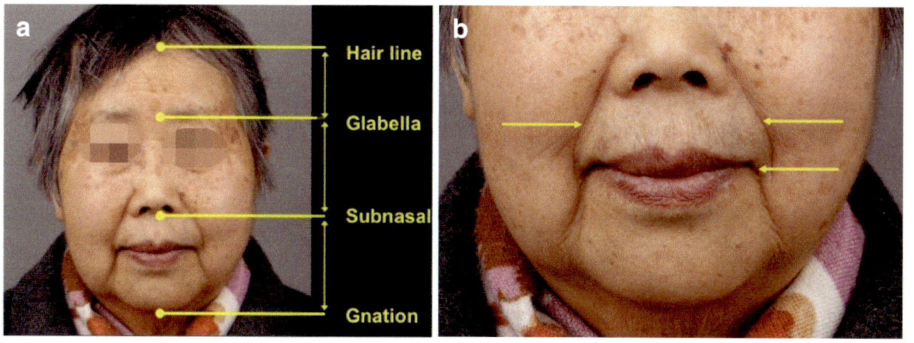

Fig. 6.84 Facial analysis. (**a**) Facial frontal view. (**b**) Lower facial 1/3 frontal view

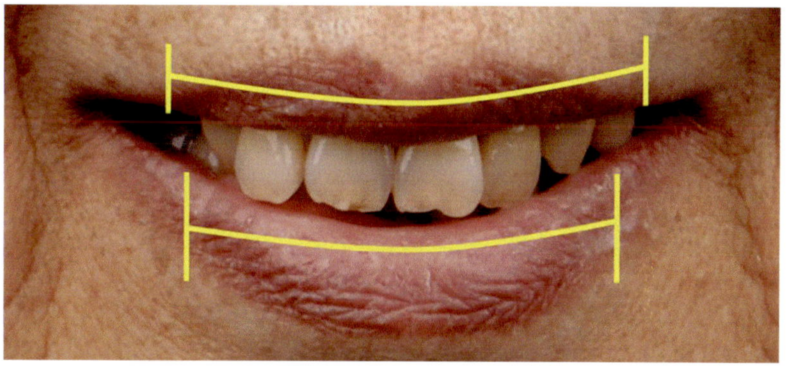

Fig. 6.85 Esthetic teeth are A4–B4

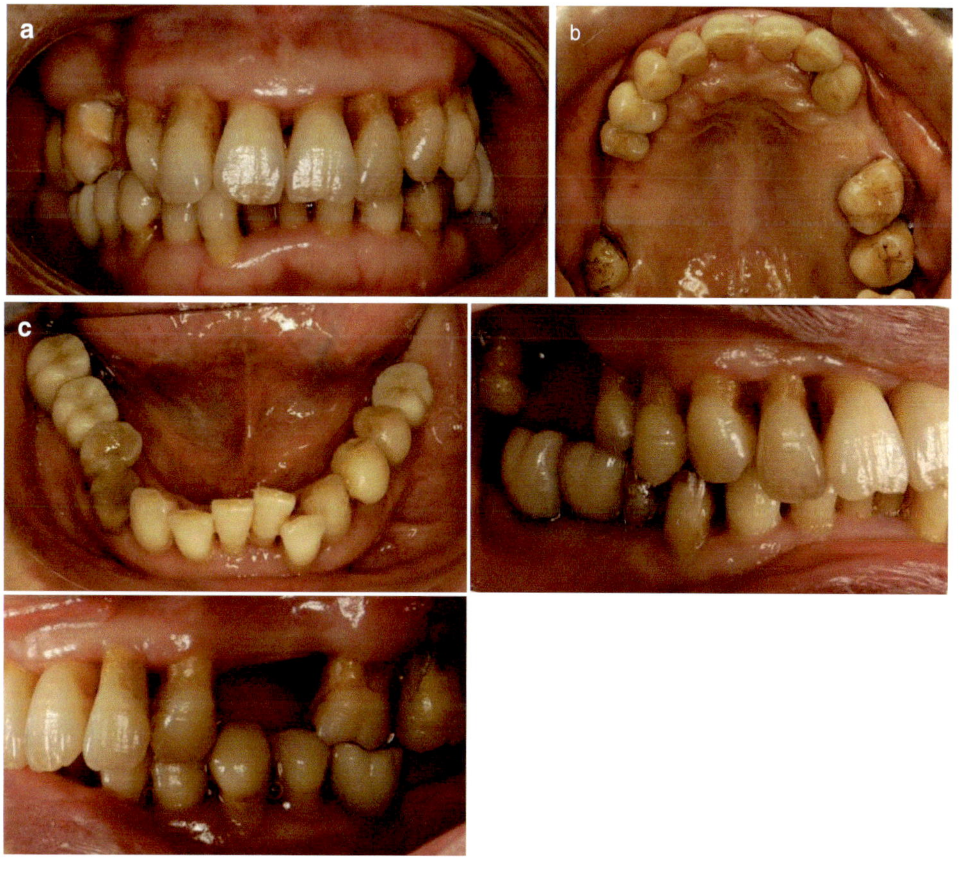

Fig. 6.86 Intraoral analysis. (**a**) Deep overbite and overjet of anterior teeth. (**b**) Missing teeth: A4, A5, B6, B7. (**c**) C6, D6 and D7 in mandibular are dental implants

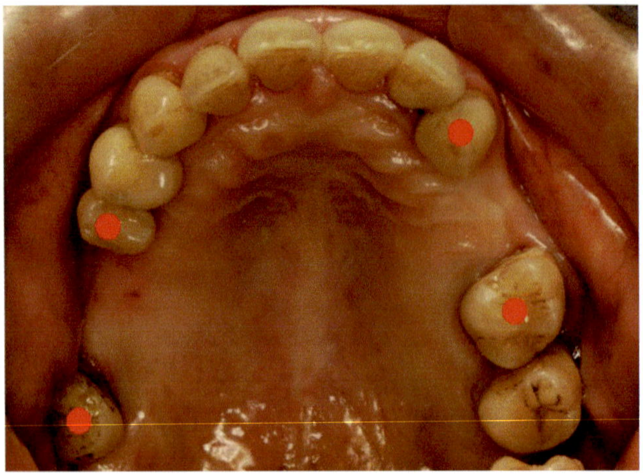

Fig. 6.87 Putting e-clasps on A3, A6, B5, and B8

2. *RPD analysis design and manufacturing*

   Framework design: A short buccally retained clasp and a lingual rest are placed on A3, three-arm clasps are put on A6 and B8, and a C clasp is designed on B5. We consider two designs of the major connector in the palate: posterior palatal bar or U palate plate (Figs. 6.88 and 6.89). Combined with the patient's oral condition and comfort, we choose the posterior palatal bar (Fig. 6.90). Trying in of the framework is shown in Fig. 6.91.

3. *After restoration*

   The final restoration is shown in Figs. 6.92, 6.93, and 6.94. The patient is contented.

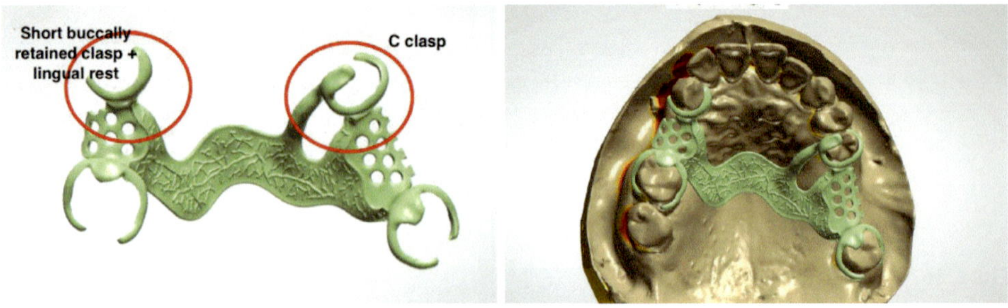

Fig. 6.88 Design one: posterior palatal bar

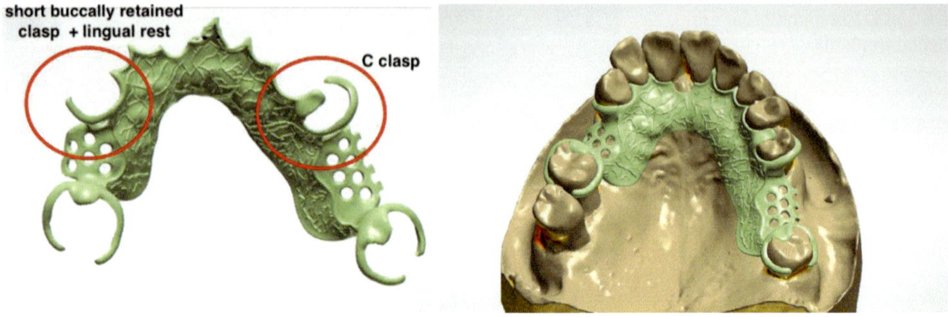

Fig. 6.89 Design two: U palate plate

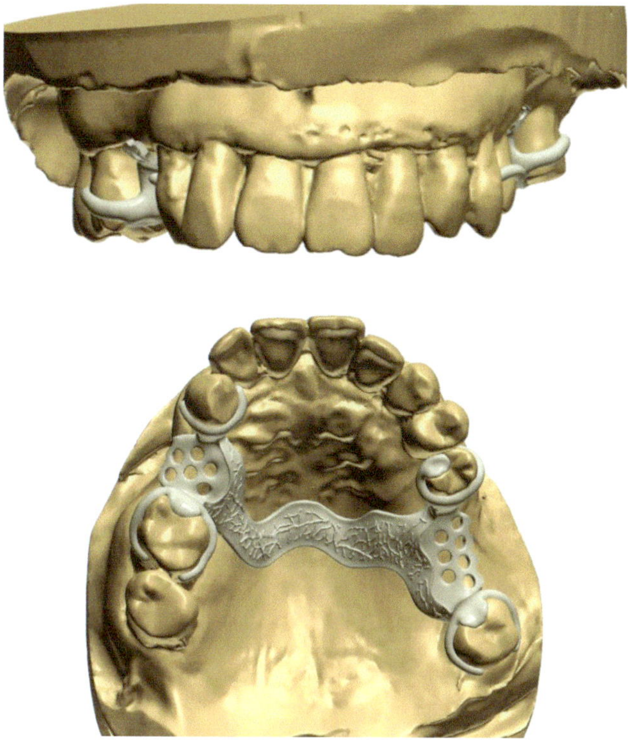

Fig. 6.90 Maxillary framework design

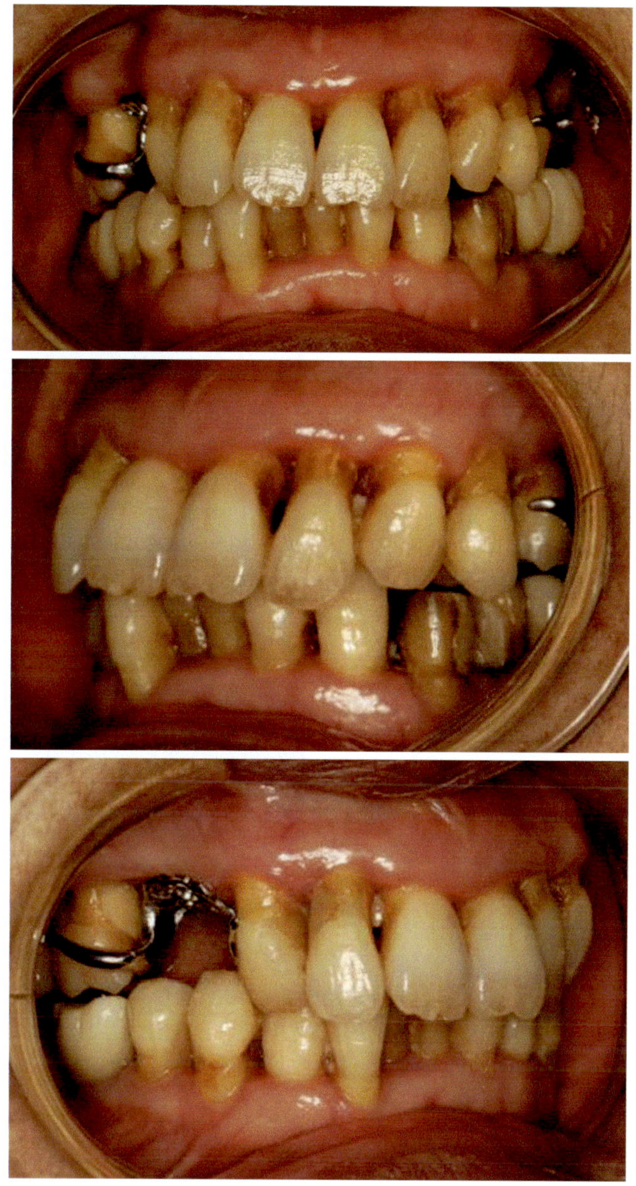

Fig. 6.91 Trying in of the framework

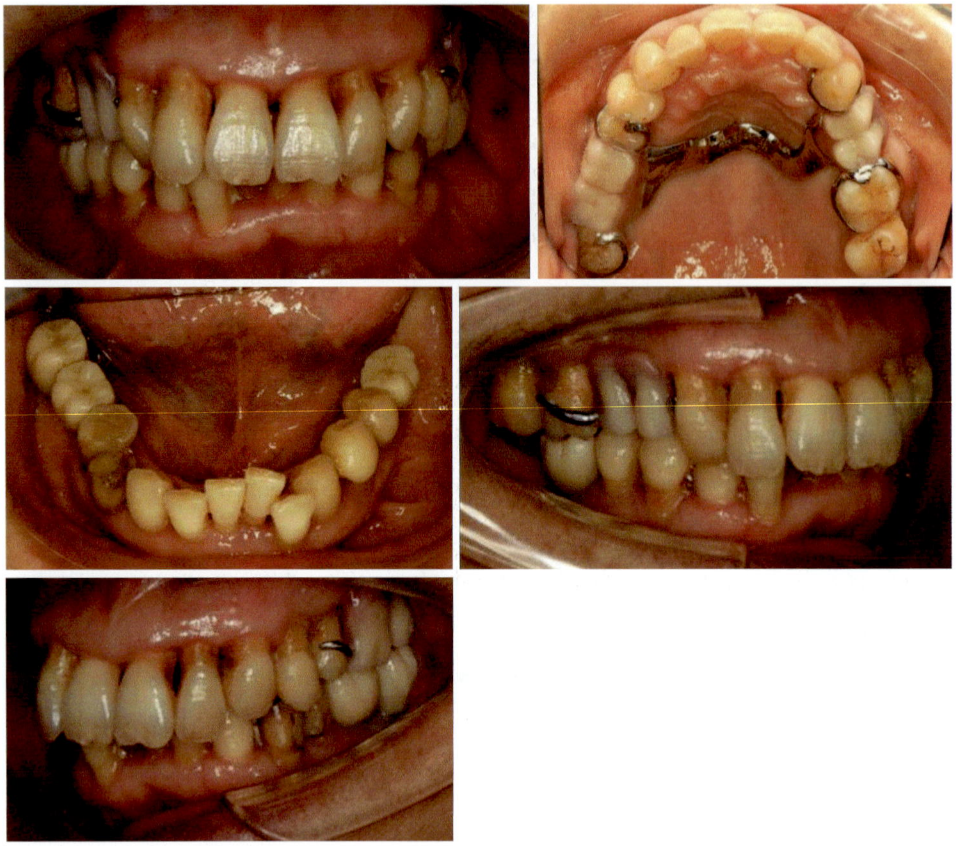

Fig. 6.92 Intraoral view with denture

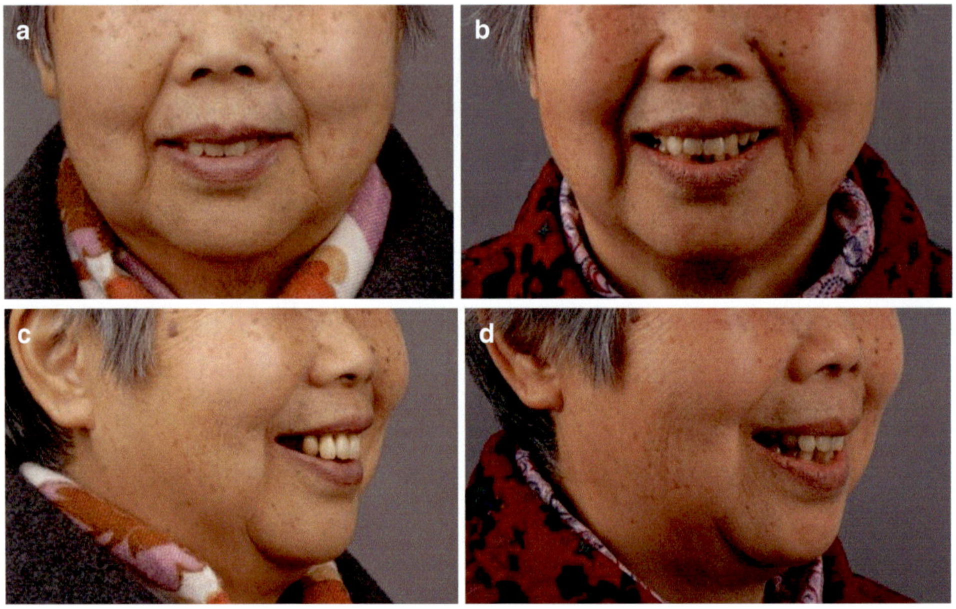

Fig. 6.93 Comparison before and after restoration. (**a**) Lower facial 1/3 frontal view before restoration. (**b**) Lower facial 1/3 frontal view after restoration. (**c**) Lower facial 1/3 lateral view before restoration. (**d**) Lower facial 1/3 lateral view after restoration

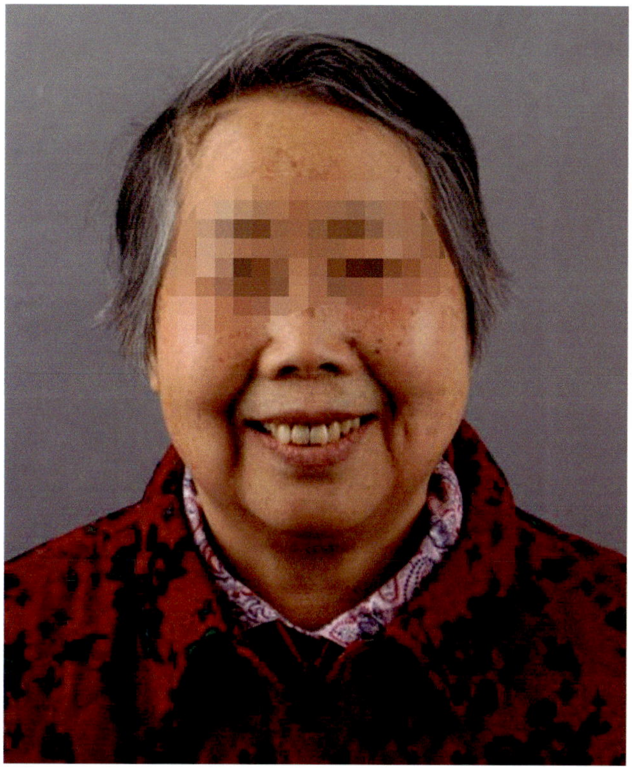

Fig. 6.94 Facial frontal view with denture

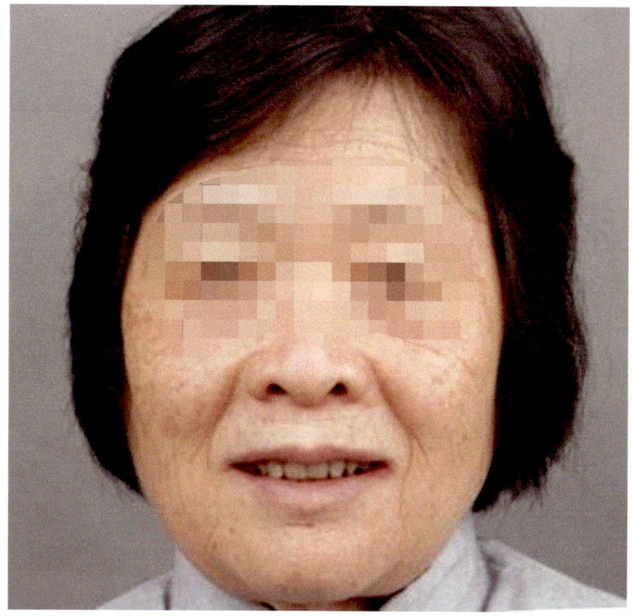

Fig. 6.95 Facial frontal view when smiling

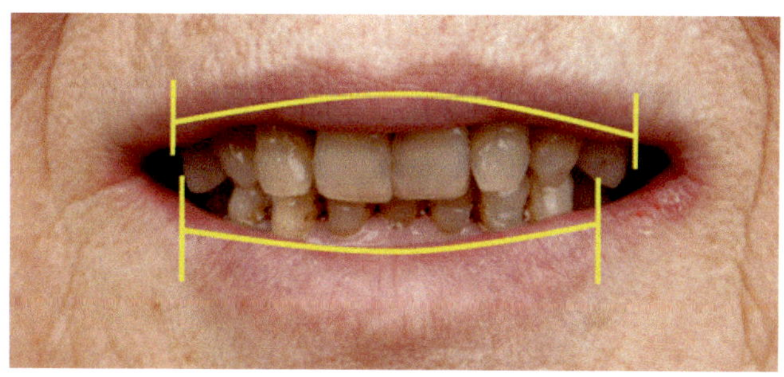

Fig. 6.96 Esthetic teeth: A4–B4, C3–D4

6.14 Case 14

Double Lingual Bar in Digital Framework RPD Design for Patient with Unilateral Free-End Edentia in the Lower Jaw

1. *Before restoration*

   A woman, 49 years old.

   Smile analysis: The patient has a middle smile line and deep overbite (Fig. 6.95). The esthetic teeth are A4–B4 and C3–D4 (Fig. 6.96).

   Dentition analysis: Missing teeth on maxilla are A5–A7. Due to the tight occlusion, there is no space for repair (Fig. 6.97). Missing teeth on mandible are D5–D7 in D area. And the anterior overbite and overjet are deep (Fig. 6.98). The patient finally chose e-clasp RPD for restoration, and we design e-clasps on D4, C6, and C7.
2. *RPD analysis design and manufacturing*

   Mandibular framework design: Opposite embrasure clasps are designed on C6 and C7, respectively, and a C clasp is designed on D4. The double lingual bar is designed on the lingual side of the anterior teeth, which is conducive to the self-cleaning of the patient's mouth (Fig. 6.99). Trying in of the framework is shown in Fig. 6.100.
3. *After restoration*

   The final effect is shown in Figs. 6.101 and 6.102.

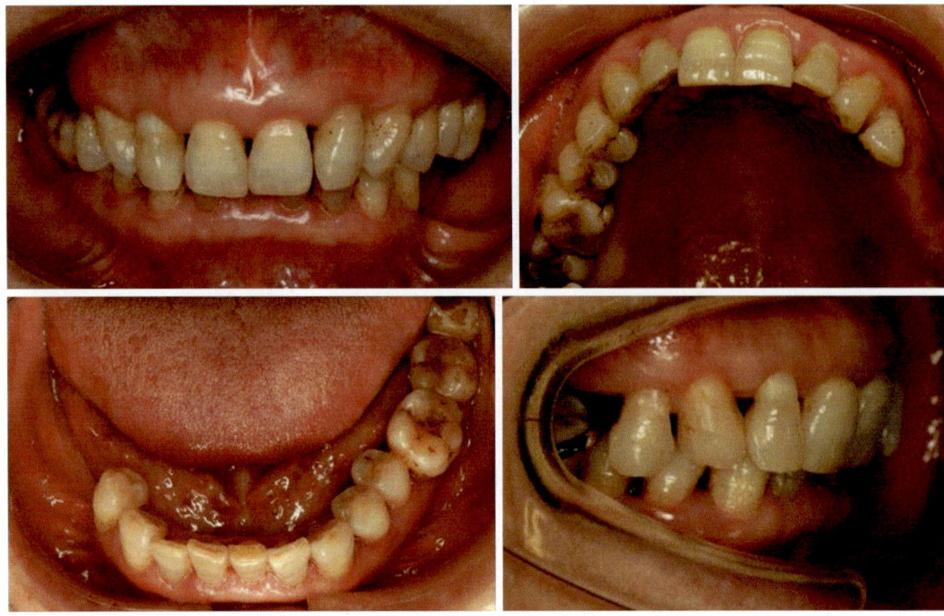

Fig. 6.97 Missing teeth on maxilla are A5–A7, and due to the tight occlusion, there was no space for repair

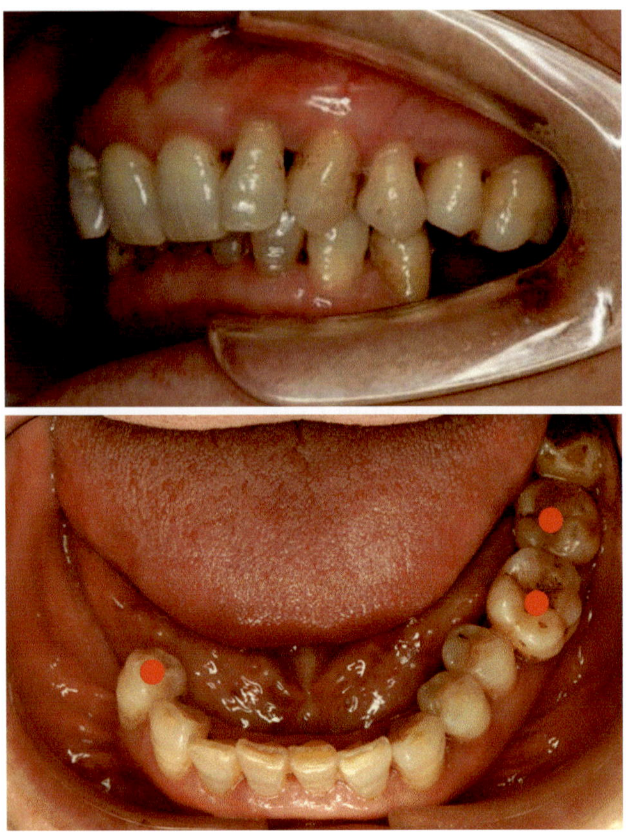

Fig. 6.98 Missing teeth on mandible are D5–D7. We design e-clasps on D4, C6, and C7

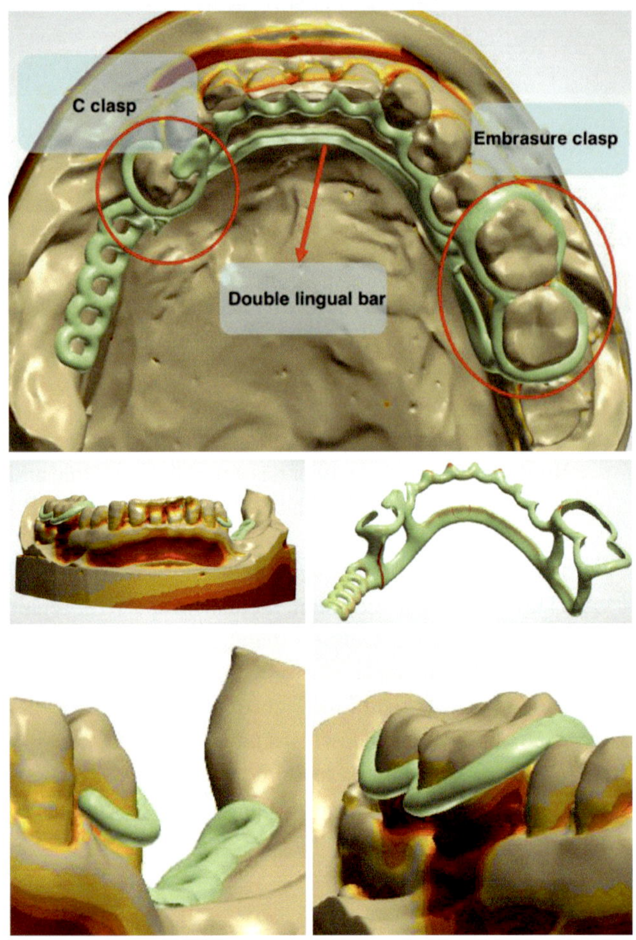

Fig. 6.99 Mandibular framework design: opposite embrasure clasps are designed on C6 and C7, respectively, and a C clasp is designed on D4

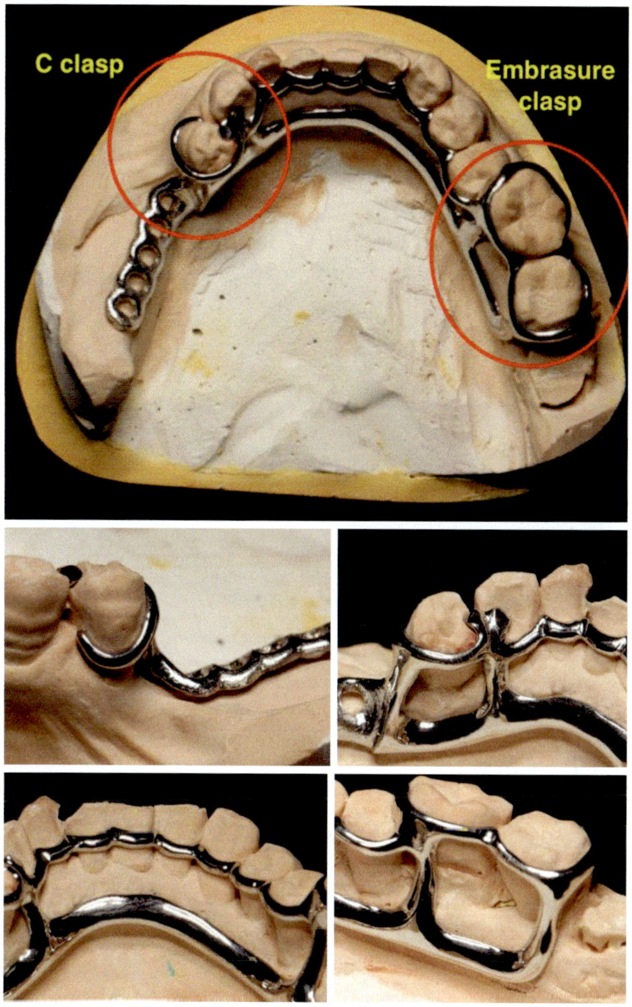

Fig. 6.99 (continued)

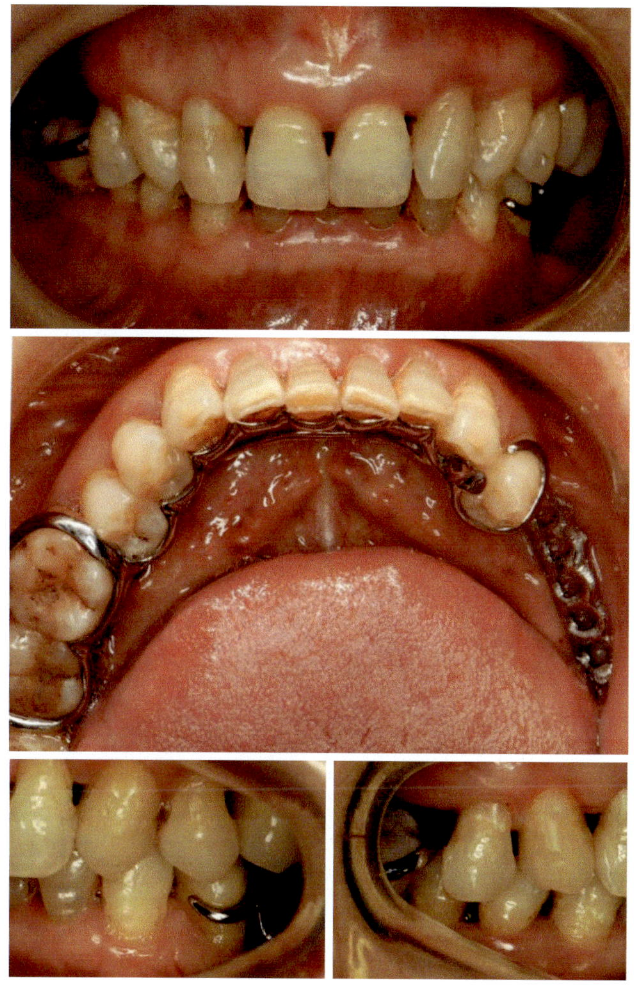

Fig. 6.100 Trying in of the framework

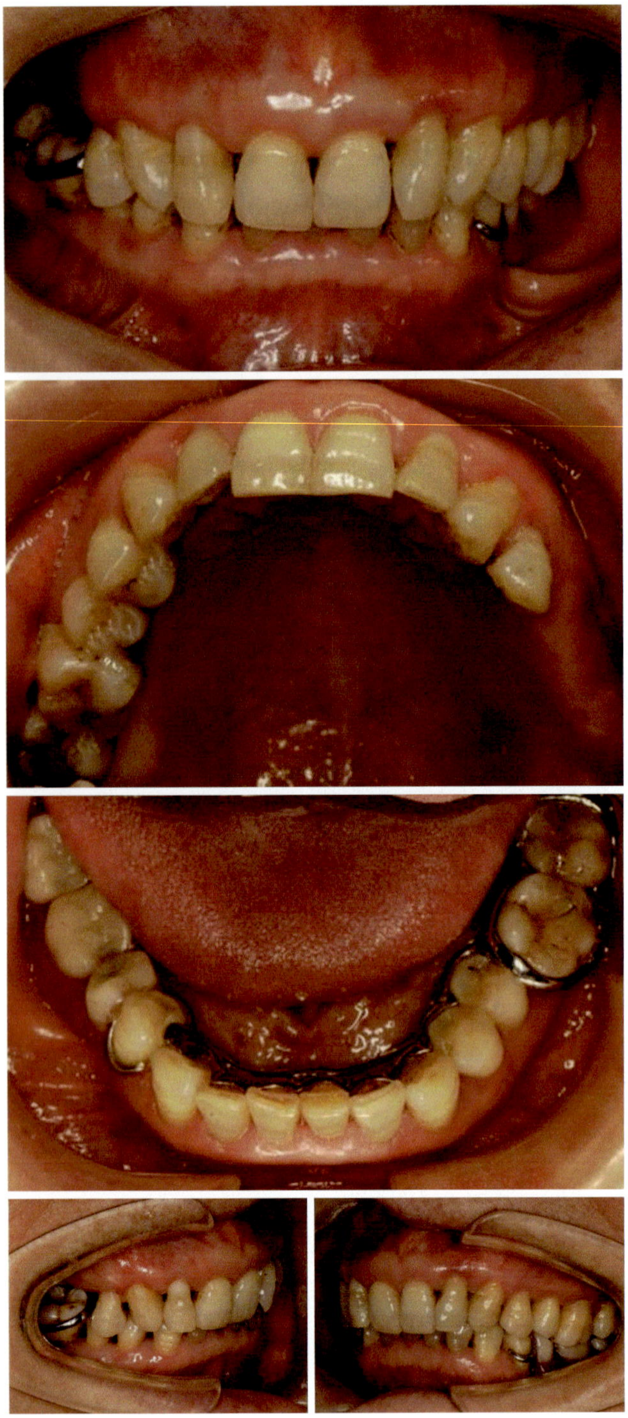

Fig. 6.101 Intraoral view with denture

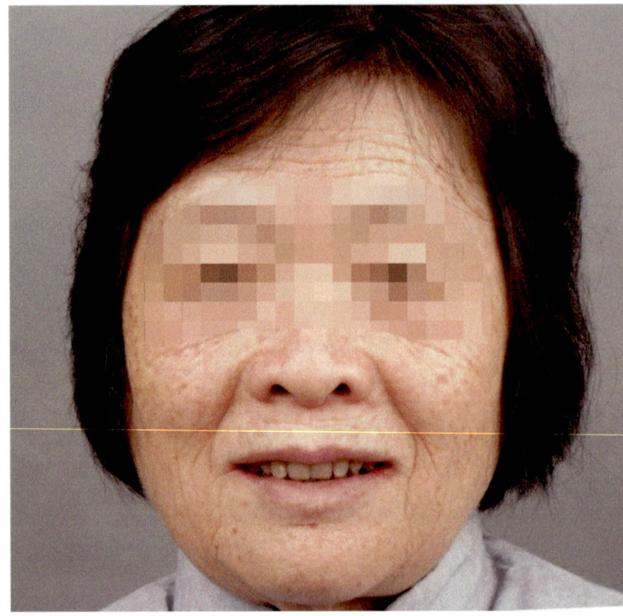

Fig. 6.102 Frontal view with denture

6.15 Case 15

E-Clasps in Digital Framework RPD Design Without Tooth Preparation for Patient with Bilateral Maxillary Free-End Edentia

1. *Before restoration*

   A woman, 58 years old.

   Smile analysis: The patient shows a short distance of lower facial 1/3 in the frontal view (Fig. 6.103). And according to Zhang's smiling exposed zone before restoration, she has an average smiling line. The maxillary esthetic teeth are A5–B5 (Fig. 6.104).

   Dentition analysis: The maxillary missing teeth are A4–7 and B6–7. And there are apparent spaces among the anterior teeth, tight occlusion of remaining teeth, severely worn teeth, deep anterior overbite, and average anterior overjet. Besides, the teeth are in a good, clean condition, and the remaining teeth are not loose (Figs. 6.105 and 6.106).

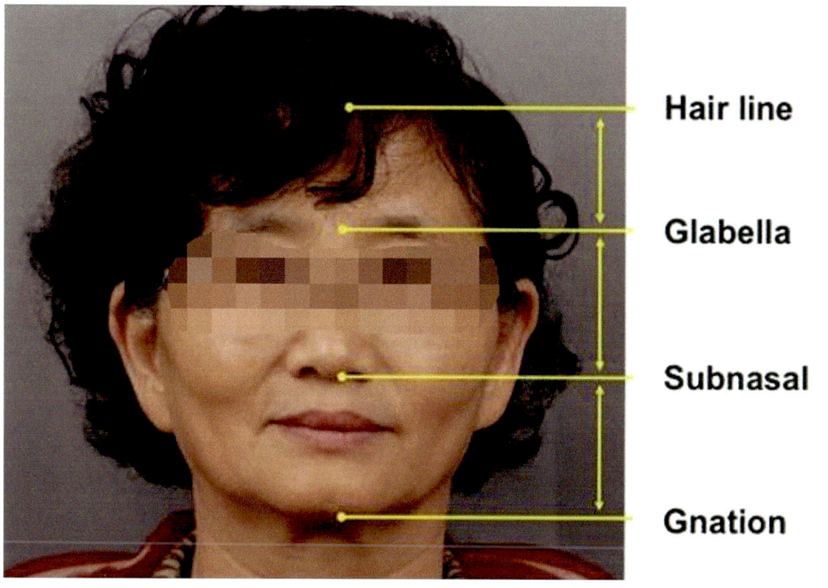

Fig. 6.103 Facial analysis. Normal proportion of the three courts and short height of lower facial 1/3

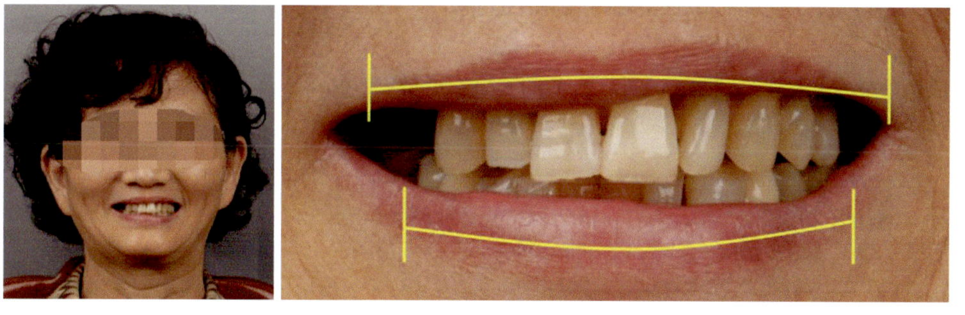

Fig. 6.104 Smiling analysis; the esthetic teeth are A5–B5. Smiling exposed area has tooth defect in A area

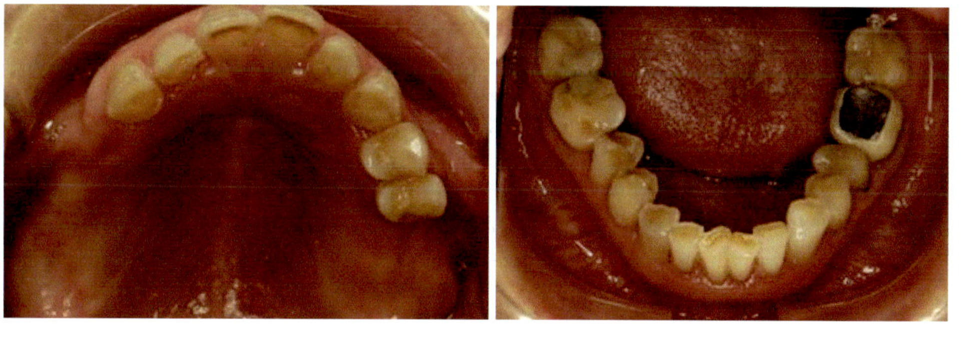

Fig. 6.105 Dentition analysis

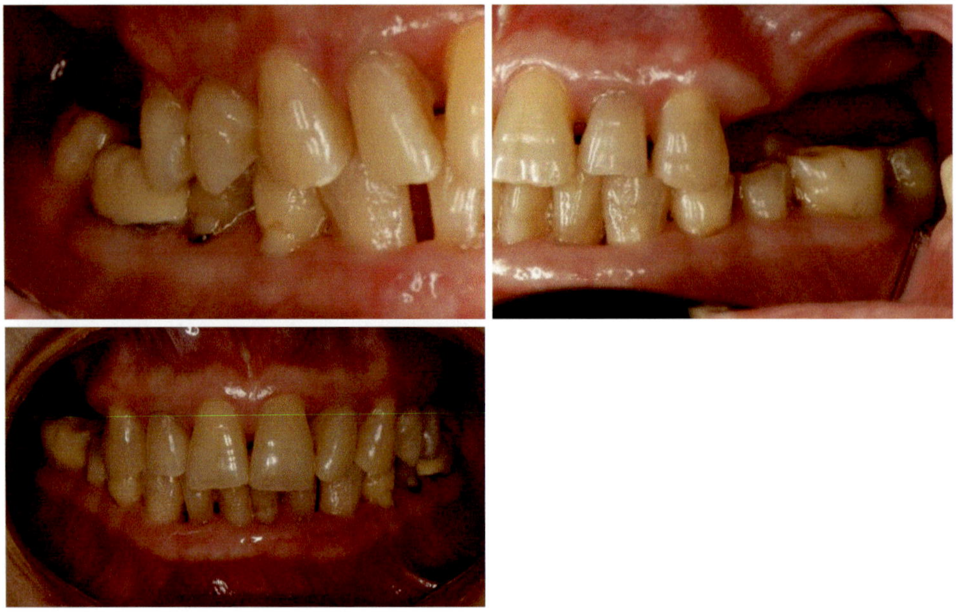

Fig. 6.106 Tight occlusion in the frontal and lateral view

As a teacher, the patient has high requirements for esthetics and pronunciation due to professional reasons, and she is afraid of surgical implantation schemes. She hopes that the restoration scheme is simple, minimally invasive, and reversible and the effect evaluation after restoration can achieve a more natural appearance. After examination, we find that the position of the posterior missing tooth on maxilla is relatively backward. So the lips and the buccal axial ridge of the abutments could be used to hide the cervical clasp. However, grinding is unacceptable for the incisors of anterior teeth, and the occlusal surfaces of posterior teeth are severely worn, and the teeth are hypersensitive. All in all, it is difficult to restore.

The lingual surfaces of maxillary anterior teeth, incisors of mandibular anterior teeth, and the occlusal surfaces of posterior teeth are severely worn, and there are apparent spaces among A3–B4.

2. *RPD analysis and manufacturing*

   The maxilla is Kennedy I dentition defect. A3, B3, and B5 are chosen as abutments, and they are all in good condition. However, not much teeth can be prepared because of tight occlusion, and the opposite is natural teeth. In order to obtain good support and stability, we design full palate plate as major connector for the upper jaw, and put short buccally retained clasps on A3 and B3. A minor connector is designed closed to the natural gap between B3 and B4 to reduce food impaction, and a three-arm clasp with good retention is designed on B5. Because tooth grinding is unacceptable, only one rest can be designed on the distal side of B5 using the existing small gap (Fig. 6.107). After the metal framework is completed (Fig. 6.108), try it in the mouth (Fig. 6.109), record the occlusal relationship, and then try the wax pattern (Fig. 6.110).

3. *After restoration*

   The final repair effect is shown in Figs. 6.111 and 6.112. The patient is satisfied.

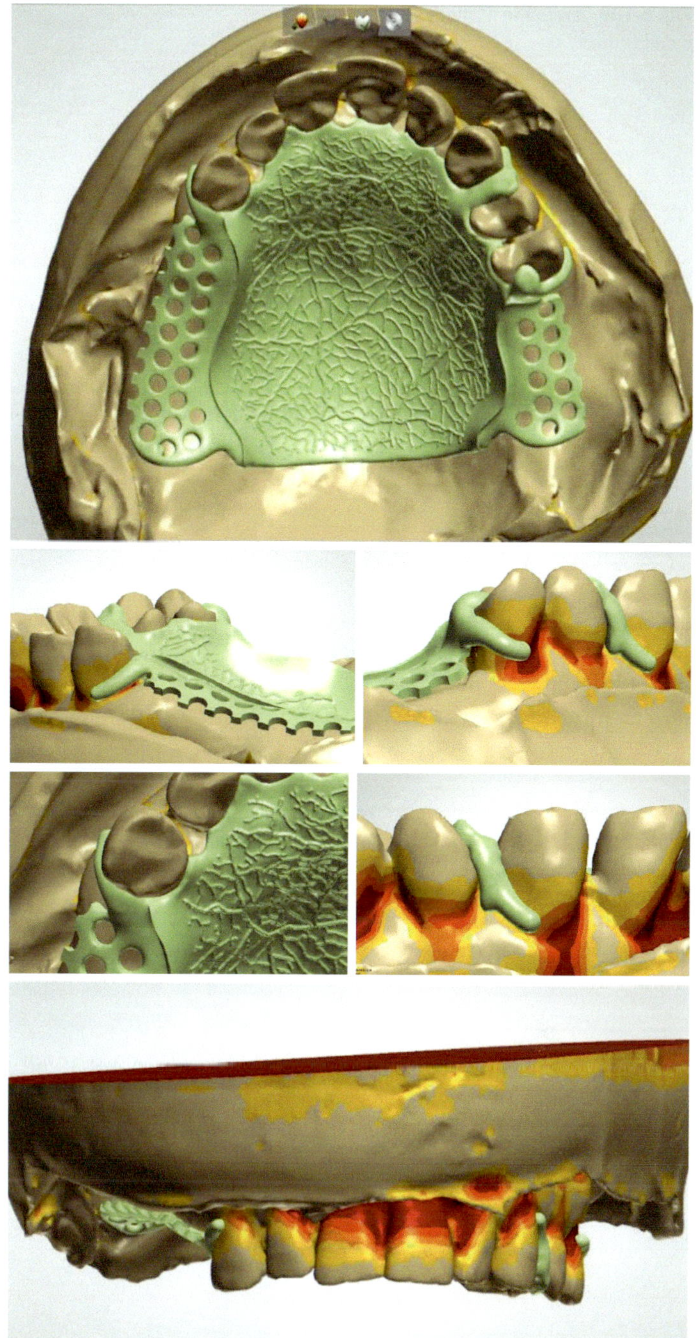

Fig. 6.107 Bilateral free-end edentia in A and B area; A3, B3—short buccally retained clasps. The arm of clasp does not cross the buccal axial rigid, and the clasp tip is hidden in the buccal view. A minor connector between B3 and B4 is thickened as anti-impact device

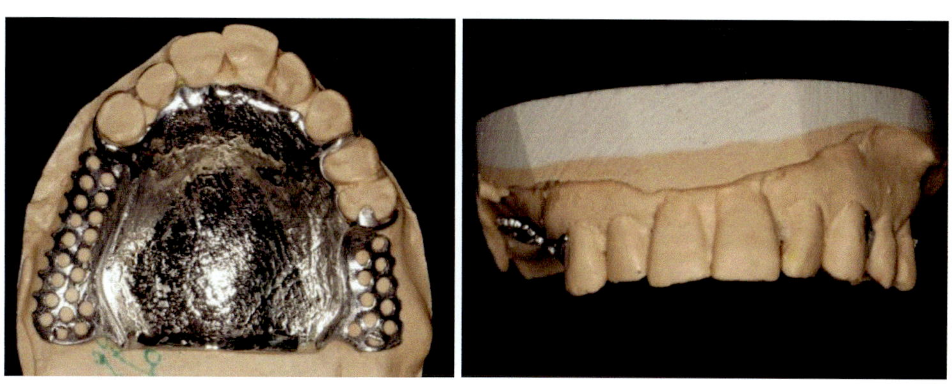

Fig. 6.108 Laser printing and polishing of the metal framework

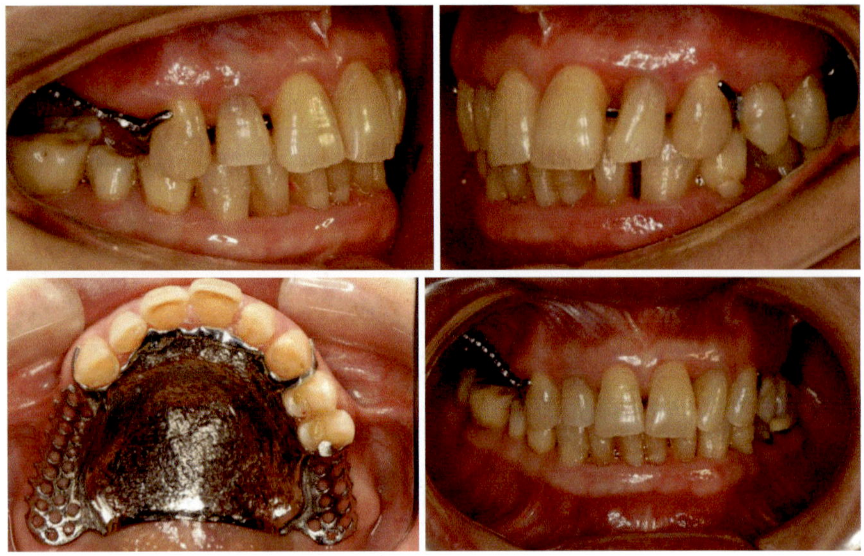

Fig. 6.109 Trying in of the metal framework

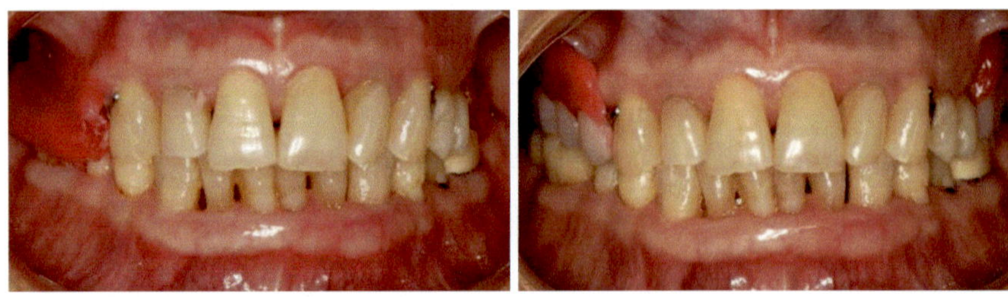

Fig. 6.110 Occlusal relationship recording and trying in of the wax pattern

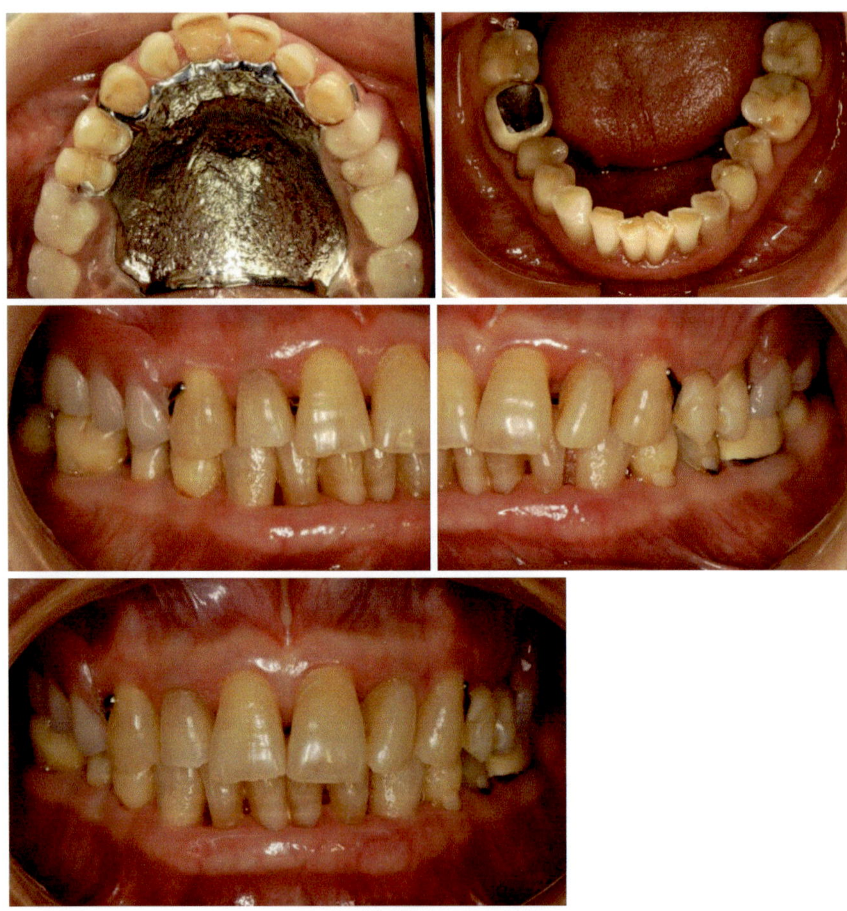

Fig. 6.111 Intraoral view with denture

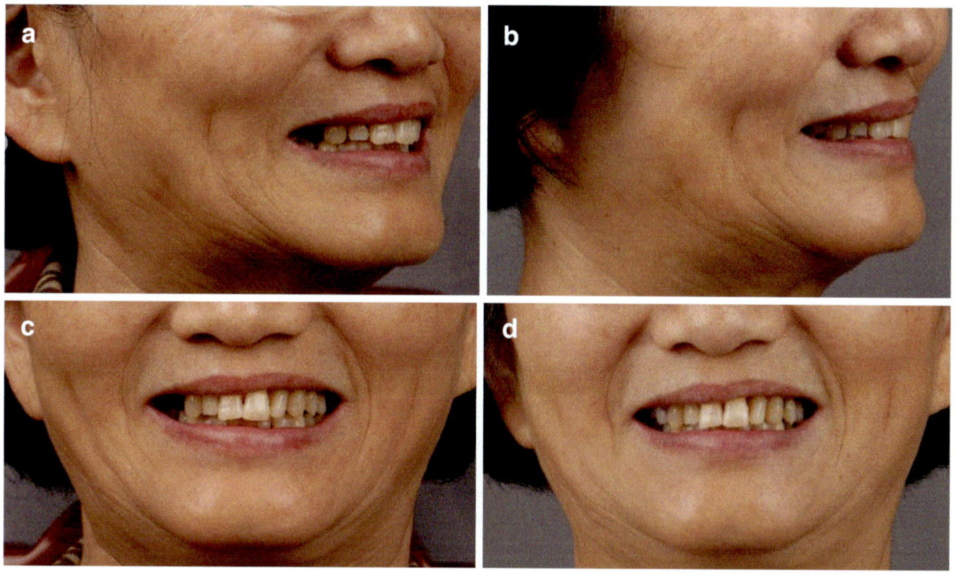

Fig. 6.112 Comparison before and after restoration. (**a**) Lower facial 1/3 lateral view before restoration. (**b**) Lower facial 1/3 lateral view after restoration. (**c**) Lower facial 1/3 frontal view before restoration. (**d**) Lower facial 1/3 frontal view after restoration

6.16 Case 16

E-Clasps in Digital Framework RPD Design for Patient with Bilateral Free-End Edentia on Maxilla and Mandible and Rare Remaining Teeth

1. *Before restoration*

   Smile analysis: A woman, 70 years old. In the lower facial 1/3 frontal view, the patient shows the loss of fattiness, apparent nasolabial groove, and mentolabial sulcus (Fig. 6.113). Due to the loss of the maxillary anterior teeth, only lower teeth can be seen when smiling (Fig. 6.114). The aging face seriously affects her appearance.

   Dentition analysis: There are only A4 and B6 left in the maxilla. And B6 is with mesial amalgam filling and defect of distobuccal cusp and serious root exposure. However, the patient is unwilling to pull the teeth. There are only C3, D3, and D5 in the lower jaw, and there is no contacted teeth in the mouth. Residual roots A5, B3, and D4 have been treated with root canal therapy, which the patient is also unwilling to remove. There are apparent tooth extraction sockets of 4, 5, and 7 in B area, and the last tooth extraction has been completed for 9 months (Fig. 6.115).

   Due to the large number of missing teeth, the RPD are mainly supported by the mucous membrane. Besides, the area of the main bearing area in B area is limited. So the remaining abutments and covered area should be used to disperse the occlusal stress as full as possible. In consideration of severe tooth root exposure in the upper jaw, a lingual self-cleaning area beneath the clasp should be allowed for oral cleaning.
2. *RPD analysis design and manufacturing*

   For the upper jaw, we design a full palate plate, a RPT clasp in A area, and a three-arm clasp on B4, leaving lingual self-cleaning area for all abutments (Fig. 6.116). For the lower jaw, we design a lingual plate, short buccally retained clasps on both C3 and D3, a three-arm clasp on D5, and three rests in the lower jaw to disperse stress (Fig. 6.117). After the metal framework is completed (Fig. 6.118), try it in the mouth (Fig. 6.119), then record the occlusal relationship, and try the wax pattern in the mouth (Fig. 6.120).
3. *After restoration*

   The final repair effect is shown in Figs. 6.121 and 6.122. The patient is satisfied.

Fig. 6.113 Facial analysis. Loss of fattiness in the lower face 1/3, deep nasolabial groove and mentolabial sulcus. Typical aging face of the elderly after teeth loss

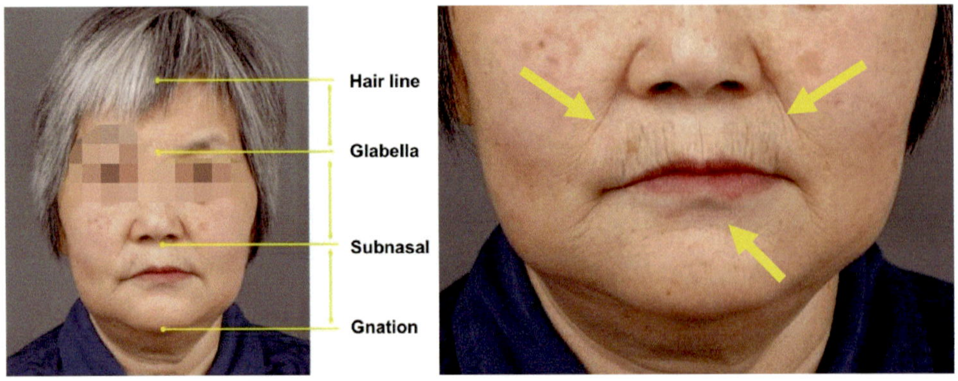

Fig. 6.114 Smile analysis. Most of the anterior teeth are missing, and only two remaining mandibular anterior teeth can be seen when smiling

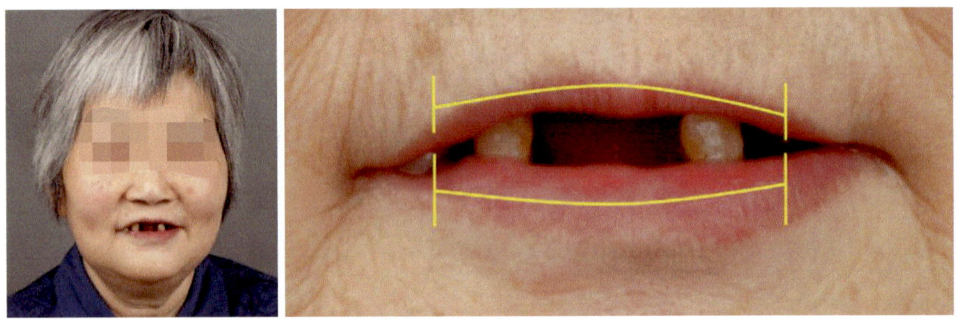

Fig. 6.115 Dentition analysis. Large number of residual roots, large tooth exposure, poor cleaning

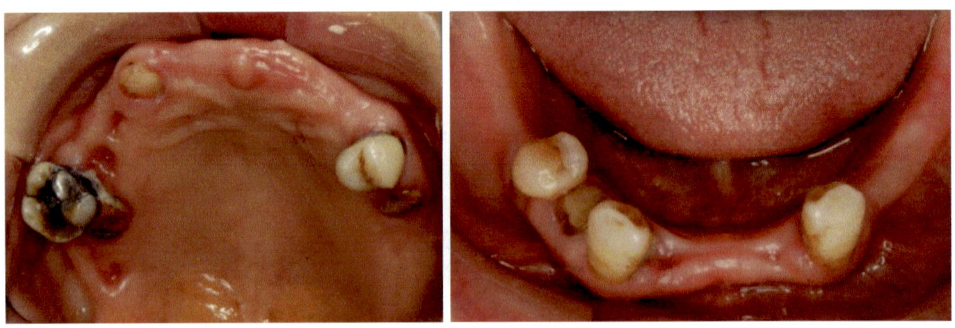

Fig. 6.116 Maxillary framework design. A4—RPT clasp, B6—three-arm clasp, The lingual side does not cover gingiva, which is good for cleaning

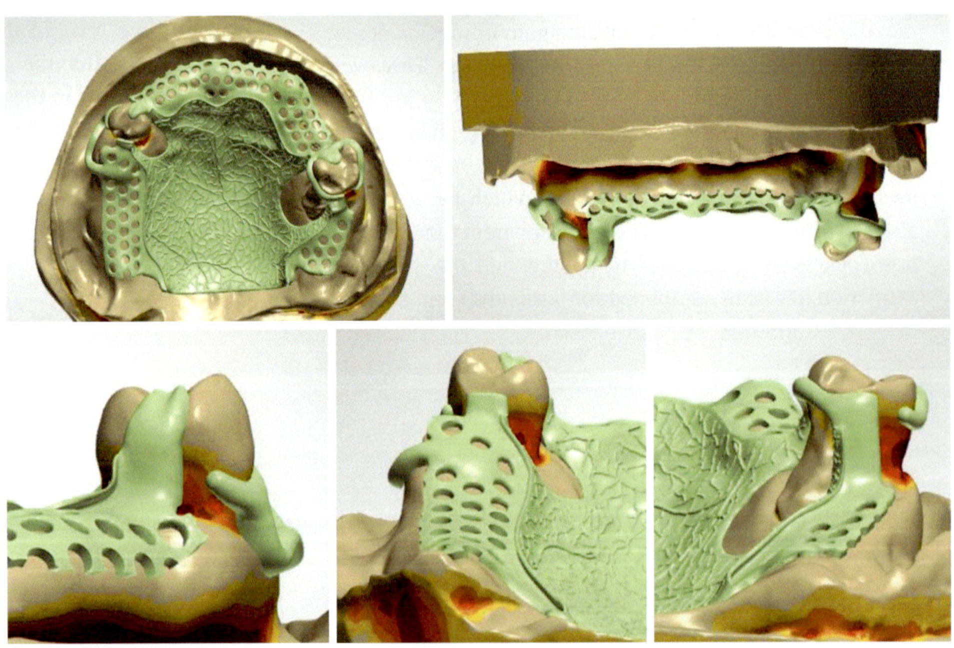

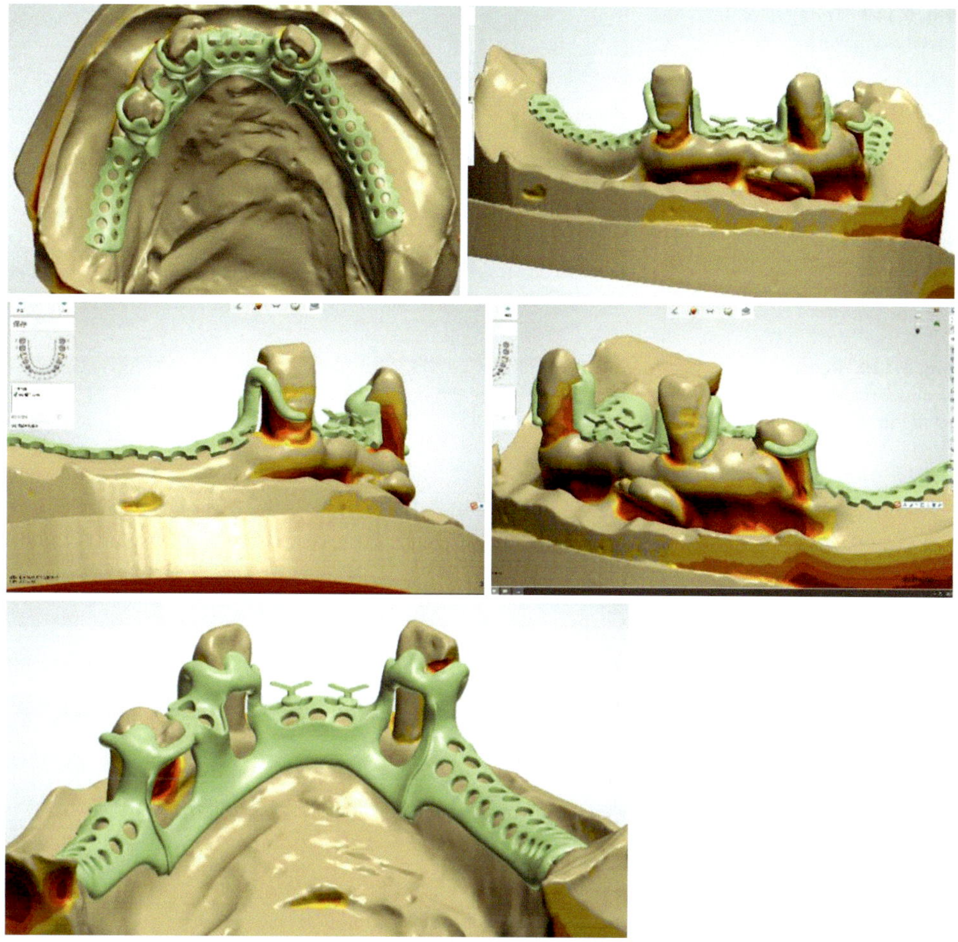

Fig. 6.117 Mandibular framework design. C3, D3—Short buccally retained clasps, D5—three-arm clasp, lingual Self-cleaning area

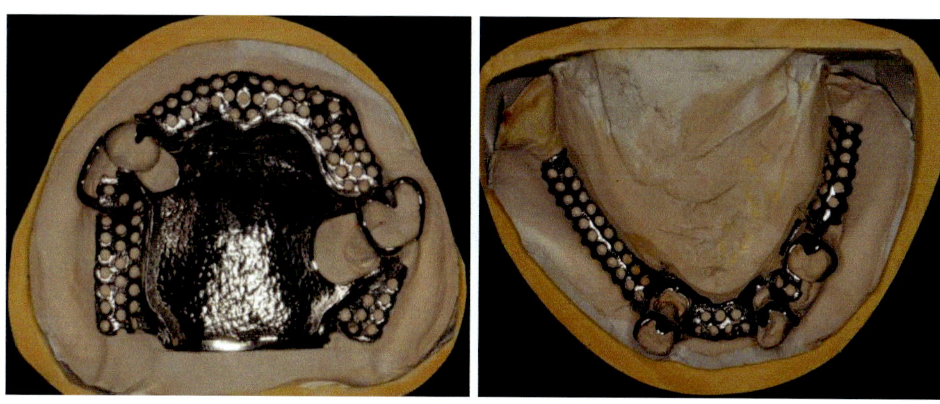

Fig. 6.118 Laser printing and polishing of metal framework

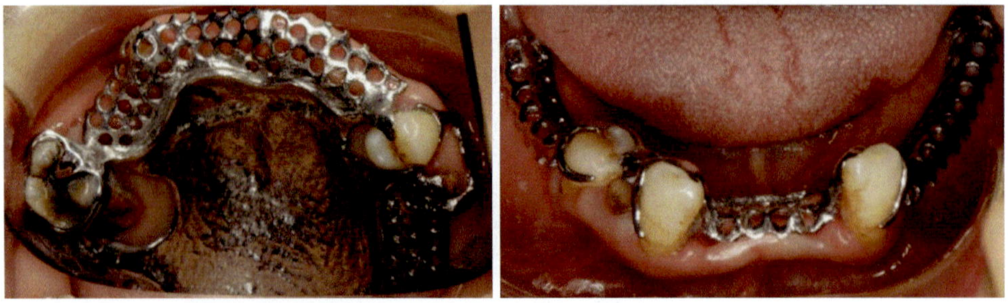

Fig. 6.119 Trying in of the metal framework

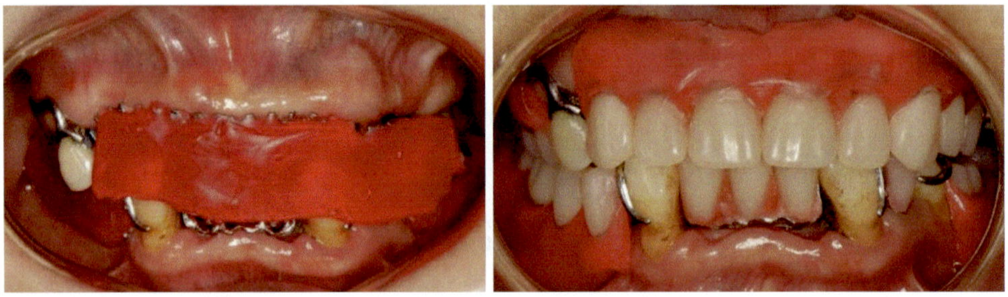

Fig. 6.120 Recording occlusal relationship and trying in of the wax pattern

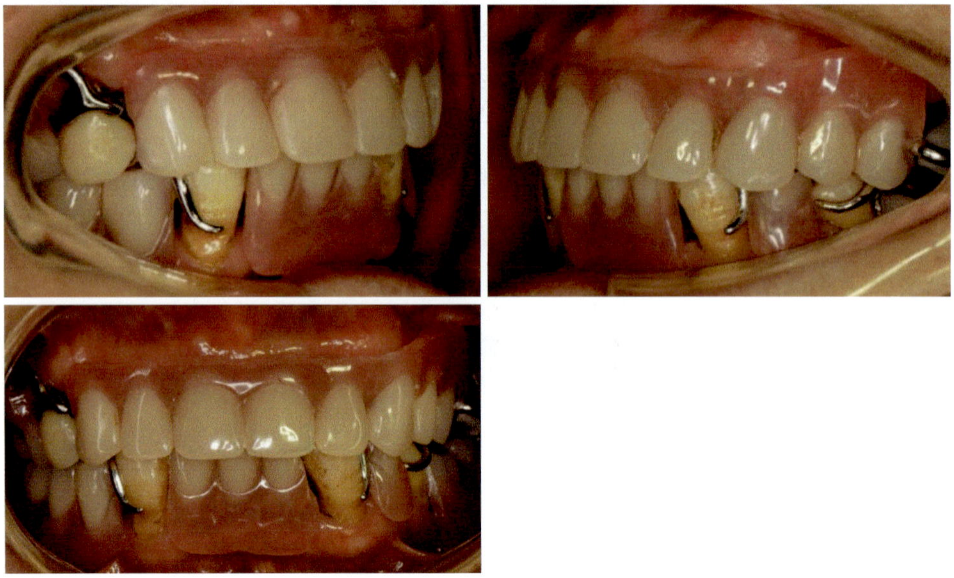

Fig. 6.121 Intraoral view with denture

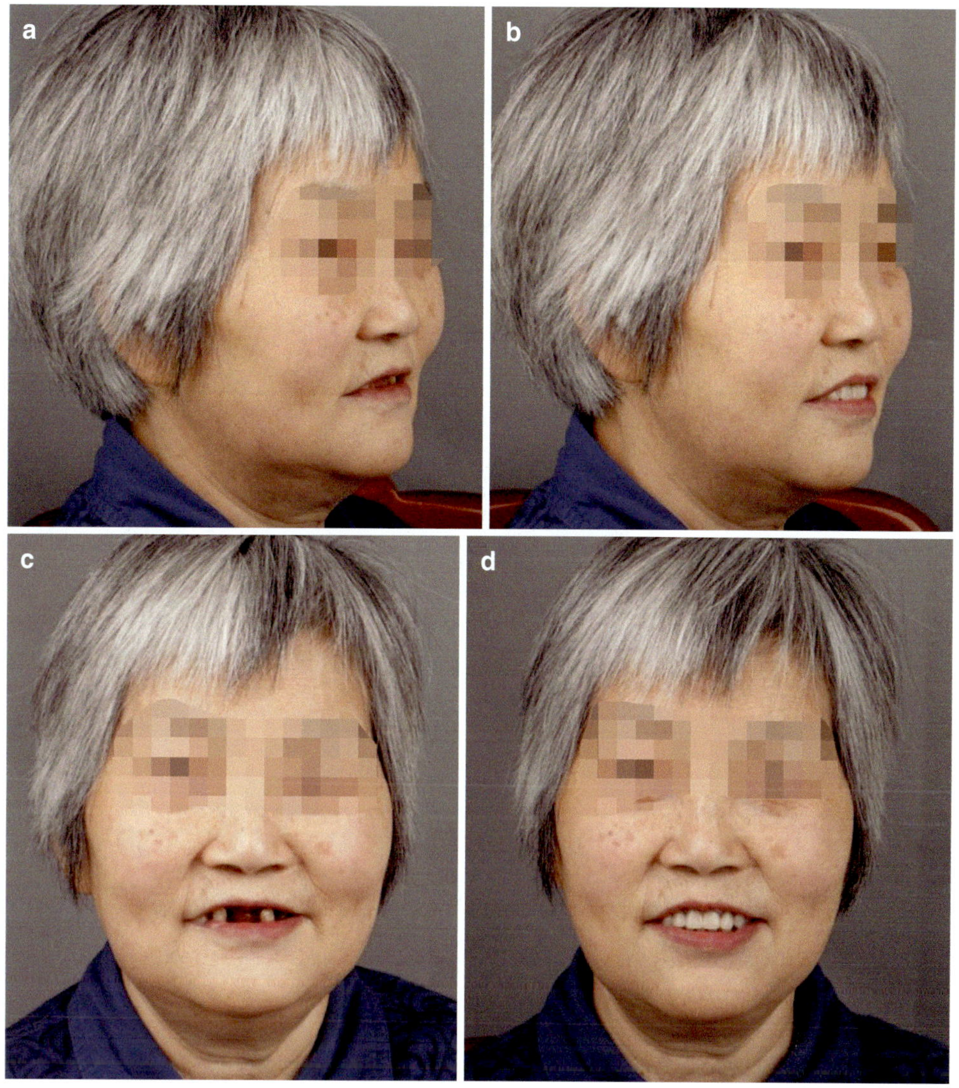

Fig. 6.122 Comparison before and after restoration. The face collapse has been greatly improved. The fattiness of the lower facial 1/3 is restored. And the metal clasp is completely hidden. Finally the patient shows a younger smile. (**a**) Facial lateral view before restoration. (**b**) Facial lateral view after restoration. (**c**) Facial frontal view before restoration. (**d**) Facial frontal view after restoration

6.17 Case 17

E-Clasps in Digital Metal Framework RPD Design for Patient with Unilateral Free-End Defect and Severe Abrasion

1. *Before restoration*

    A man, 85 years old. The patient with Parkinson's disease has difficulty in moving. Because the old denture was fractured while eating, he came to see the doctor and asked to replace it.

    Smile analysis: In the frontal view, we see the loss of lip fattiness, small exposure of the upper anterior teeth, large exposure of the lower anterior teeth, and apparent wear of the lower anterior teeth (Fig. 6.123).

    Dentition analysis: Most of maxillary teeth of patient are missing. The patient is with post-core porcelain crown restorations on A1 and B1, whose labial edge becomes dark and exposed (Fig. 6.124). Besides, there are lingual porcelain layer wear and metal exposure. A2, B2, and B3 only have thin tooth wall, A3 is a residual root, and the remaining teeth A7 are in good condition. The patient has Kennedy II dentition defect on mandible, severe wear of the lower anterior teeth, and tight occlusion (Fig. 6.125). Moreover, there is a reverse and steep Spee curve on the right side (Fig. 6.126). At the same time, the patient's old denture is examined, and it is found that the old maxillary denture is broken along the metal finish line. Hygienic condition in the mouth is normal and food debris is visible.

Fig. 6.123 Facial analysis

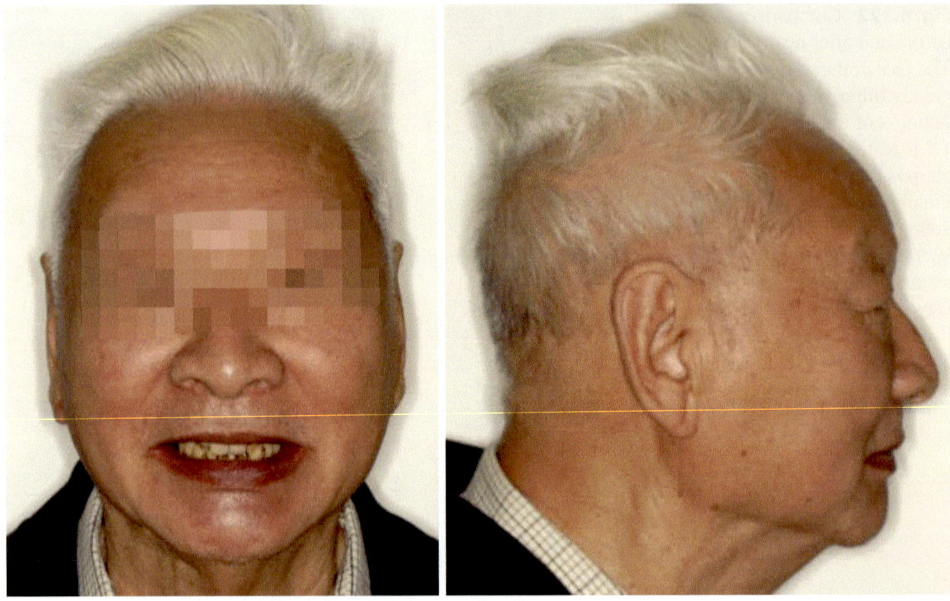

Fig. 6.124 Post-core porcelain crown restorations on A1 and B1

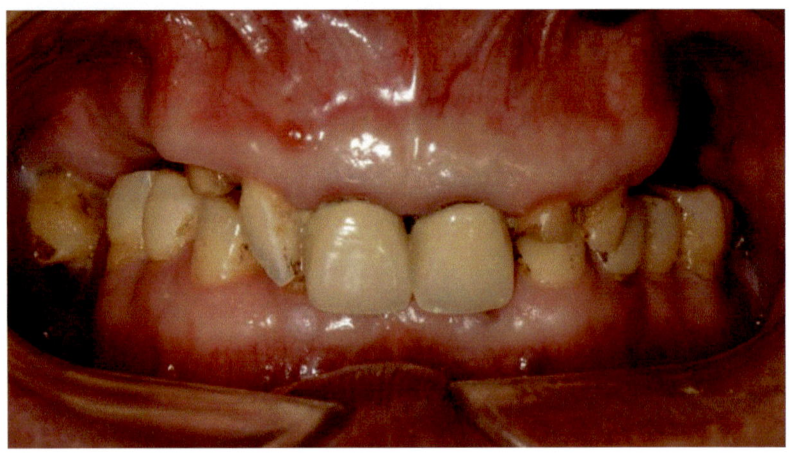

Fig. 6.125 Severe wear of the maxillary anterior teeth, lingual porcelain layer wear, and metal exposure

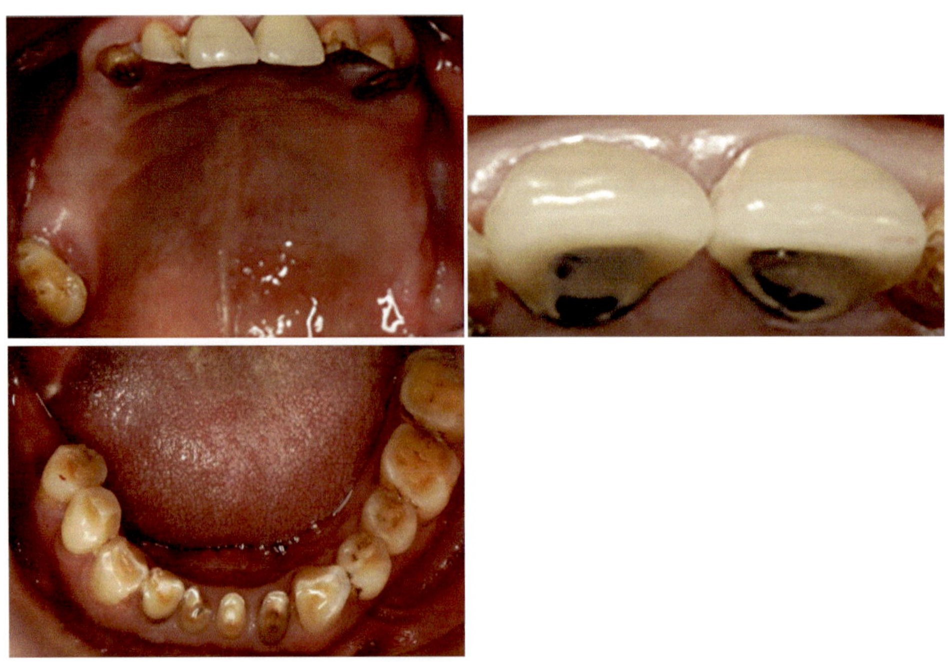

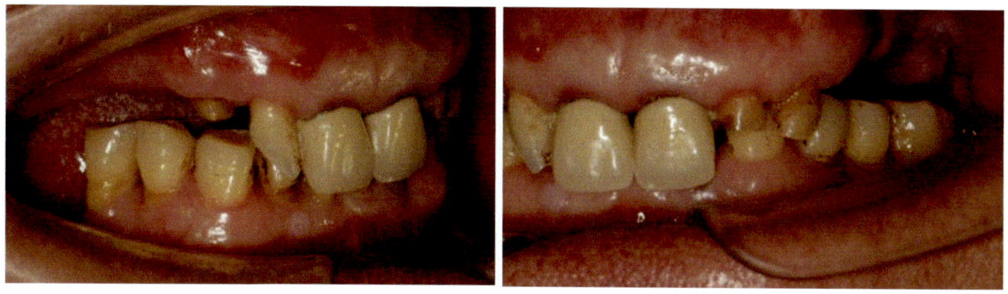

Fig. 6.126 Tight occlusion, reverse, steep Spee curve

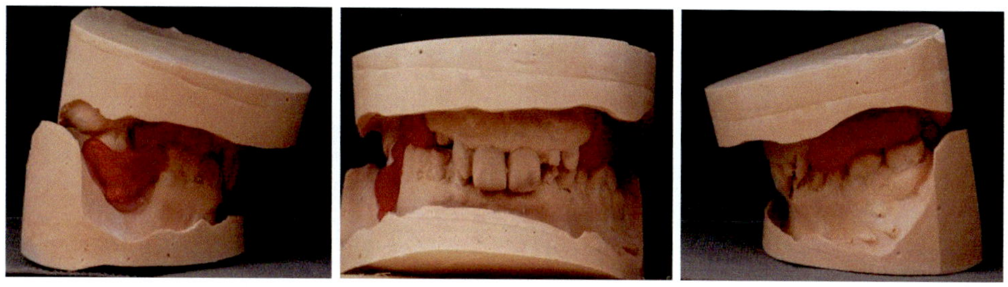

Fig. 6.127 Occlusal relationship recording

2. *RPD analysis design and manufacturing*

In the face of such an excessively deep and abnormal occlusion, it is better to correct it. However, there is no obvious symptom in the temporomandibular joint examination, and the patient consciously feels no discomfort in the current occlusion; furthermore, considering the patient's age and physical condition, we infer that the patient's joints are in a compensatory state. Therefore, conservative treatment is adopted to preserve the current occlusion relationship (Figs. 6.127 and 6.128).

In addition, another difficulty in this case is the design of the maxillary framework. Due to the patient's tight occlusion, many missing teeth in the upper jaw and abutments on one side; it is easy to form a long arm of force. In order to prevent the maxillary denture from breaking again, we choose a design of an integrated maxillary denture with metal occlusal surface. However, there are fewer remaining teeth in the upper jaw, and some of them have serious defect. How not only to ensure the retention, support, and stability of the maxillary dentures under the existing condition, but also to facilitate the removal and placement of patient with Parkinson's disease is the challenge in this case.

In consideration of the patient's old age and physical inconvenience, the number of follow-up visits should be minimized and the visit time shortened. Therefore, we decided to complete the manufacturing of denture at one time after obtaining the impression and the occlusal relationship under the premise of ensuring the quality.

There are few remaining teeth in the upper jaw. First, a three-arm clasp is placed on A7. The bodies of B2 and B3 are too thin to bear the force. The remaining body of A2 are relatively larger, so a short-arm clasp is designed to close the gap between A2 and A3. We use a lingual base plate to counteract and the residual root A3 as support. Occlusal surfaces of artificial teeth are made of metal, and only the buccal side is filled with glue (Fig. 6.129). In order to ensure the mucosal retention, the palate plate is extended to 2 mm behind the palatine fovea, and the postdam area is depicted. The design of the mandibular framework is shown in Fig. 6.130, the occlusal design is shown in Fig. 6.131, and the final RPD is shown in Fig. 6.132.

3. *After restoration*

The final repair effect is shown in Figs. 6.133 and 6.134. The patient is satisfied.

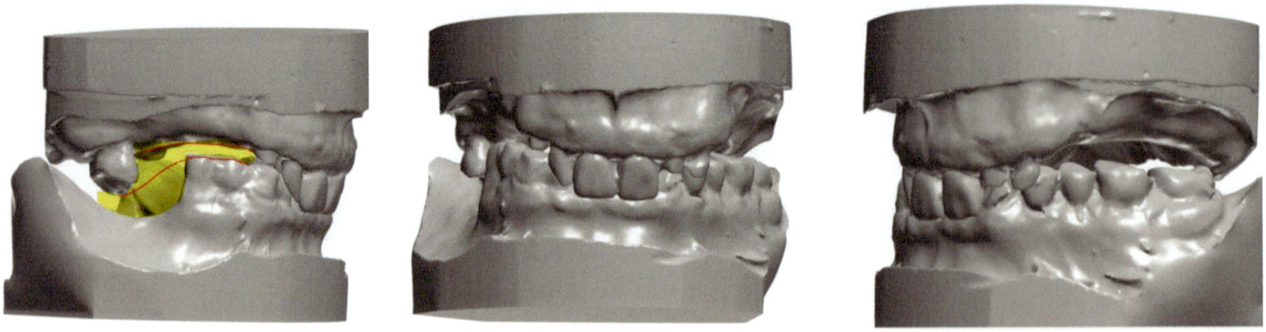

Fig. 6.128 Tight occlusion

Fig. 6.129 Framework design. (**a**) Maxillary framework design: design a short-arm clasp to close the gap between A2 and A3 and a lingual base plate to counteract, and then use A3 residual root as support. Occlusal surfaces of artificial teeth are made of metal and the buccal side is filled with glue. (**b**) Maxillary framework detail. Integrated maxillary design, no weak points

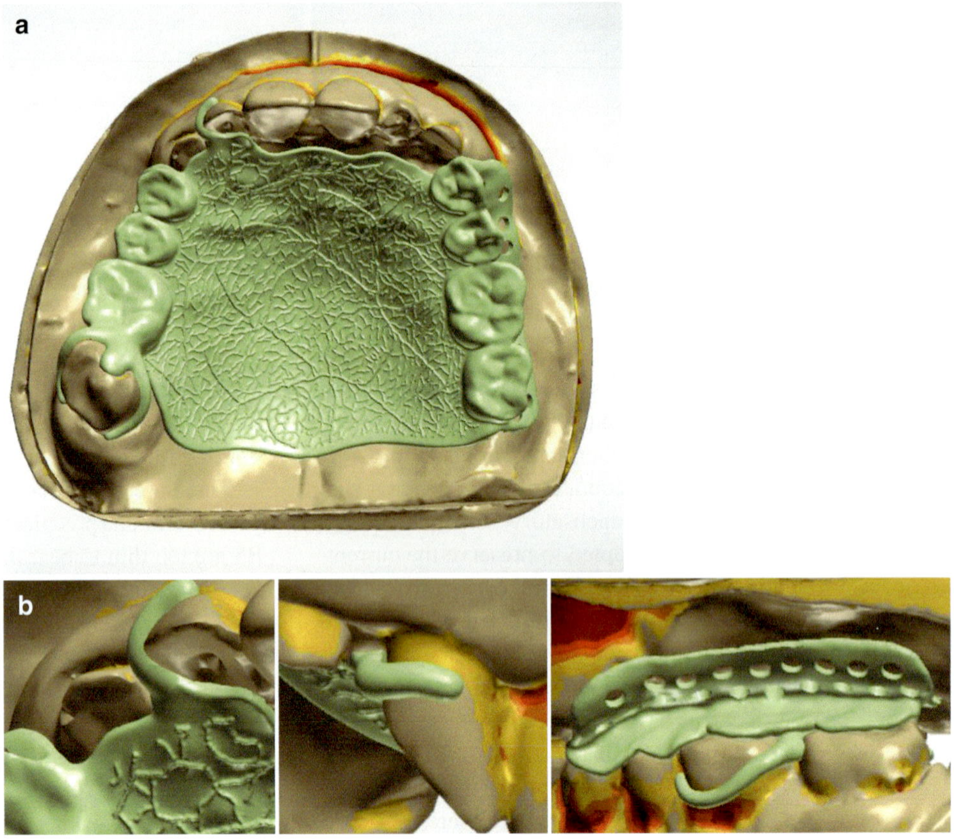

Fig. 6.130 Mandibular framework design and details: the structure is an example for easy wearing and self-cleaning

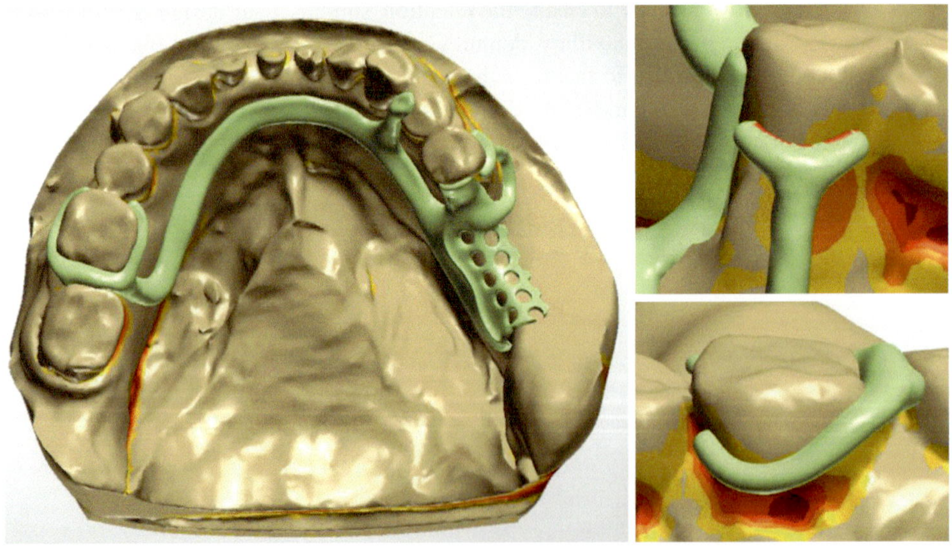

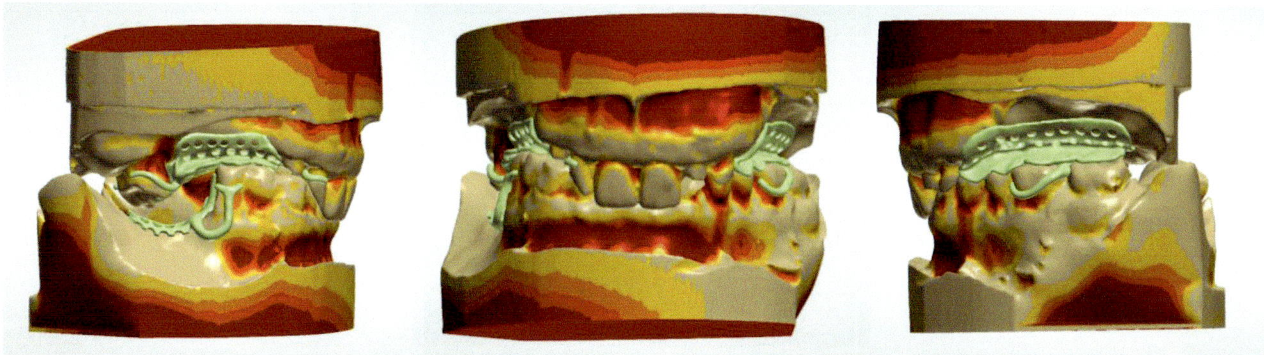

Fig. 6.131 Overall occlusal design

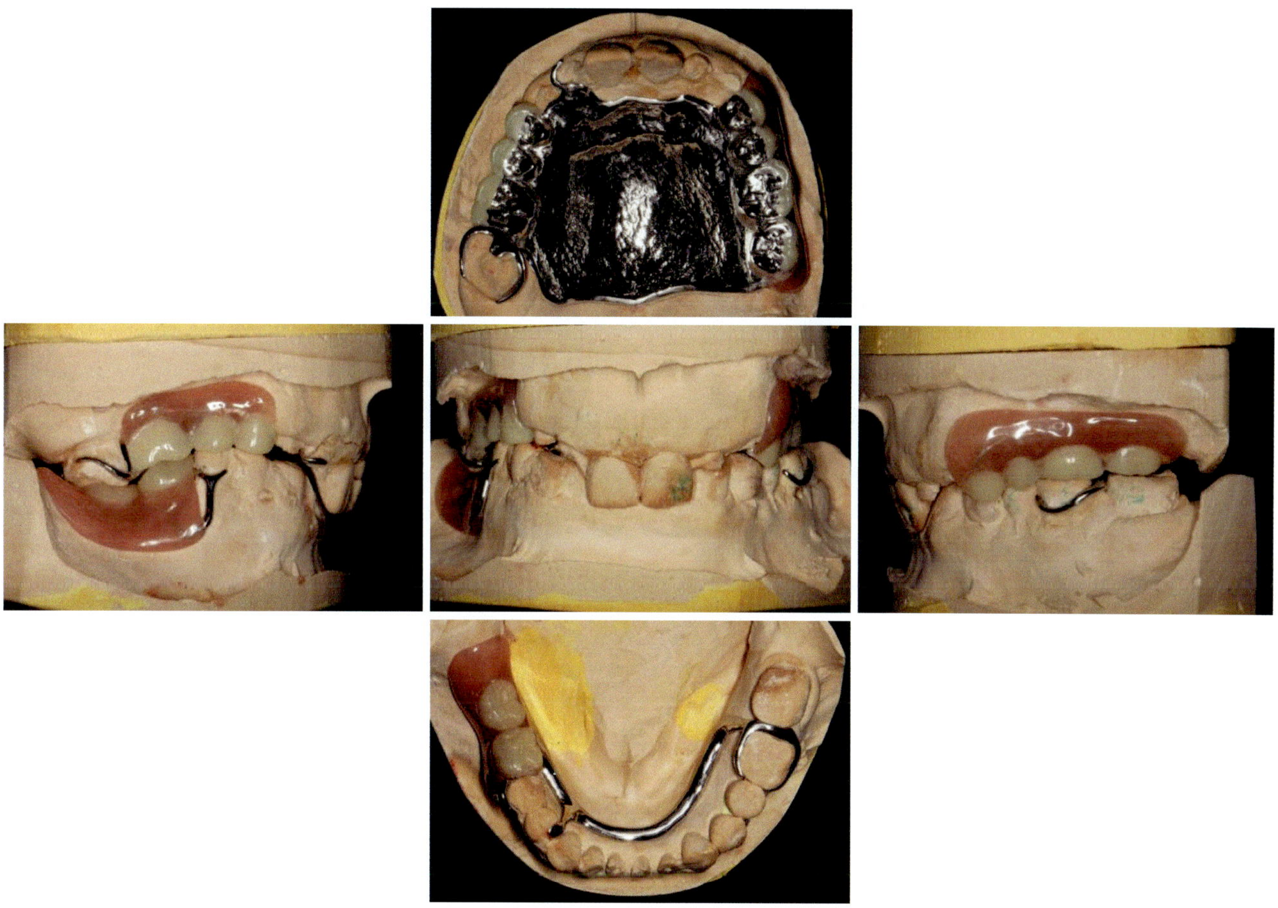

Fig. 6.132 The final denture

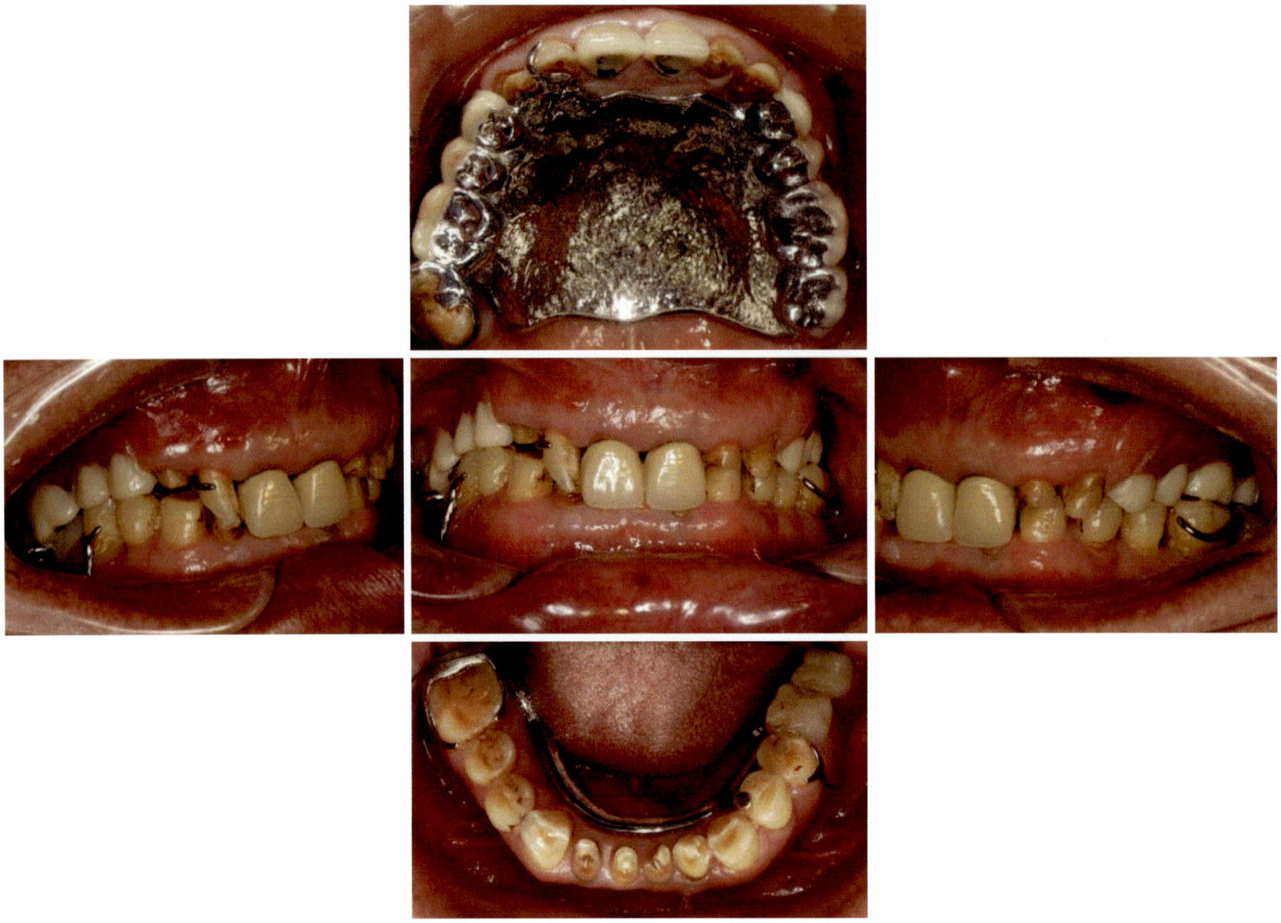

Fig. 6.133 Intraoral view with denture. Be in position after adjusting the occlusion, then instruct the patient to perform try-in and removal exercises and adjust the retention force appropriately

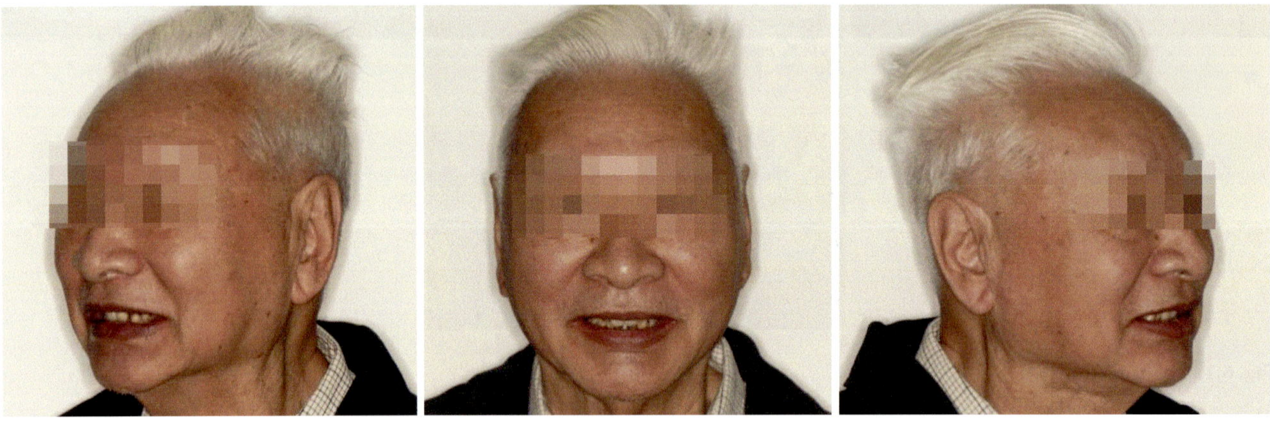

Fig. 6.134 Facial view with denture. No metal exposure after wearing the denture. The denture with suitable occlusion, and good retention is comfortable and easy to be removed. Finally the patient shows a satisfactory smile

6.18 Case 18

Multi E-Clasp Combination in Digital Framework RPD Design for Patient with Non-free-End Edentia on the Maxilla and Mandible

1. *Before restoration*

A man, 45 years old.

Smile analysis: The patient shows the absence of maxillary central incisors in the frontal view (Fig. 6.135). According to a small amount of gum exposure when smiling, the patient has an average-high smile line, and his smile is unnatural (Fig. 6.136).

Dentition analysis: The patient's missing teeth are A1, A4–A7, B1, B4–B7, C1–C2, C5, and D5–C7. The patient has deep anterior overbite, normal anterior overjet (Fig. 6.137), as well as poor periodontal condition. C3 and C4 are II°loose, and the remaining teeth are I°loose. Therefore, in the subsequent design, attention should be paid to avoiding the gingiva to facilitate self-cleaning.

In order to improve the pink and white esthetic effect of the anterior area, we proposed a removable and fixed combined restoration scheme (Fig. 6.138). However, because the patient came from out of town and his time was limited, the anterior teeth fixed and removable combined program was abandoned. After we informed the patient about the esthetic risks through the esthetic dental assistant, the patient still accepted.

2. *RPD analysis design and manufacturing*

The upper jaw is Kennedy class III non-free-end edentulous. Short buccally retained clasps are placed on A4 and B4, and traditional three-arm clasps are placed on A8 and B8. Anterior palatal bar with posterior palatal bar is used as major connectors, and the gingiva should be avoided (Fig. 6.139). Check for no metal exposure using the esthetic dental assistant (Fig. 6.140).

There are many missing teeth in D area of the lower jaw. A mesial rest and a T clasp are placed on C4, which reduces the lateral force. A distal rest is placed on the abutment C8 to prevent excessive distal sinking. Since the undercut of C8 is concentrated on the lingual-mesial surface, we designed a ring clasp to take advantage of the undercut. In D area, a C clasp is designed on D4, and a united short-arm clasp is placed on D7 and D8, which can play the role of a splint. Avoid the gingiva when designing the connector (Fig. 6.141). After the framework is completed (Fig. 6.142), we arrange artificial teeth (Fig. 6.143), and try the wax pattern on (Fig. 6.144).

3. *After restoration*

It can be seen that the final anterior teeth esthetic effect is not perfect, but the patient expressed acceptance (Figs. 6.145 and 6.146).

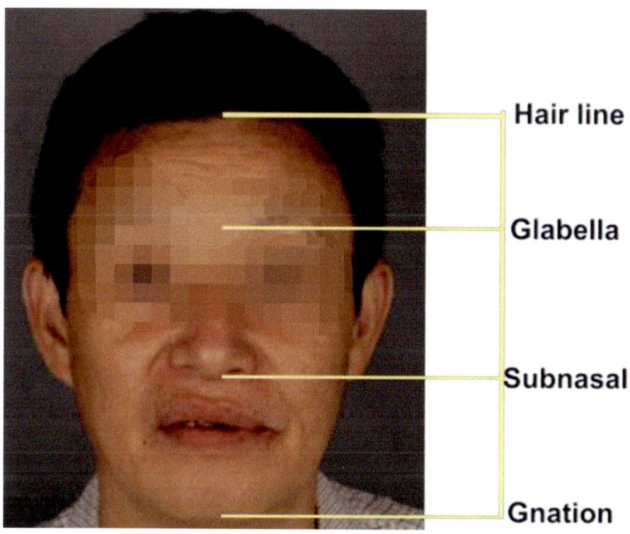

Fig. 6.135 Three courts with normal proportions and asymmetric face

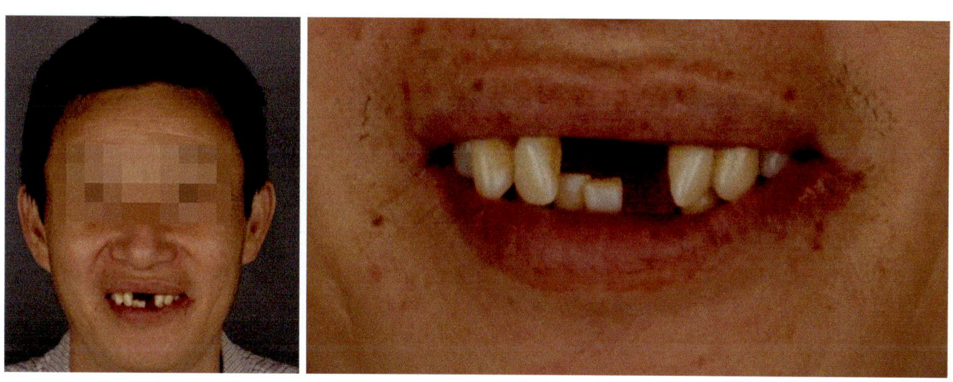

Fig. 6.136 Esthetic teeth are A3–B3; the cervix of A3 and B3 is covered by upper lip2

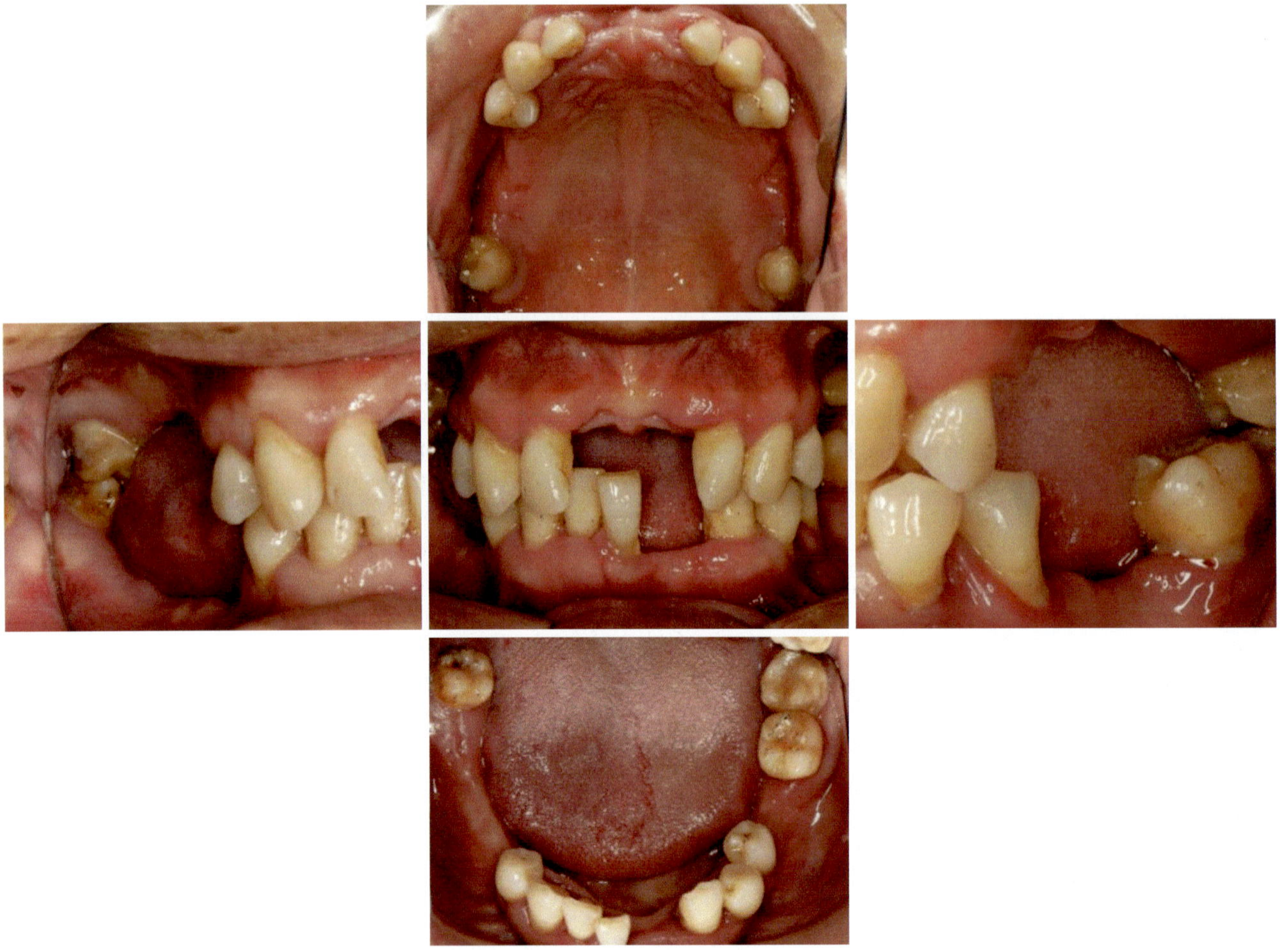

Fig. 6.137 Intraoral view

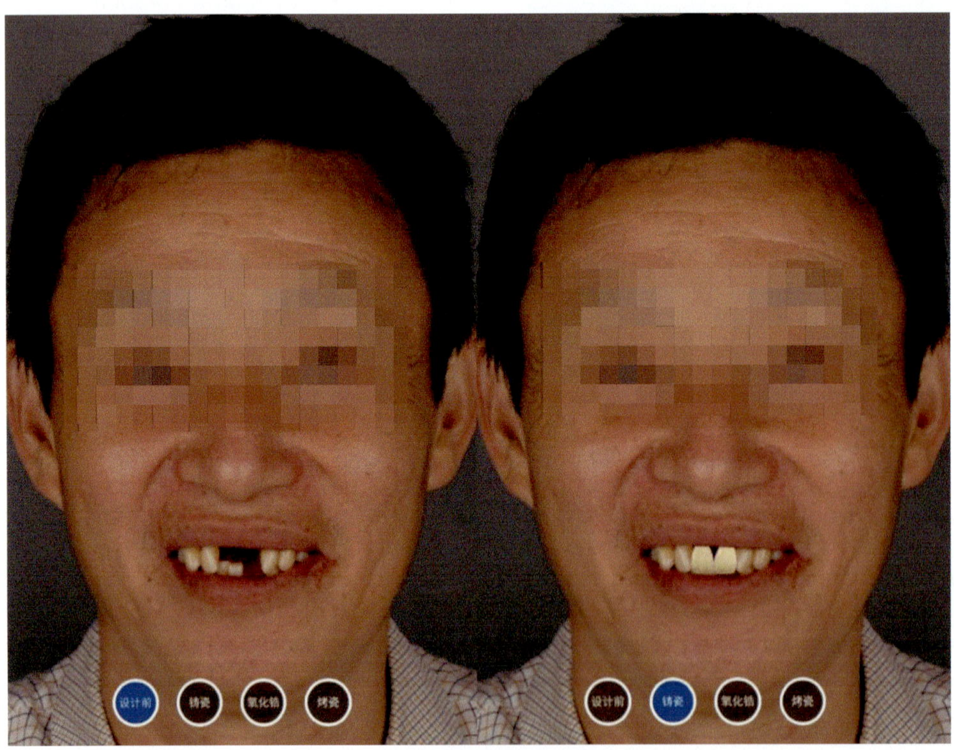

Fig. 6.138 Informing patients of esthetic risks through intraoral preview technique

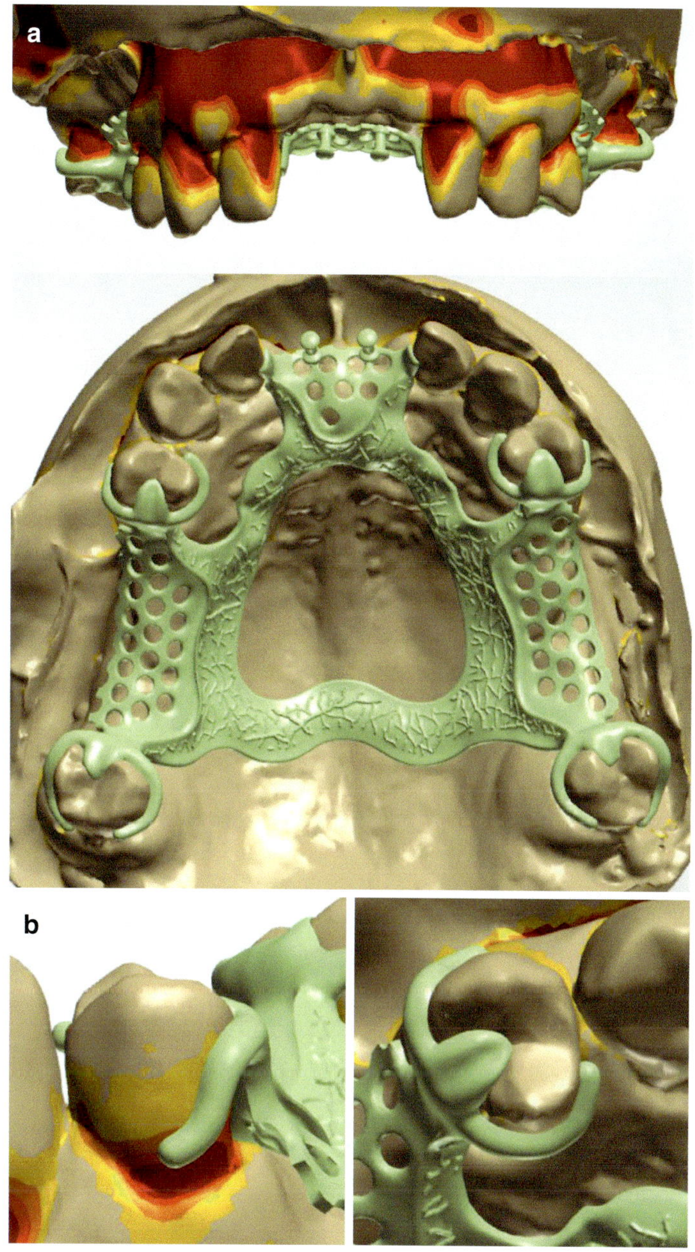

Fig. 6.139 Maxillary framework design. (a) Labial and occlusal view. (b) A4-short buccally retained clasp

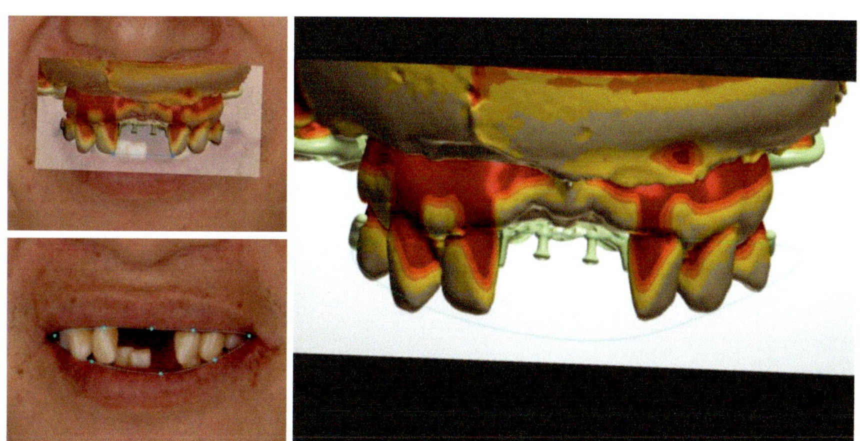

Fig. 6.140 Check for no metal exposure with the esthetic dental assistant

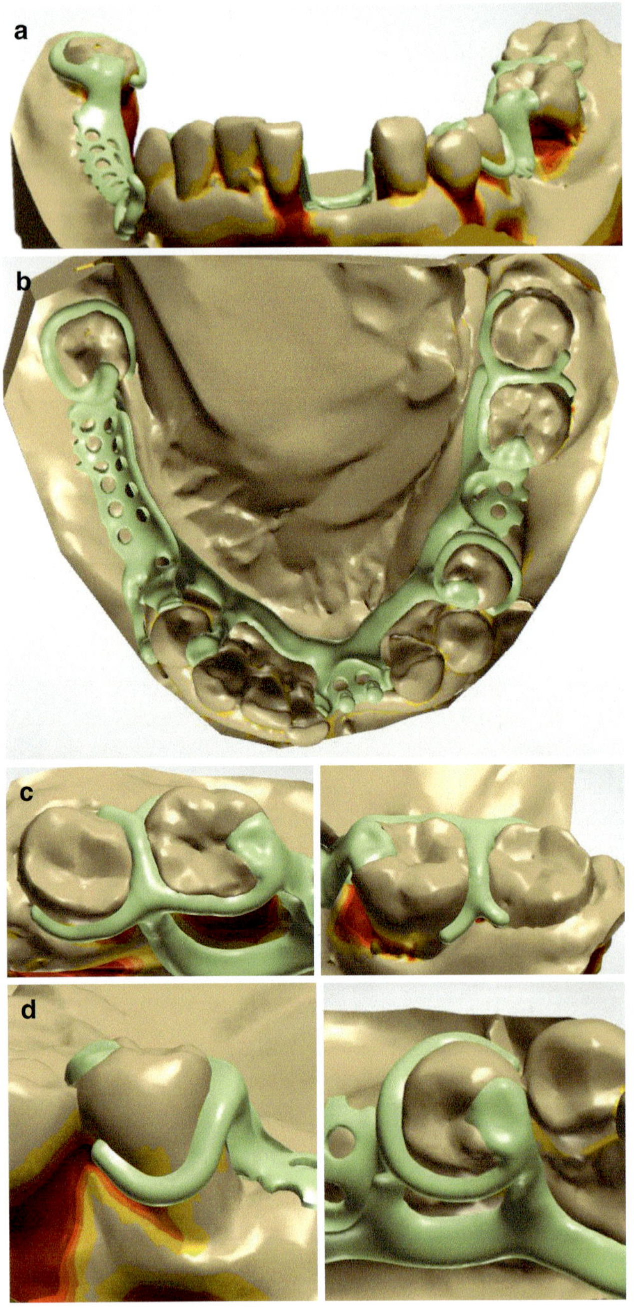

Fig. 6.141 Mandibular framework design. (**a**) Buccal view. (**b**) Occlusal view. (**c**) D7, D8-united short-arm clasp. (**d**) D4-C clasp. (**e**) C8-ring clasp

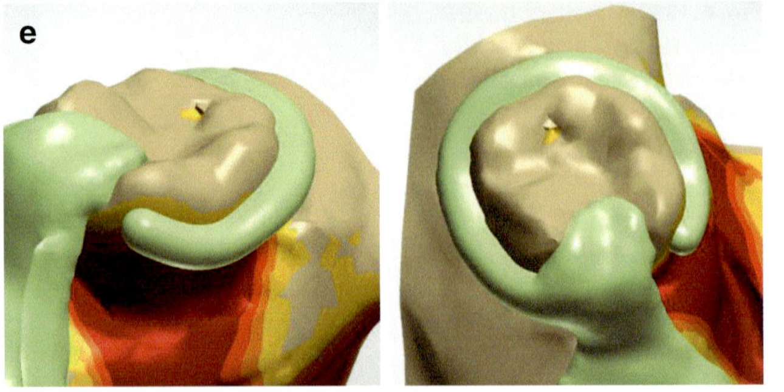

Fig. 6.141 (continued)

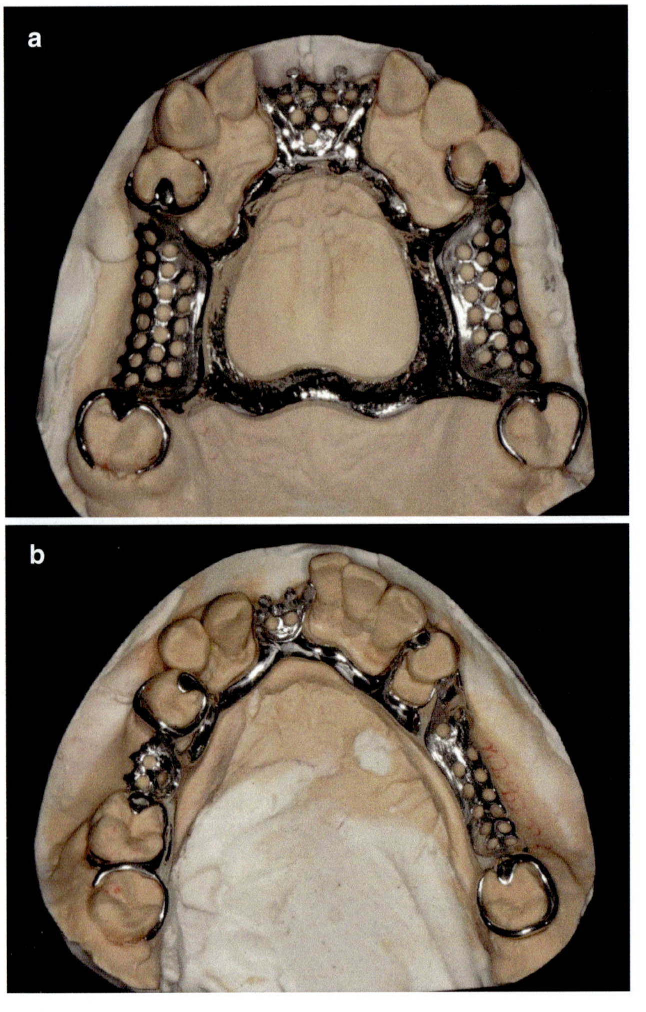

Fig. 6.142 Grinding and polishing after the framework forming. (**a**) Maxillary framework completion. (**b**) Mandibular framework completion

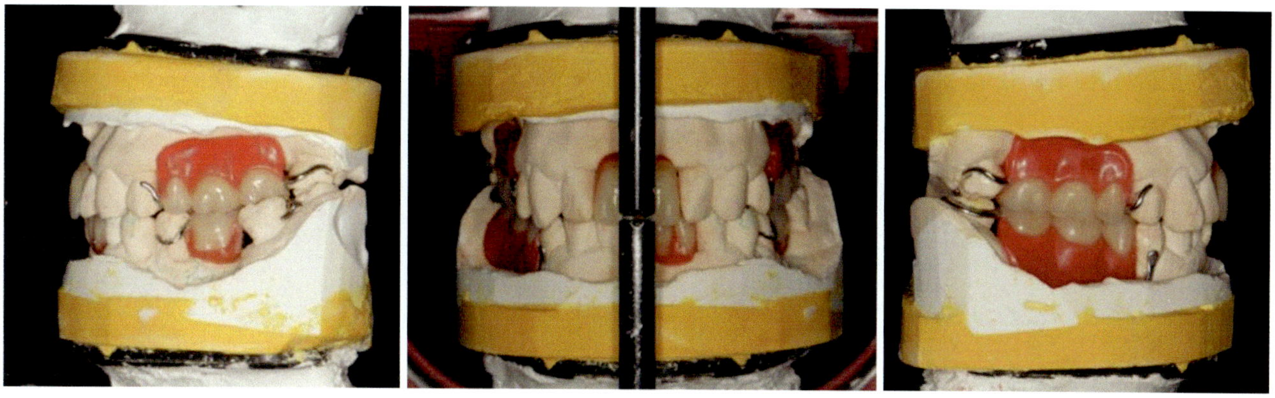

Fig. 6.143 The teeth arrangement and wax pattern

Fig. 6.144 Trying in of the wax pattern

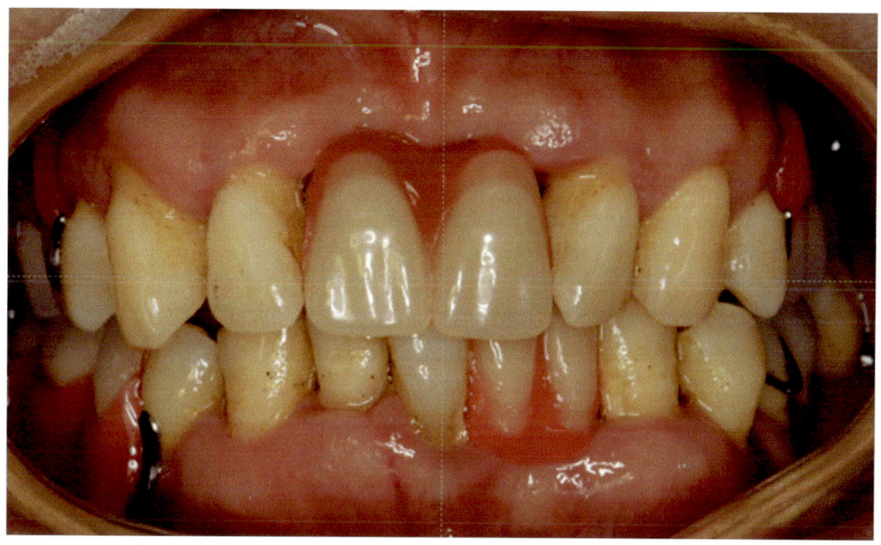

Fig. 6.145 Comparison before and after restoration in the facial frontal view

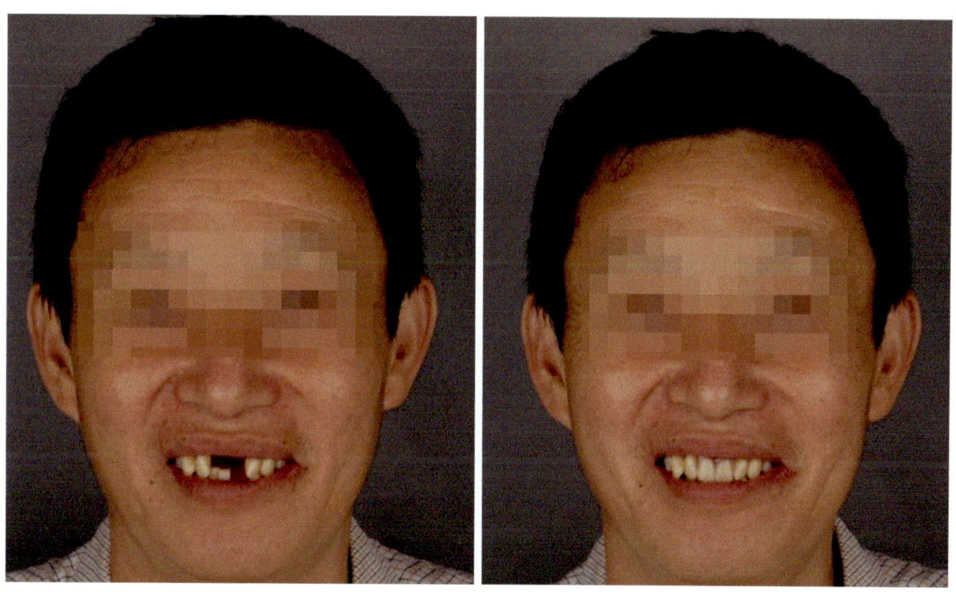

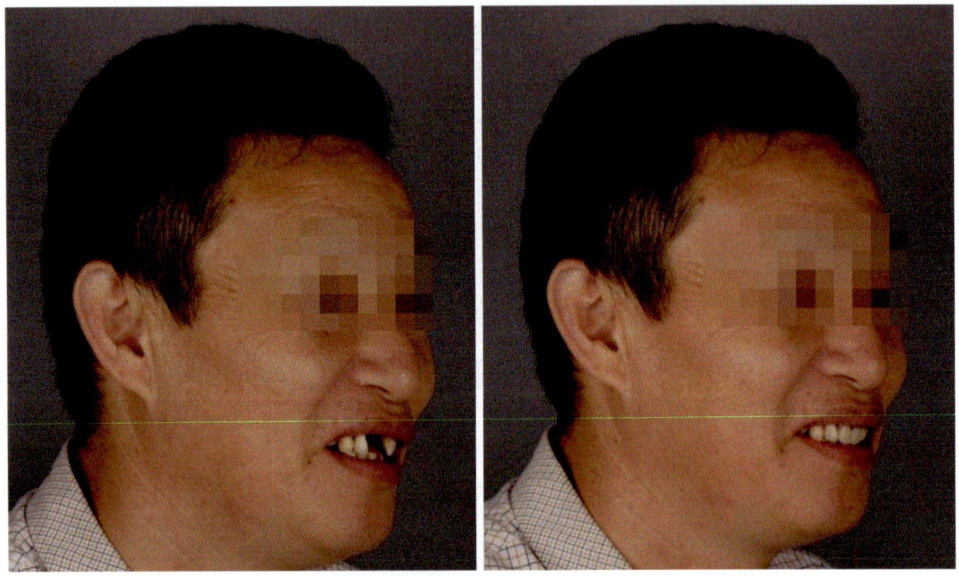

Fig. 6.146 Comparison before and after restoration in the facial lateral view

6.19 Case 19

E-Clasps Combined with Deformed Occlusal Rest in Digital Framework RPD Design to Correct Spee Curve

1. *Before repair*

   A woman, 60 years old. Maxillary and mandibular dentition defects have been for more than 30 years.

   Smile analysis: The patient's face is symmetrical with a relatively normal proportion, and the height of basifacial 1/3 is acceptable (Fig. 6.147). The patient has a low smile line, whose upper teeth cannot be exposed when smiling. The esthetic teeth are C4–D3 with the visible cervix of teeth (Fig. 6.148).

   Dentition analysis: The patient with Kennedy III dentition defect in the upper and lower jaw has deep overbite (Fig. 6.149). And there is no bounce or pain in the temporomandibular joints. Her oral hygiene is average.

2. *RPD analysis design and manufacturing*

   We design a lingual bar as the maxillary major connector to reduce globus sensation. Short buccally retained clasp is placed on the abutments A5, B4, C4, and D2 to reduce the clasp exposure when smiling. A combined clasp is placed on B6 and B7 to ensure the retention of the maxillary framework.

   Because the remaining teeth of the lower jaw are worn, the contour of the retaining teeth is utilized for clasp design as full as possible. The undercut of C4 is concentrated on the lingual surface, so a three-arm clasp with lingual retentive arm and buccal resistant arm is designed. At the same time, taking advantage of the existing gap between D2 and D3, a short buccally retained clasp is placed on D2. A distal adjacent surface plate is placed on D3 to enhance friction retention. Because the crown of C7 is short, metal occlusal surface is designed on C7 to restore a certain occlusal curve. The major connector design of the mandible framework adopts a lingual plate to ensure the stability of the framework (Fig. 6.150); try the wax pattern in the mouth after teeth arrangement (Fig. 6.151). When the patient is satisfied, complete the restoration (Fig. 6.152).

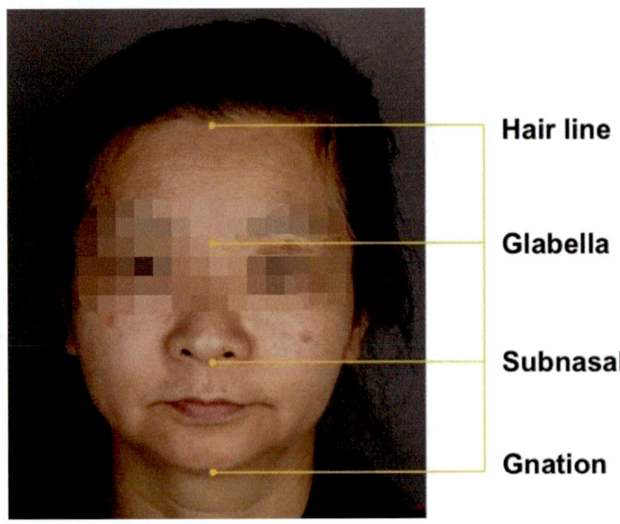

Fig. 6.147 Facial analysis. Normal proportion of the three courts and proper height of lower facial 1/3

3. *After restoration*

   The final repair effect is shown in Fig. 6.153. The clasp exposure is minimal when the patient smiles. The maxillary artificial teeth and denture base improve the facial protrusion. The patient's face is younger than the condition before restoration (Fig. 6.154). She is quite contented.

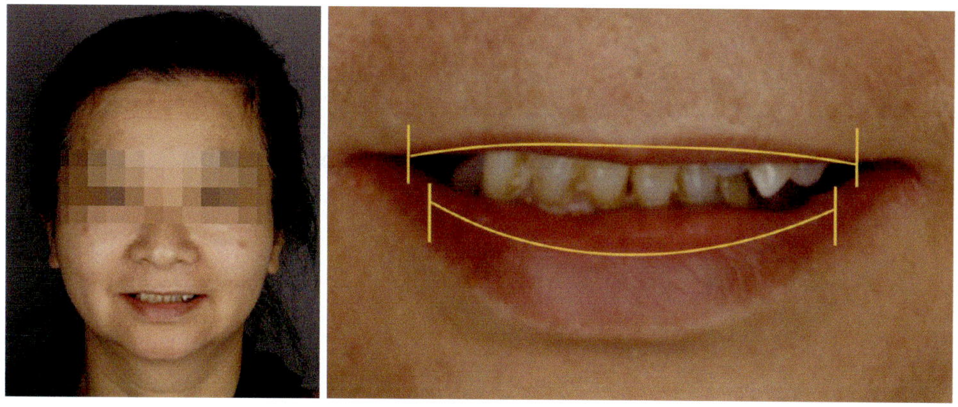

Fig. 6.148 Smile analysis. This patient is low smile line. Esthetic teeth are C4–D3

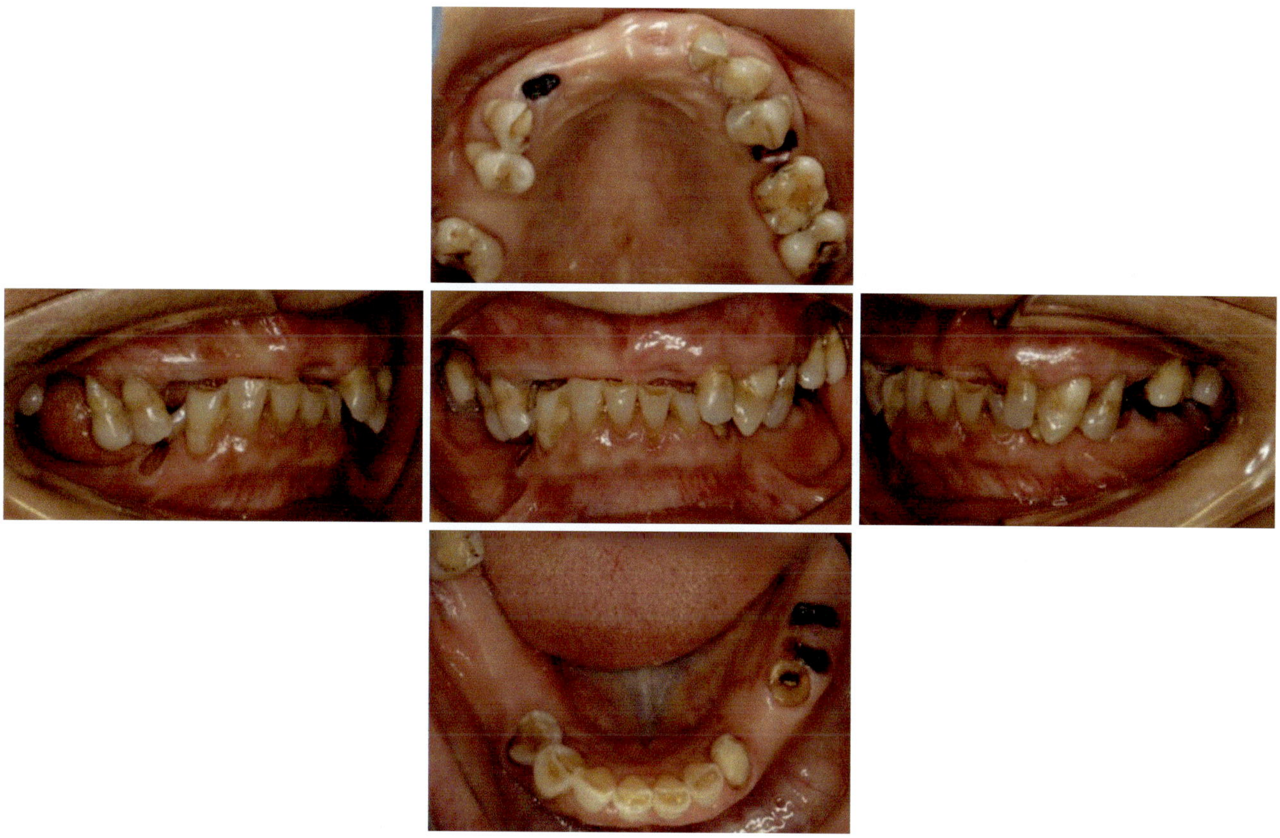

Fig. 6.149 Intraoral view

Fig. 6.150 Framework design

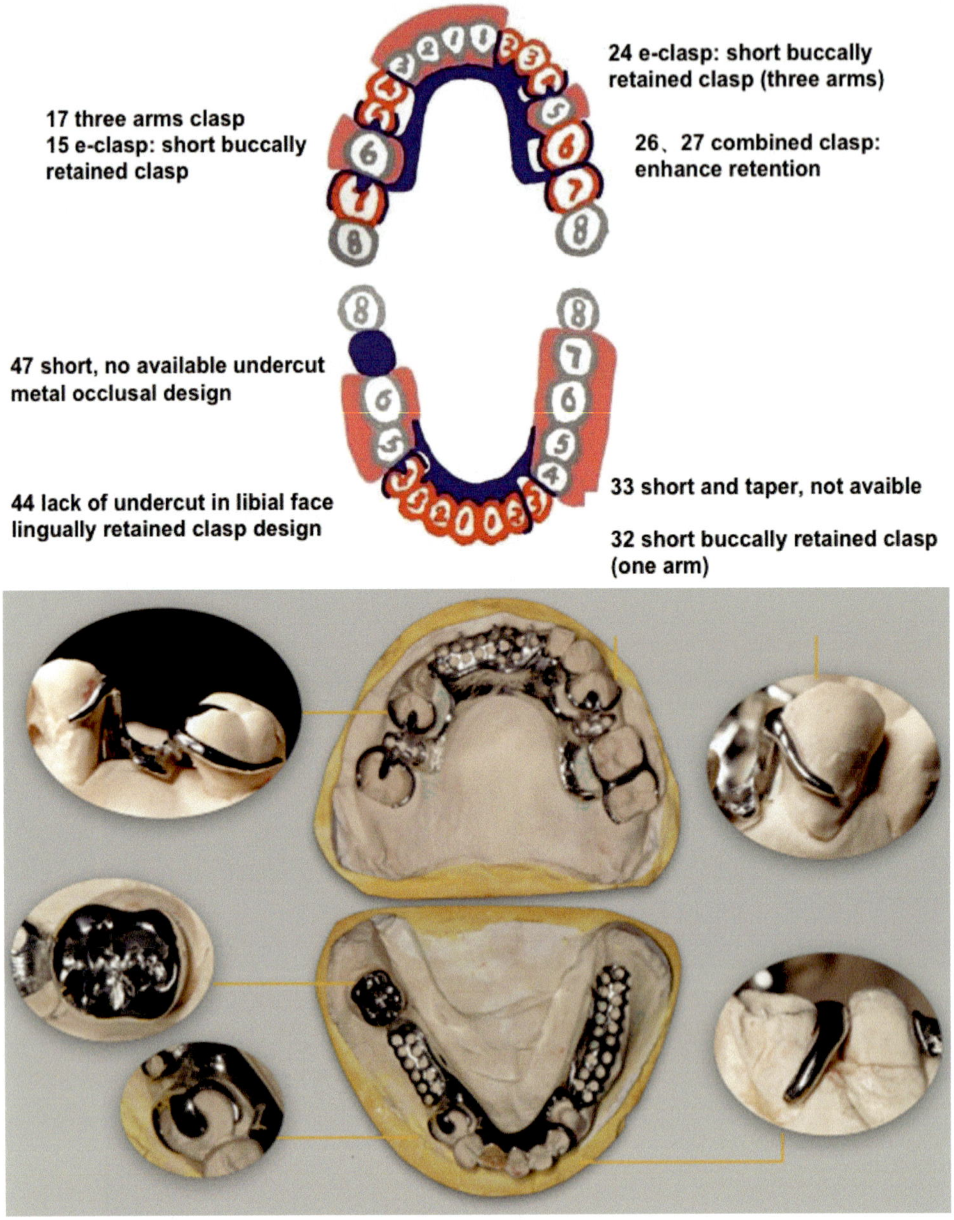

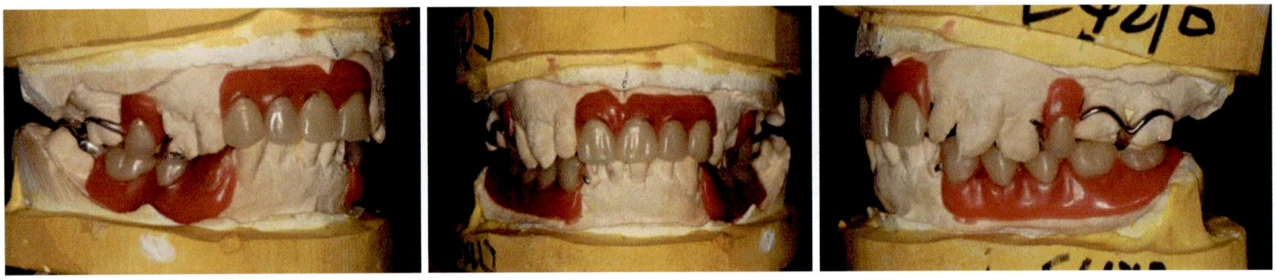

Fig. 6.151 Trying in after teeth arrangement

Fig. 6.152 Restoration completion

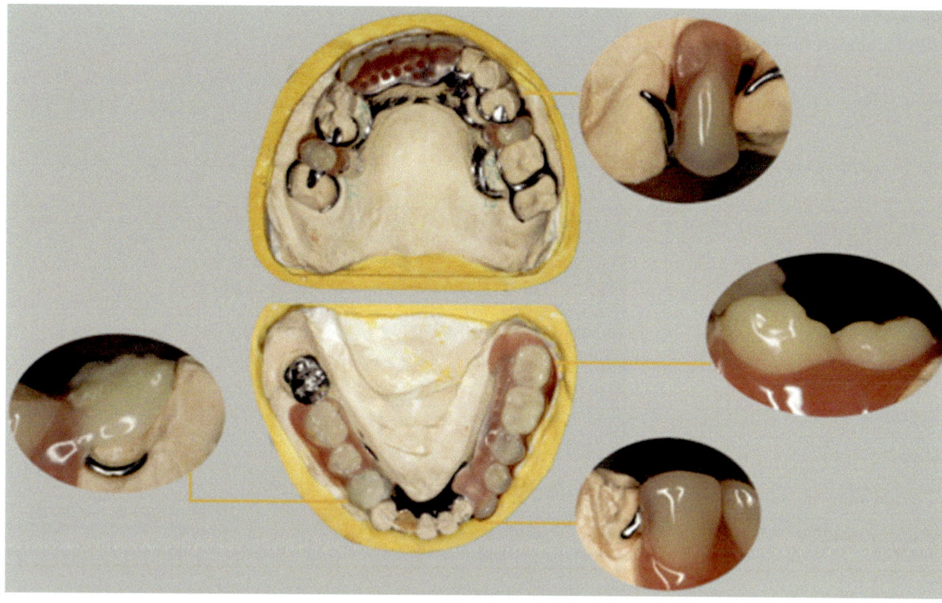

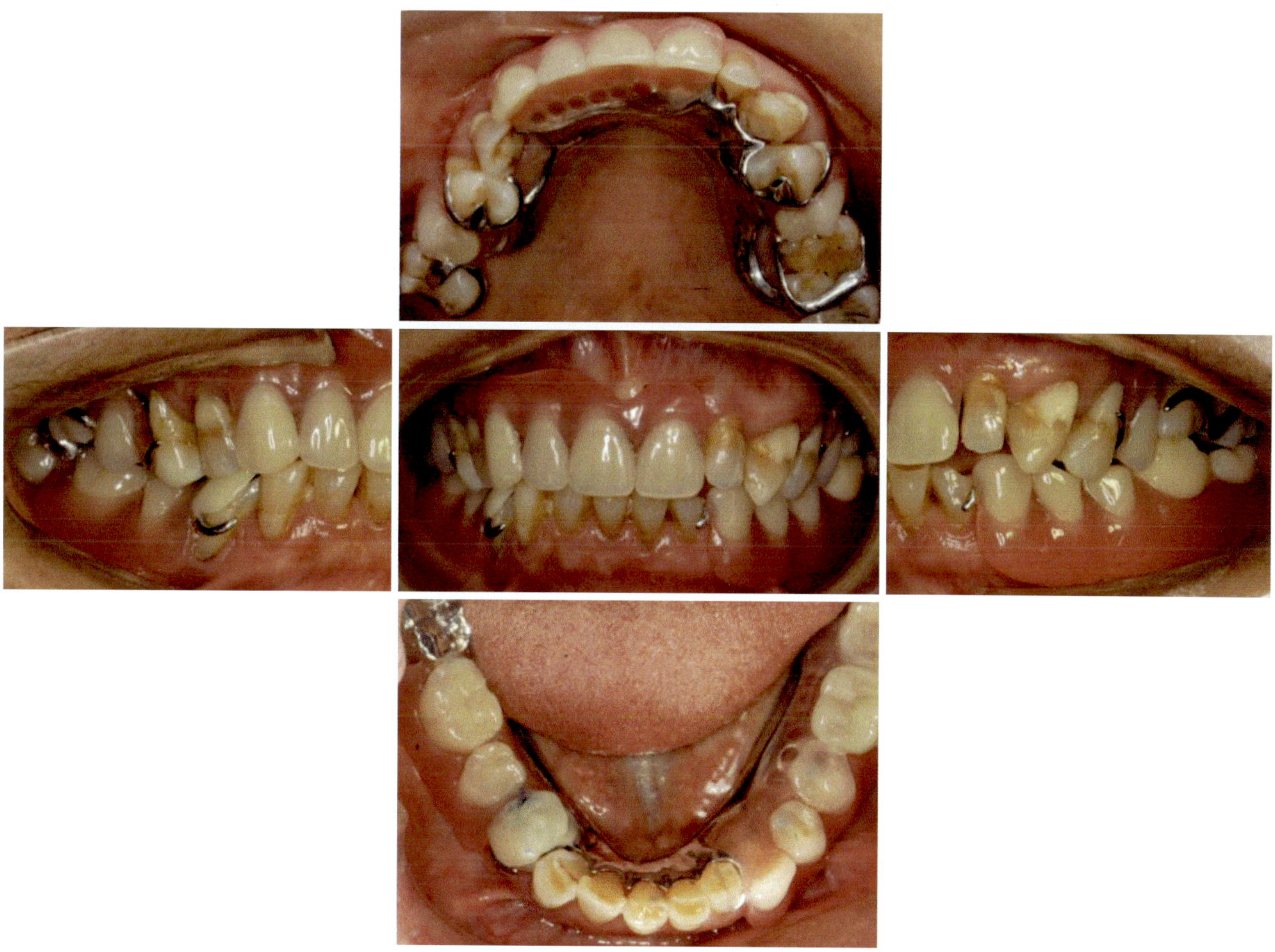

Fig. 6.153 Intraoral view with denture

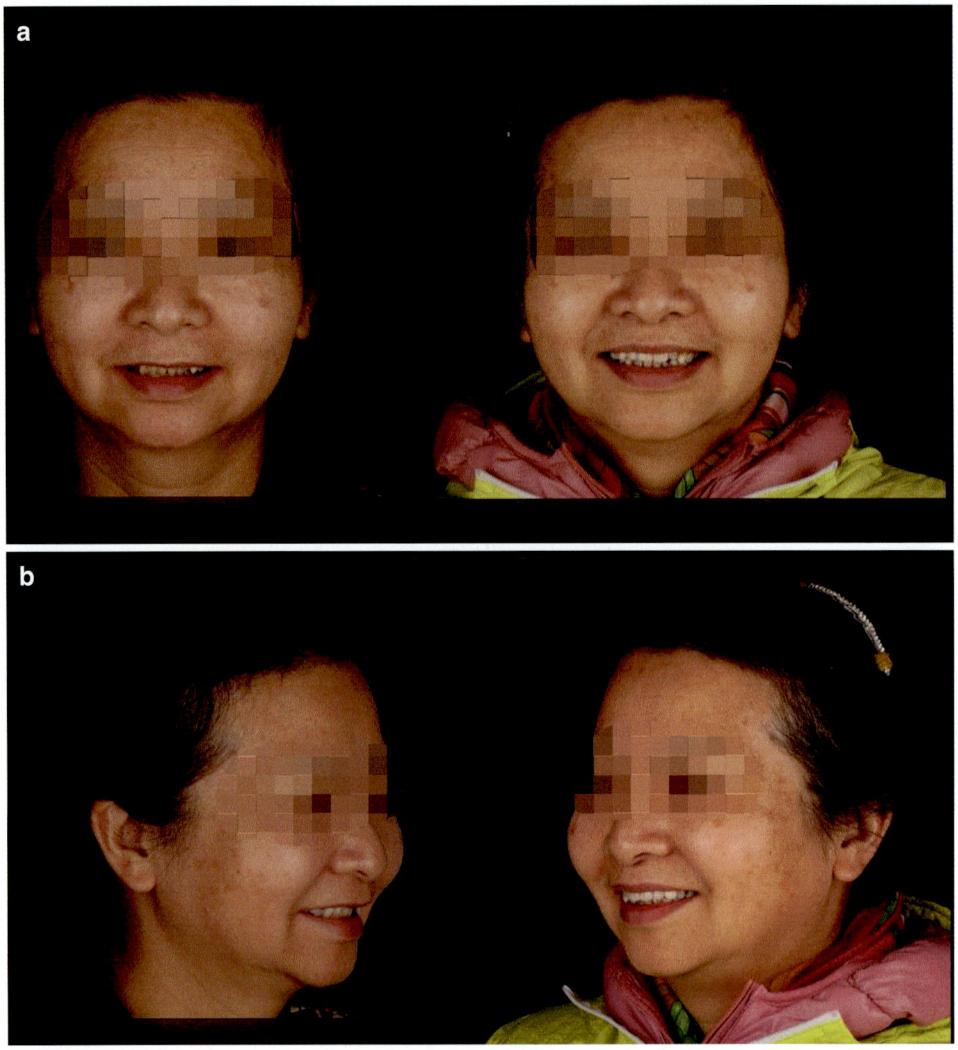

Fig. 6.154 Comparison before and after restoration. (**a**) Facial frontal view. (**b**) Facial lateral view

6.20 Case 20

E-Clasps Combined with Metal Occlusal Surface in Digital Framework RPD Design for Patient with Dentition Defect and Insufficient Restoration Space

1. *Before restoration*

   A male, 52 years old. Ten years ago, the patient underwent maxillary and mandibular prosthesis. Due to the partial fracture of the denture clasp, the denture was unstable. Now, he requires restoration.

   The patient has a scar on the left cheek, mouth-opening limitation, and poor oral hygiene condition. The patient has Kennedy III dentition defect on the maxilla and Kennedy IV dentition defect on the mandible. There is a residual root B4 and deep overbite. His occlusion is so tight that the left mandibular teeth contact on the maxillary alveolar ridge. The position of the alveolar ridge in the upper jaw is too close to the outside of paired jaw teeth. If the occlusal function is ensured according to the conventional teeth arrangement and occlusal design, the position of the artificial teeth will be too close to the lingual side, which affects the esthetics. Or if we arrange teeth and improve esthetics in accordance with the contour of the upper jaw, this position will lose occlusal contact, which affects function and may cause elongation of the paired jaw teeth. Therefore, in this case, the design of dentures with both esthetics and function becomes difficult. In addition, a large amount of soft tartar deposits can be seen in the patient's mouth, which indicates his poor oral hygiene (Figs. 6.155 and 6.156).

2. *RPD analysis design and manufacturing*

   In consideration of both esthetics and function of the denture, we apply the design of double dentition for B4, B5, and B6 in the upper jaw: the inner metal occlusal sur-

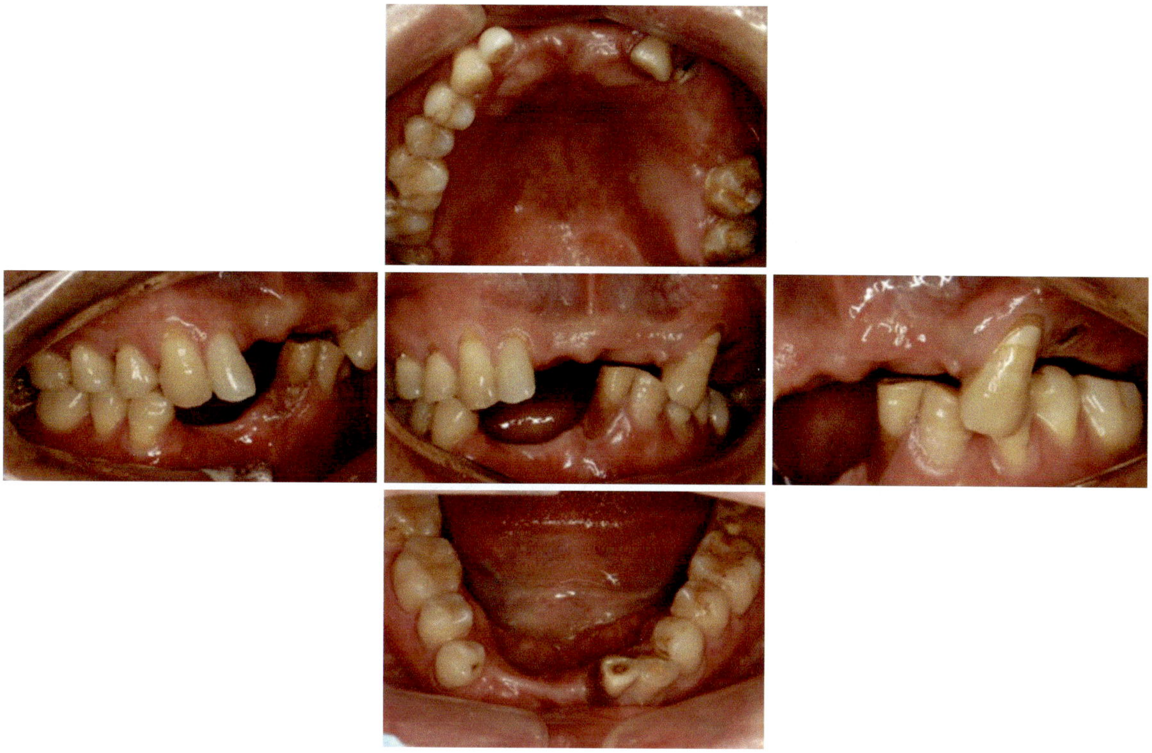

Fig. 6.155 Intraoral view

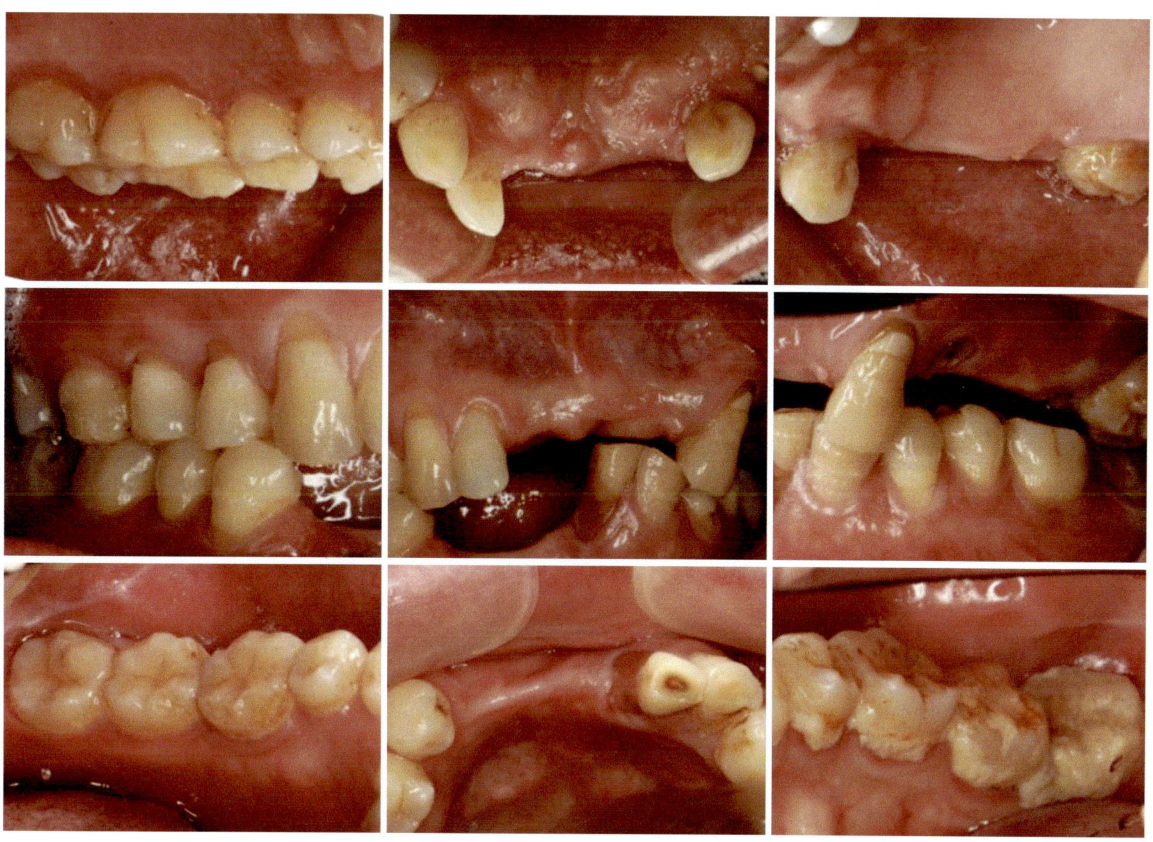

Fig. 6.156 Intraoral partial view

face to restore function and the outer plastic artificial tooth to improve esthetics. In the anterior region, a united short-arm clasp is placed on A3 and A4, and a short buccally retained clasp is placed on B3. At the same time, a three-arm clasp is placed on B7 in the posterior region to ensure the retention of the framework. A rest is set on B7, and a lingual plate is used as the major connector to ensure the entire stability. On C4 and C5, D4, and D5 in the lower jaw, united short-arm clasps are placed to ensure retention (Fig. 6.157). After the framework is completed (Fig. 6.158), try it in the mouth. The denture is in good position, the clasps fit the abutment, the retention force is moderate, and there is no movement (Fig. 6.159). The restoration is finally completed (Fig. 6.160).

3. *After restoration*

   There is little clasp exposure, and denture is retentive and stable without movement. This solution restore the patient's occlusal function while taking into account the esthetics. Finally, the patient expresses satisfaction (Fig. 6.161).

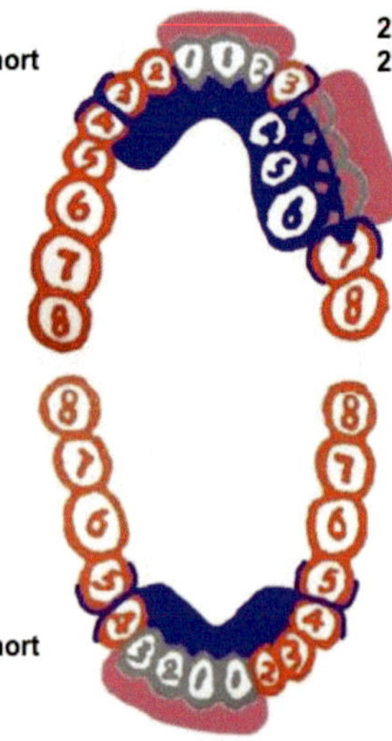

Fig. 6.157 Framework design

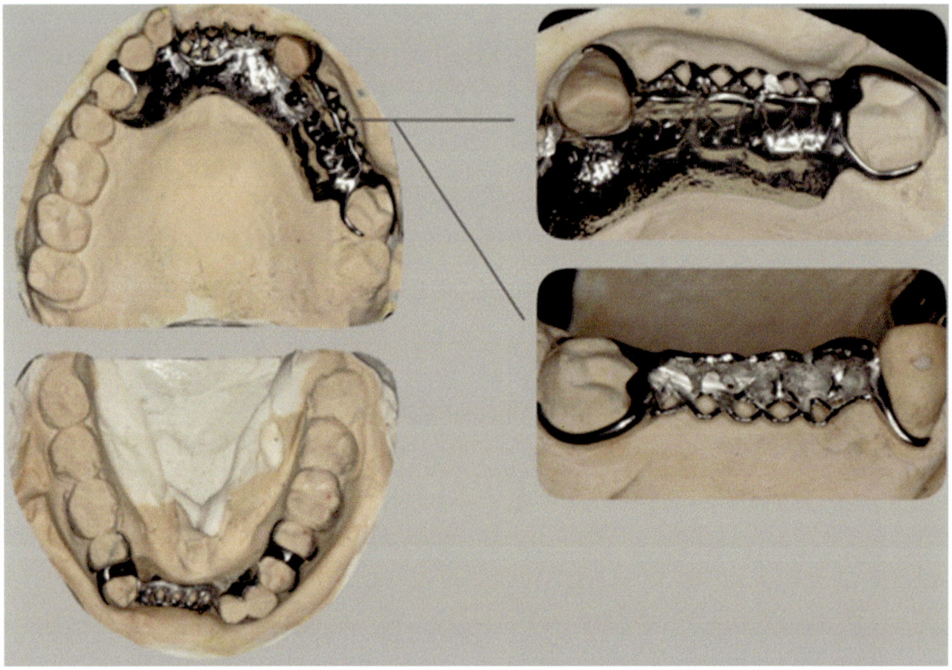

Fig. 6.158 Framework completion

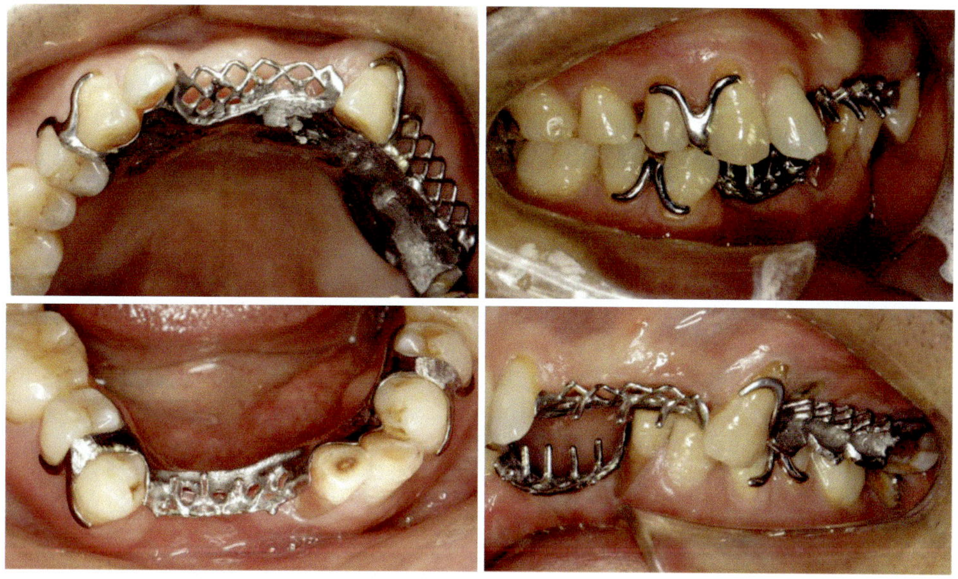

Fig. 6.159 The framework tried both on the model and in the mouth is well positioned, the clasps fit the abutment, the retention force is moderate, and it is stable without movement

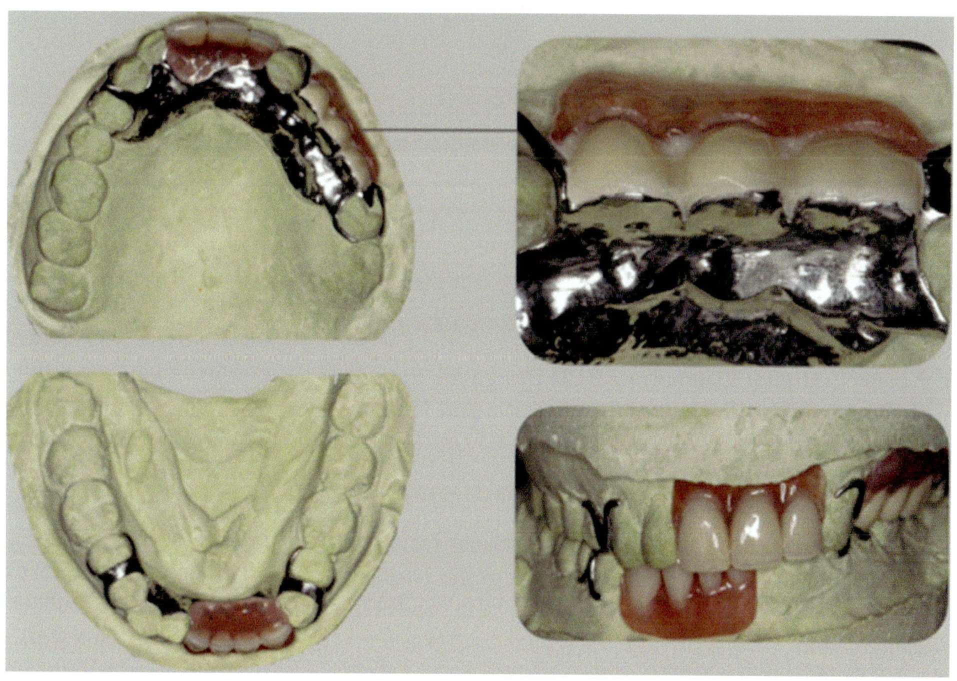

Fig. 6.160 Final restoration completion

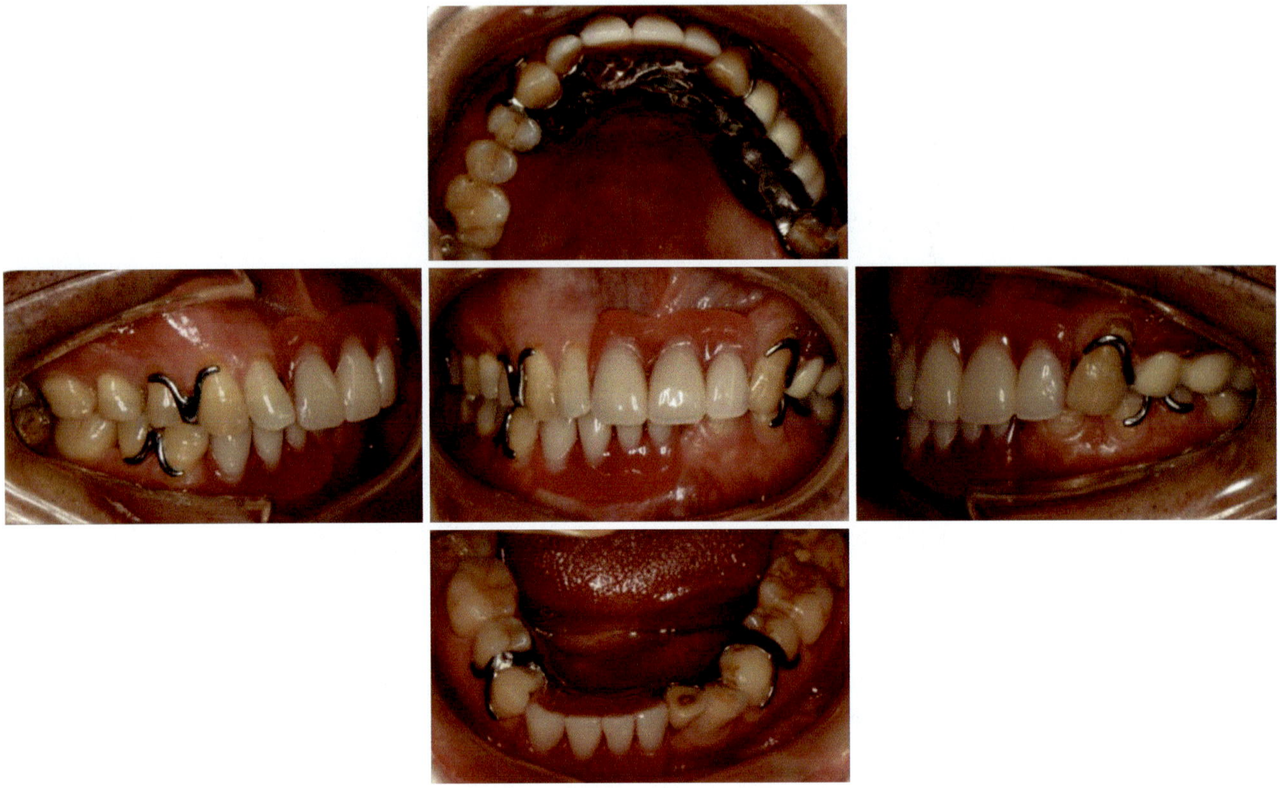

Fig. 6.161 Intraoral view with denture

6.21 Case 21

E-Clasps in Digital Framework RPD Design for Patient with Bilateral Maxillary Free-End Edentia and High Laugh Line

1. *Before restoration*

   A woman, 60 years old.

   Facial analysis: The patient has a normal facial pattern, symmetrical face, a normal height of the basifacial 1/3, and a high smile line. The esthetic teeth are A3–B3 (Fig. 6.162).

   Dentition analysis: The patient has Kennedy I dentition defect on the maxilla and Kennedy III dentition defect on the mandible. Her missing teeth are A4–A7, B4–B7, C1–C2, C5–C7, D1, and D5–D7 (Fig. 6.163). She has poor oral hygiene.

2. *RPD analysis design and manufacturing*

   Maxillary dentition is bilateral free-end edentulous. C clasps are placed on A3 and B3. Because the abutments are located in the esthetic area, in addition to considering the location of the undercut when designing the clasps, we try to place the tip of the clasp on the gingival covert location. Because there are many missing teeth and bilateral free-end loss, a full palate is designed as the major connector to disperse the force (Fig. 6.164). There is bilateral free-end edentia in the lower jaw. Combined clasps are placed on C3–C4 and D3–D4. Mesial rests are placed to reduce the lateral force on the abutment and protect the abutment (Fig. 6.165).

   When the framework is tried in the mouth, it is retentive and stable without movement (Fig. 6.166). The details of the framework are shown in Fig. 6.167. Due to free-end edentia in the upper and lower jaws, the vertical height cannot be determined. The occlusal relationship is recorded by a wax rim (Fig. 6.168). After arranging the teeth according to the occlusal relationship, the wax pattern is tried in the mouth (Fig. 6.169).

3. *After restoration*

   The final effect with denture is shown in Fig. 6.170. The denture is stable with little clasp exposure when smiling. The effect before restoration is shown in Fig. 6.171. The patient is satisfied.

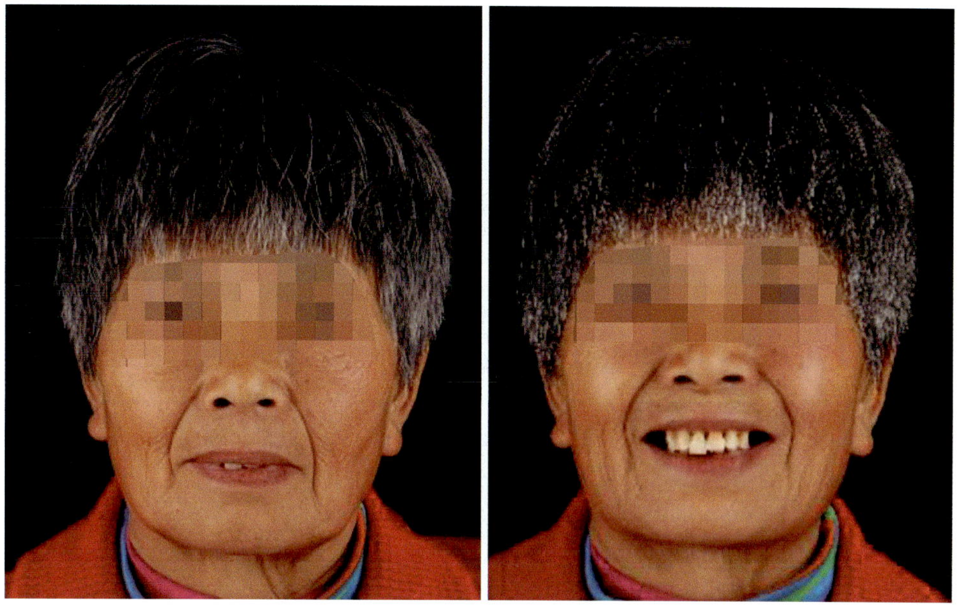

Fig. 6.162 Facial analysis

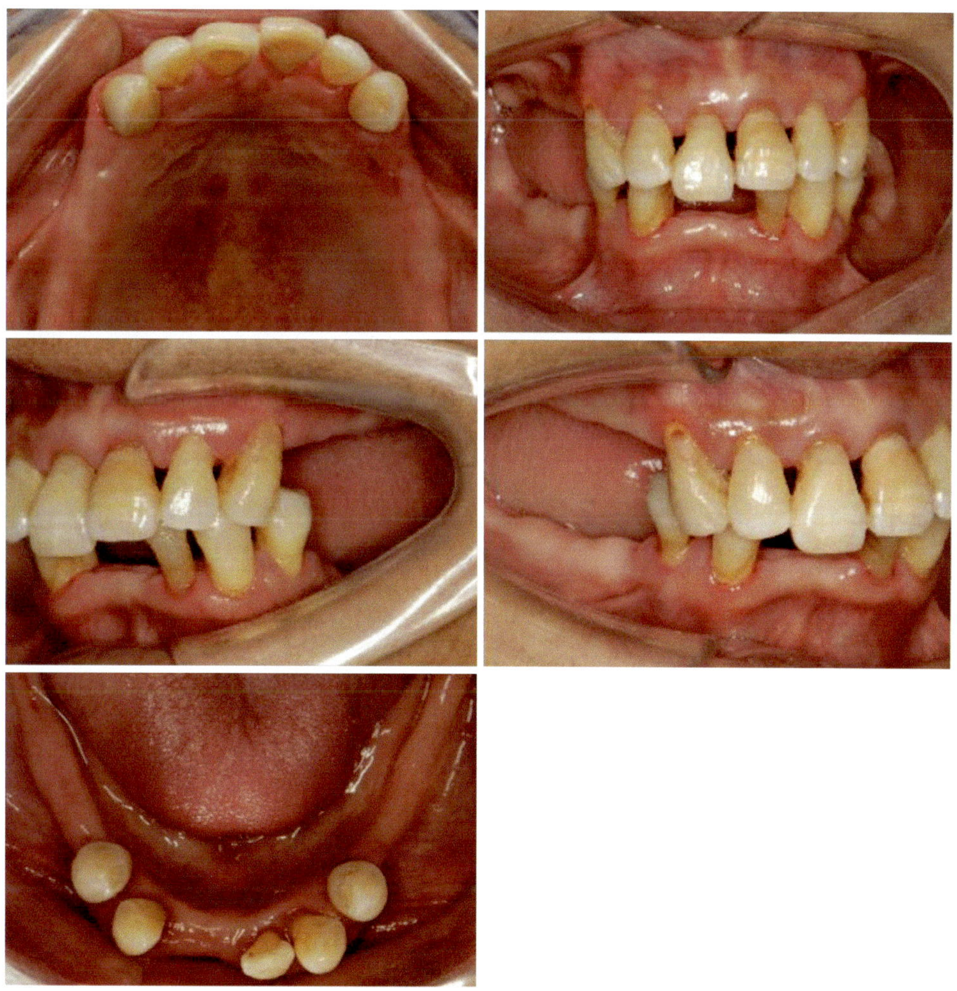

Fig. 6.163 Intraoral view

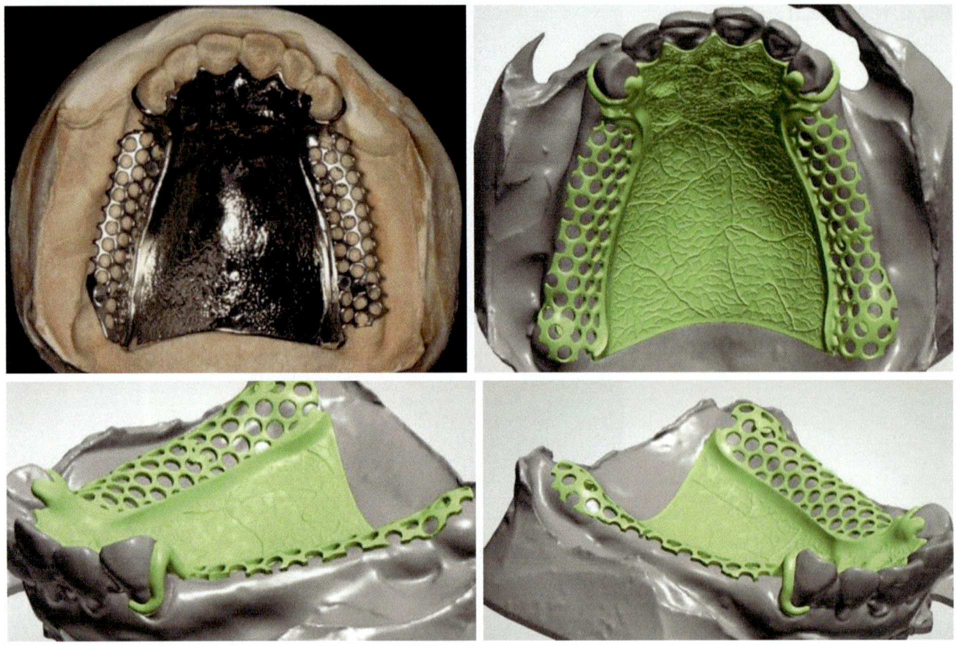

Fig. 6.164 Maxillary framework design

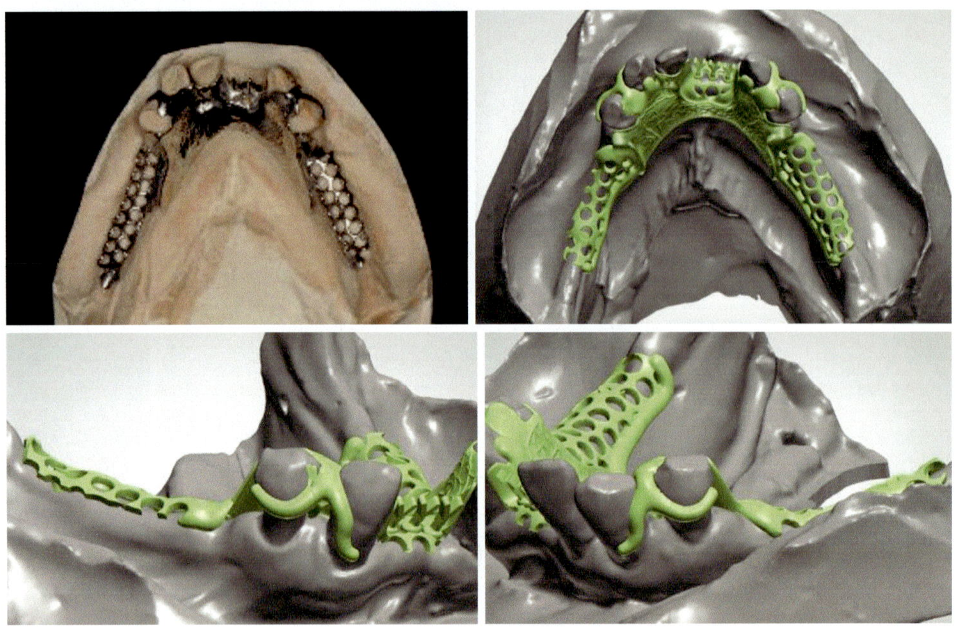

Fig. 6.165 Mandibular framework design

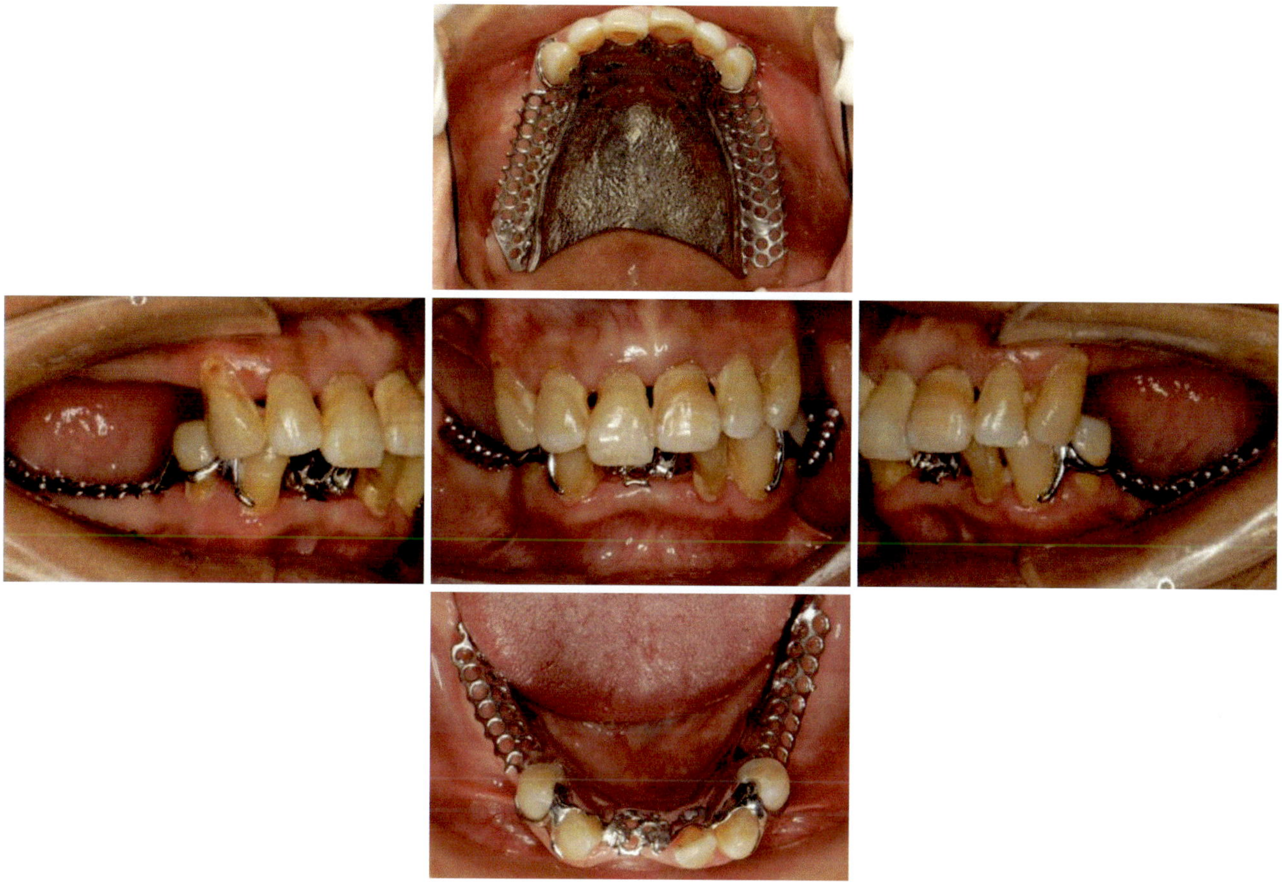

Fig. 6.166 Trying in of the framework

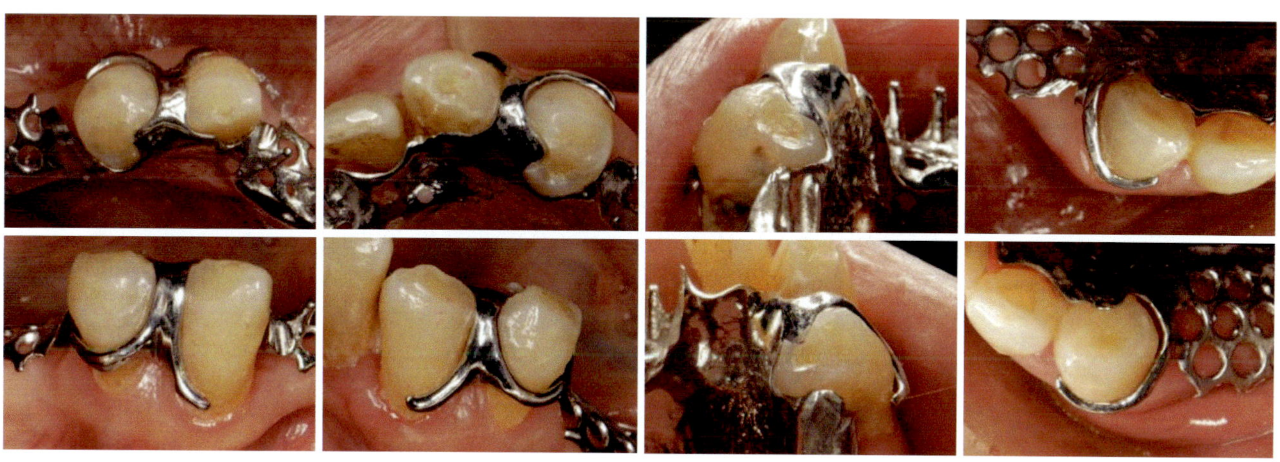

Fig. 6.167 Framework details

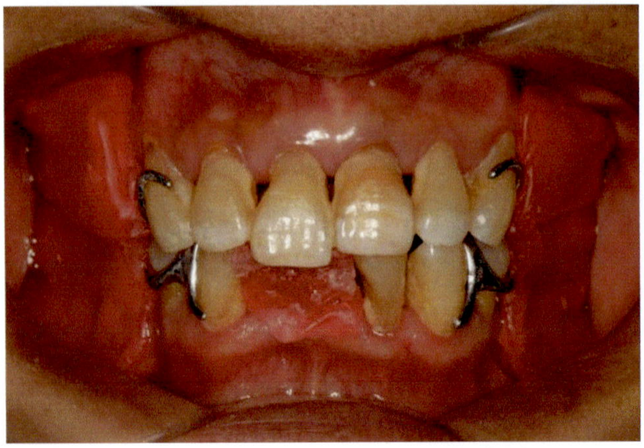

Fig. 6.168 Recording occlusal relationship by a wax rim

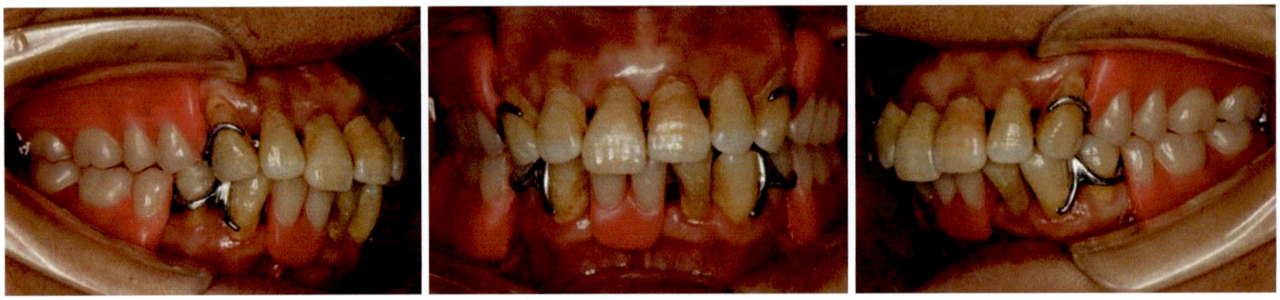

Fig. 6.169 Trying in of the wax pattern

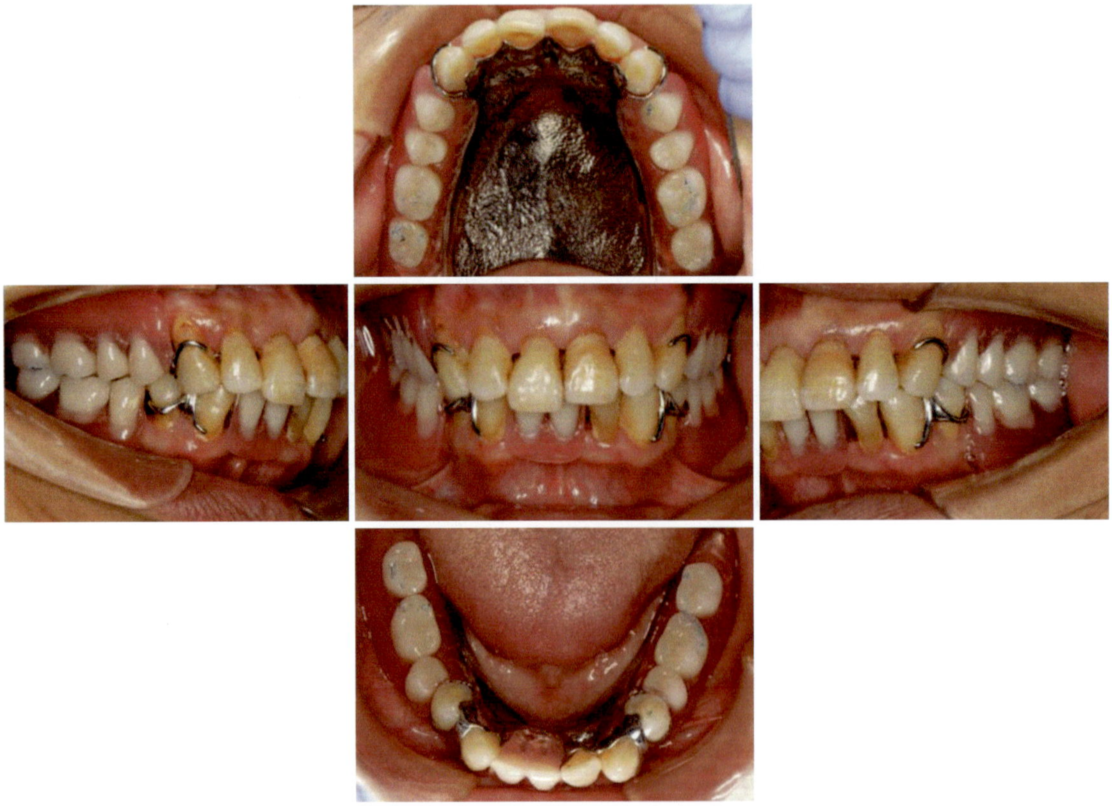

Fig. 6.170 Intraoral view with denture

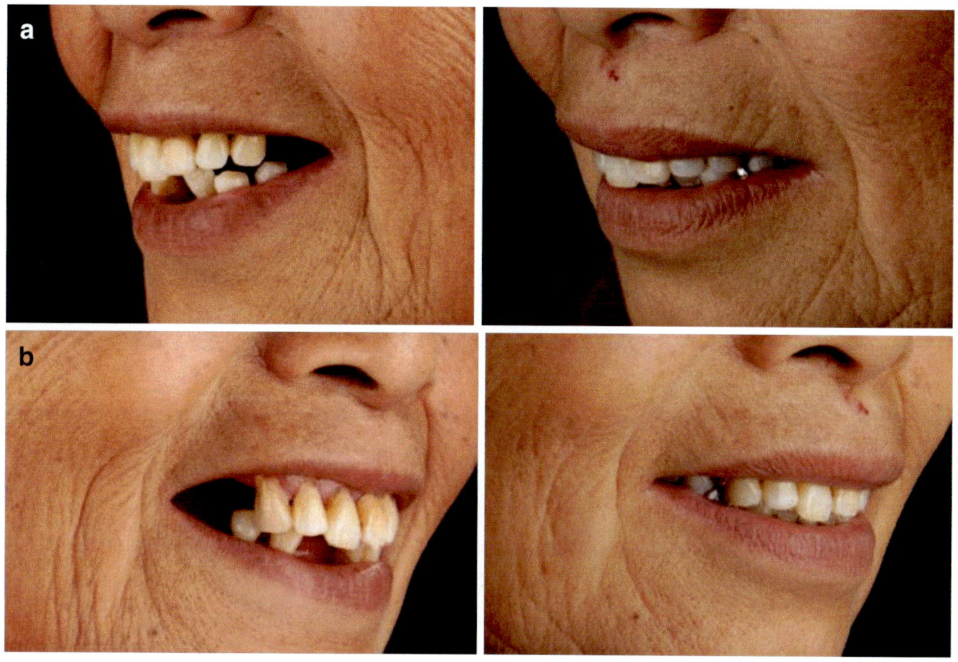

Fig. 6.171 Comparison before and after restoration. (**a**) Facial left lateral view. (**b**) Facial right lateral view

6.22 Case 22

A man, 80 years old. In the past 1 year, the denture was conscious of poor retention, stability, and masticatory function.

1. *Before restoration*
   The patient's face is symmetrical. Due to the absence of upper and lower dentition, the lower 1/3 of the face becomes shorter, and a deeper nasolabial groove can be seen (Fig. 6.172). In the mouth, the alveolar ridge of the mandible is low and flat, and the posterior tooth area is blade-shape (Fig. 6.173). There are a lot of dental calculus, plaque, and pigmentation in the old denture; the denture does not fit well, and the joint wear is serious. No joint abnormality was found after joint consultation.
2. *RPD analysis design and manufacturing*
   Because the patient requires to reduce the volume of complete denture as much as possible to reduce the foreign body sensation, the metal base is used. First, make the initial impression mold (Fig. 6.174), then make individual tray (Fig. 6.175) according to the initial model and initial relationship, use individual tray to obtain the final impression mold and final relationship (Fig. 6.176), try to arrange teeth according to the final model and final relationship (Fig. 6.177), and complete the production of restoration after trial wearing denture (Fig. 6.178).
3. *After restoration*
   See Figs. 6.179 and 6.180 for the final repair effect.

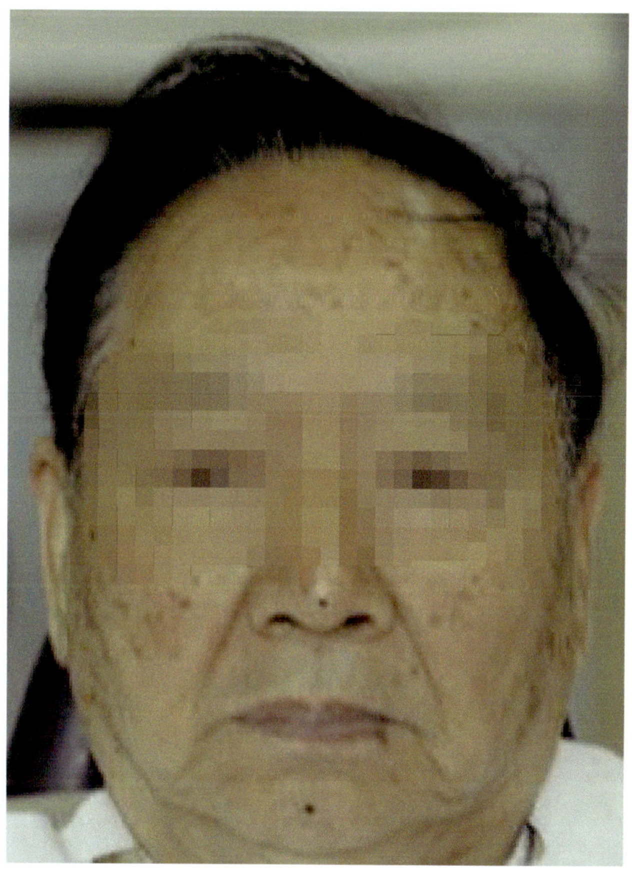

Fig. 6.172 Full-face view

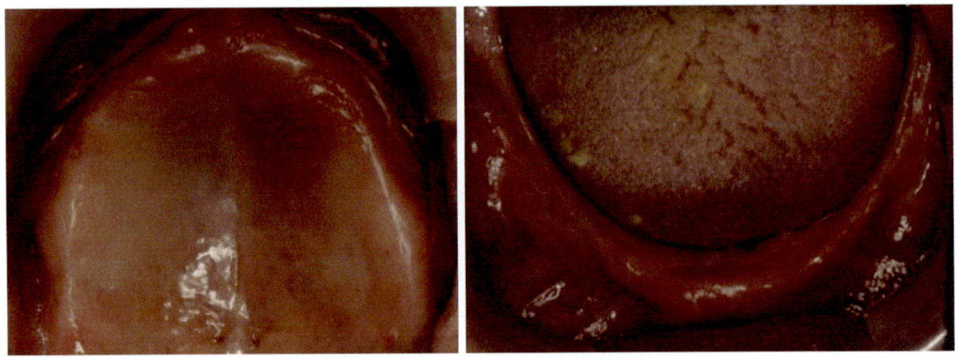

Fig. 6.173 Intraoral view

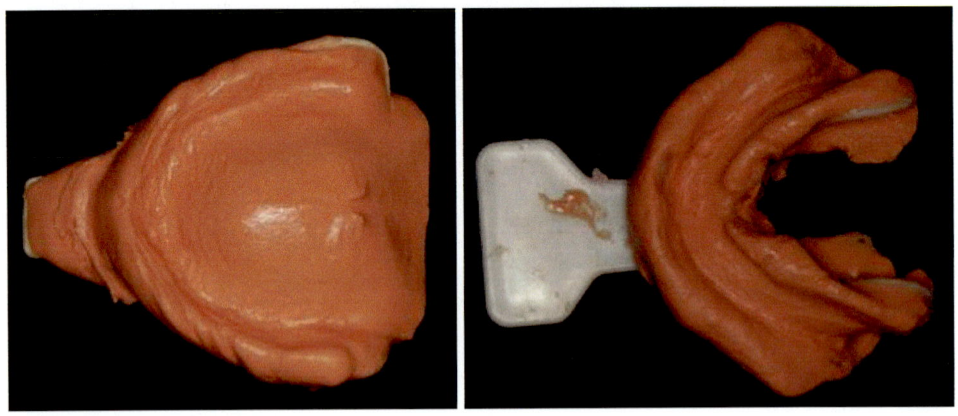

Fig. 6.174 The first impression

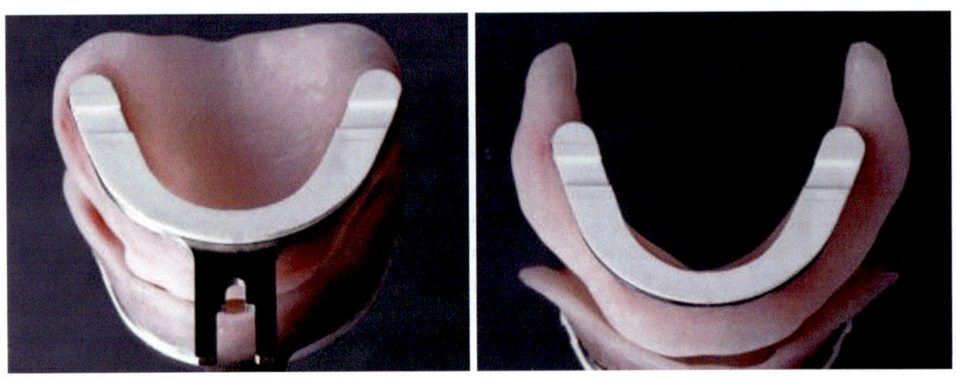

Fig. 6.175 Individual tray

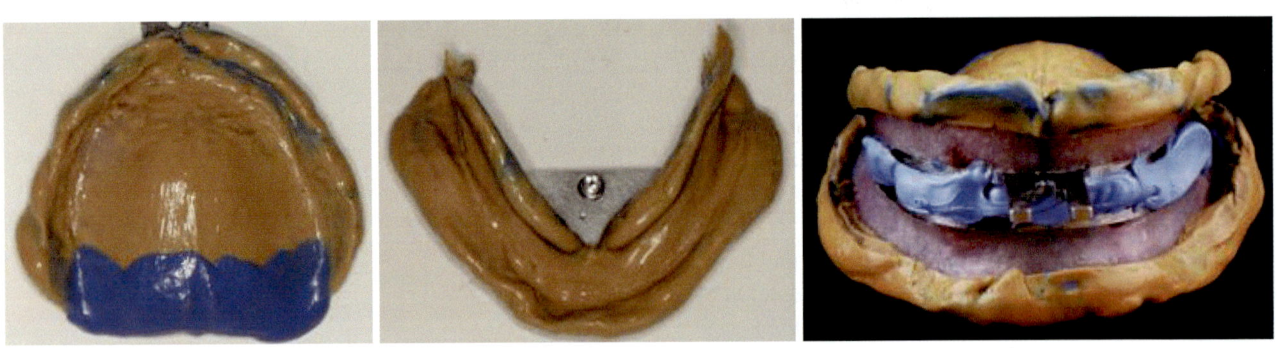

Fig. 6.176 Obtaining final impression and final relation

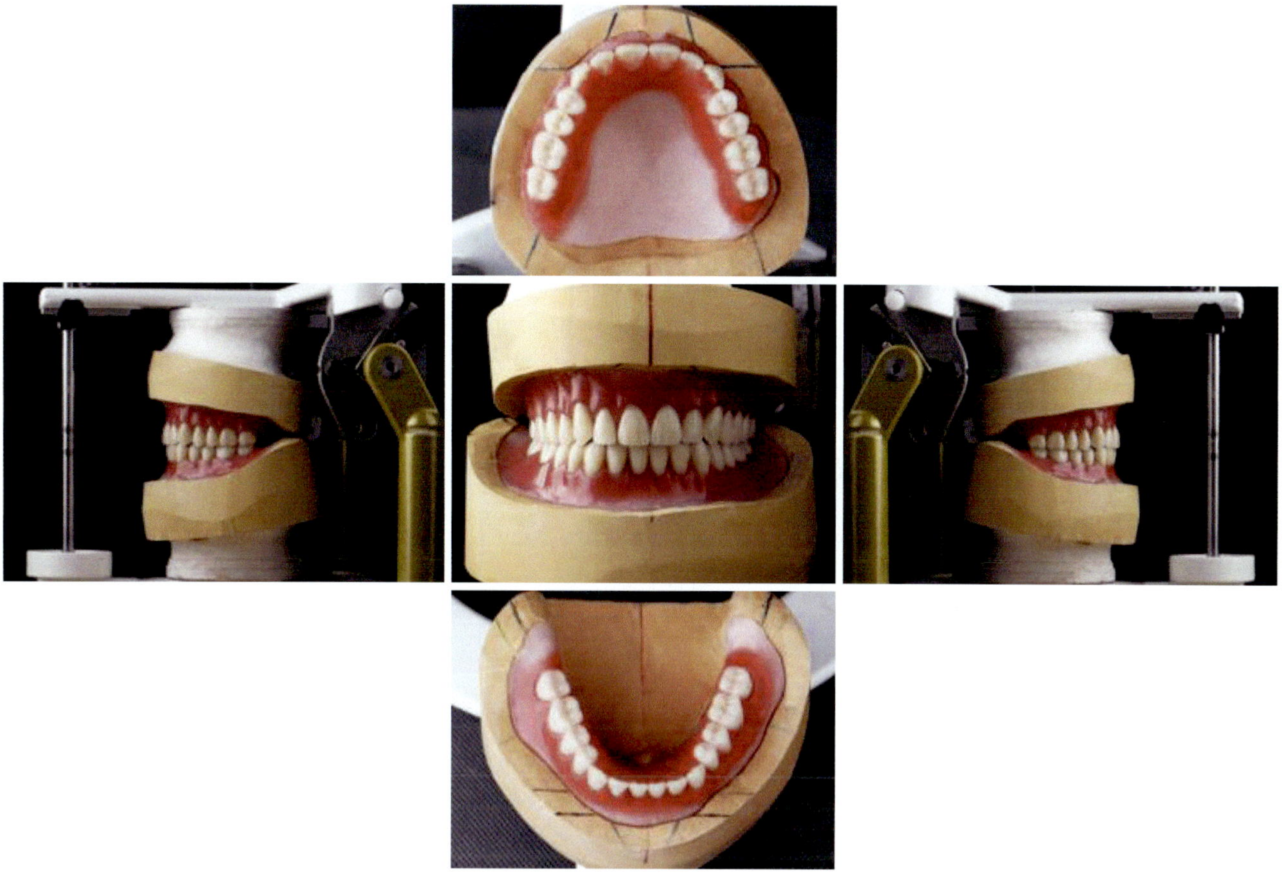

Fig. 6.177 Tooth arrangement

Fig. 6.178 Restoration completion

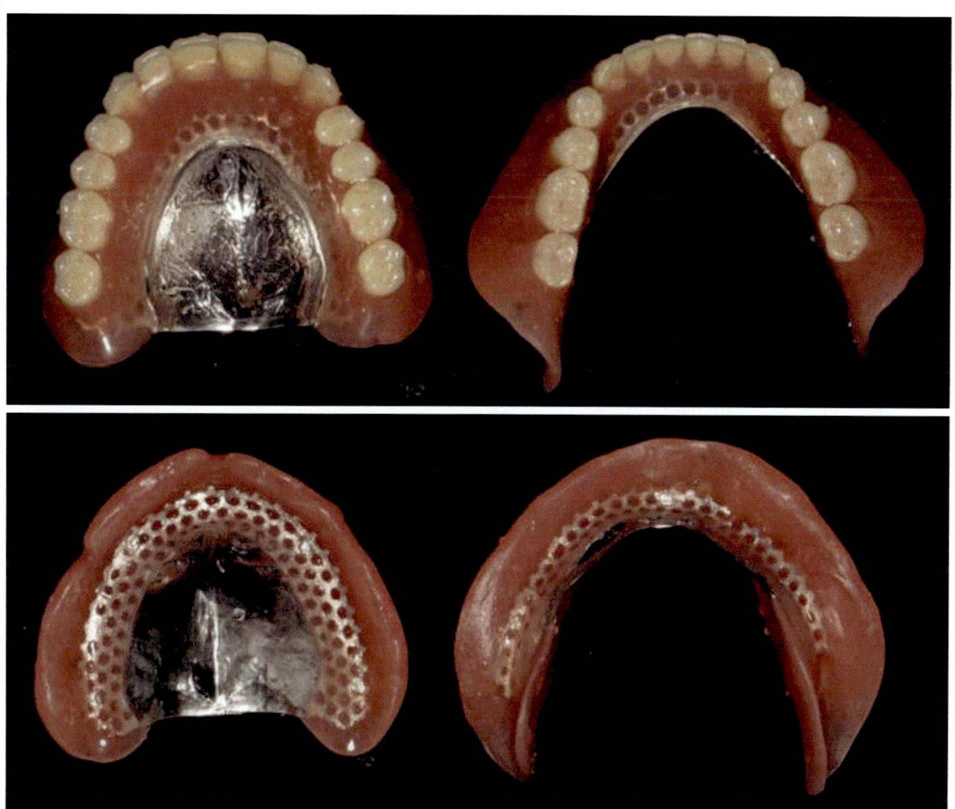

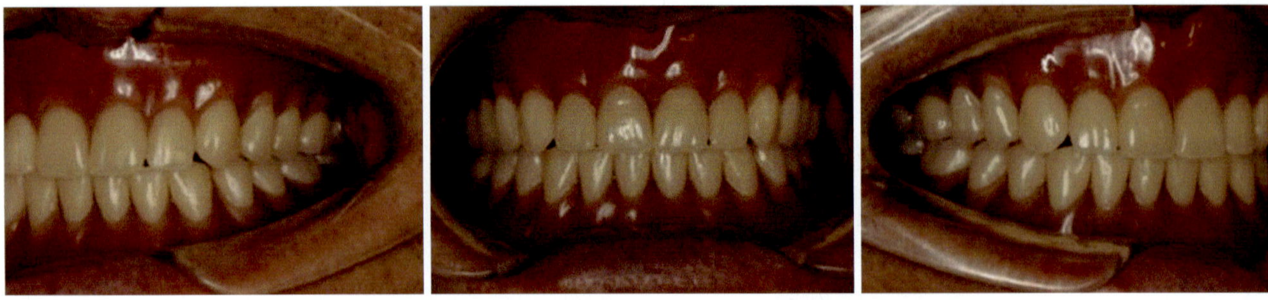

Fig. 6.179 The intraoral renderings

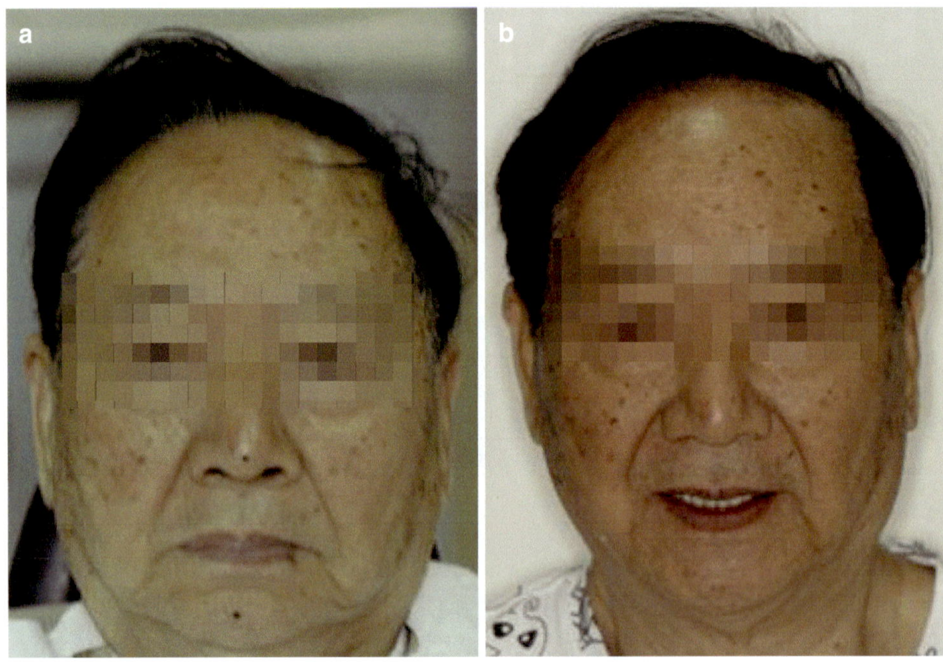

Fig. 6.180 Comparison before and after restoration. (**a**) Before restoration. (**b**) After restoration

6.23 Case 23

1. *Before restoration*

   A woman, 78 years old. Many years ago, all the teeth in the upper jaw were removed due to loose. Now, the old denture is loose, so it is required to make a new denture.

   Because the upper teeth are missing, the face collapses, the nasolabial groove is deep, and the lower teeth can be seen when smiling (Fig. 6.181), showing an aging face. The upper jaw is edentulous, the arch is sharp and round, the attachment position of frenum is high, the top of palate is shallow, and the mandibular is Kennedy III dentition defect. C4–C6 is absent in area C, and the alveolar ridge in the edentulous area is in the shape of a blade (Fig. 6.182). Oral hygiene is poor. In the design of mandibular support, it should be noted that because the complete denture is used in the opposite jaw, the mandibular denture should be as stable as possible to avoid prying. The old mandibular denture is shown in Fig. 6.183.
2. *RPD design and manufacturing*

   The upper jaw is edentulous, so single complete denture is used. For the lower jaw, the combined clasp is placed on D4D5, and the two arm clasp is placed on D7. On the side of edentulous space, the three-arm clasp is placed the distal abutment C7, and the C clasp is placed on the mesial abutment C3. The C clasp design can reduce the lateral force on the mesial abutment C3 while ensuring the retention force and preventing the denture from floating. The double lingual bar major connector design can disperse occlusal force, which has good stability, is convenient for self-cleaning, and promotes gingival health (Fig. 6.184). The design details of mandible framework are shown in Fig. 6.185. The retention of the denture is stable in wax pattern trial wearing (Fig. 6.186).

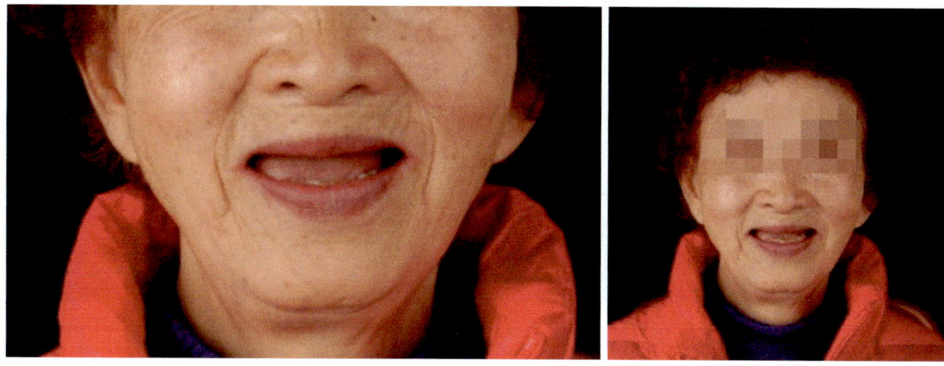

Fig. 6.181 Lower third of facial view

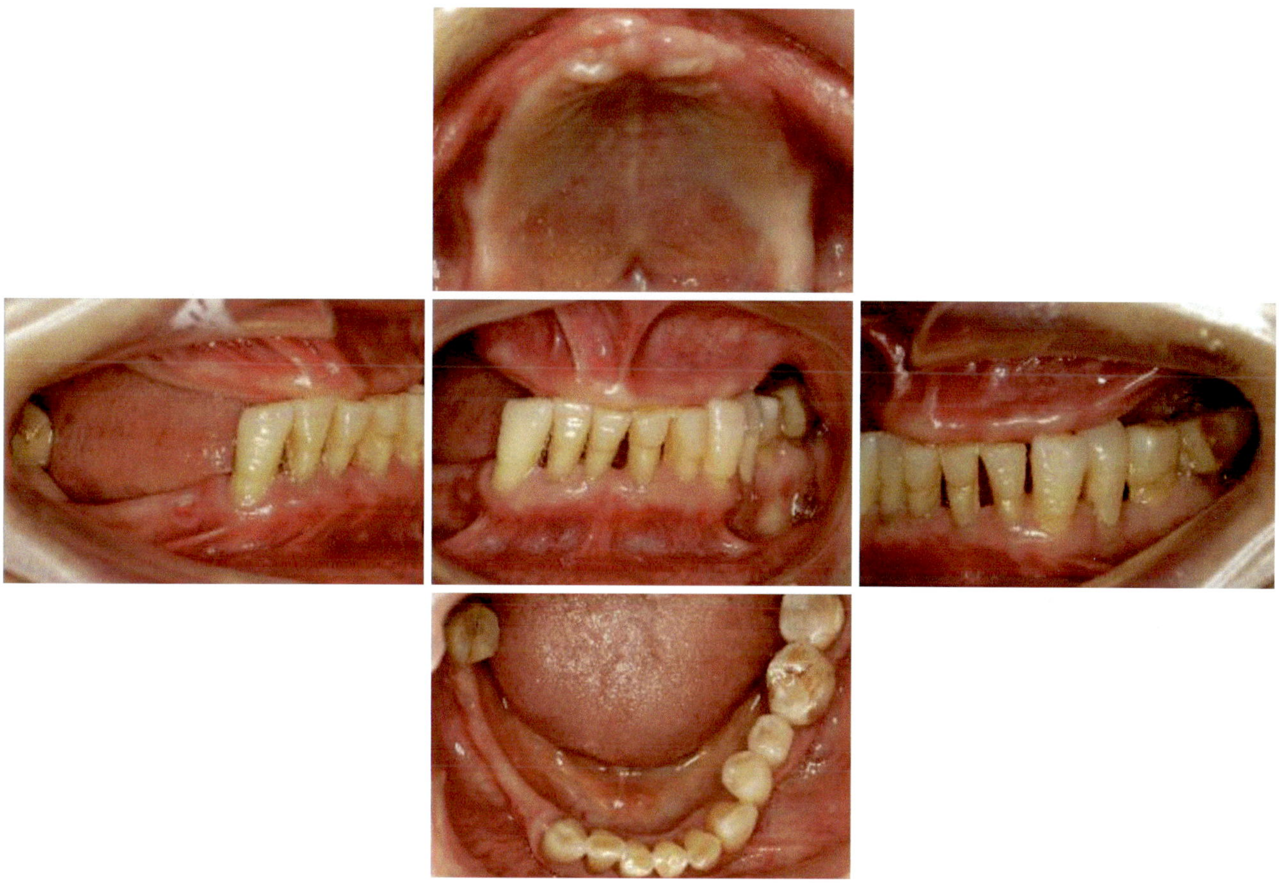

Fig. 6.182 Intraoral condition

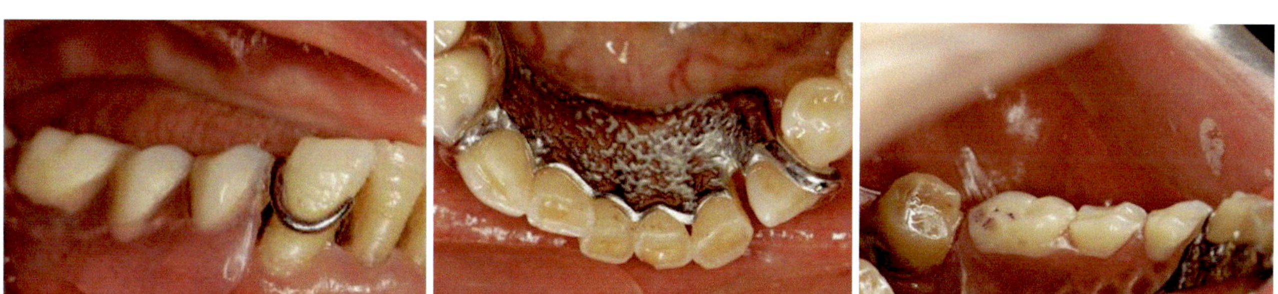

Fig. 6.183 Old mandibular denture

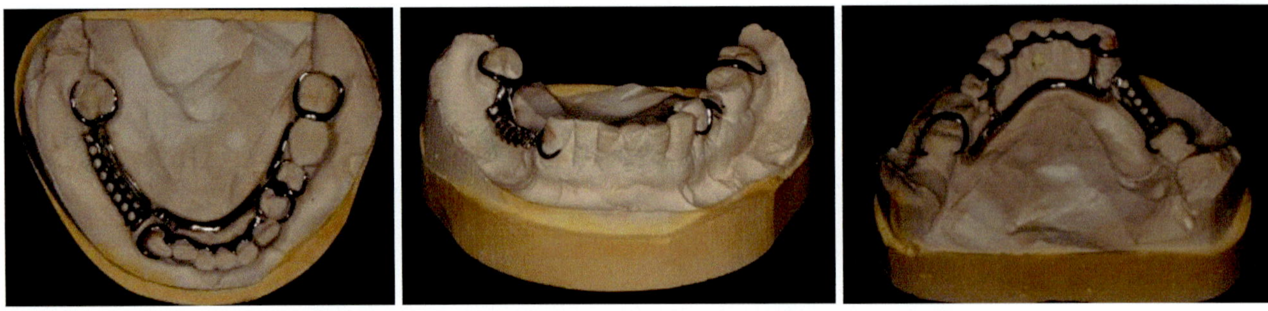

Fig. 6.184 Design of mandible framework

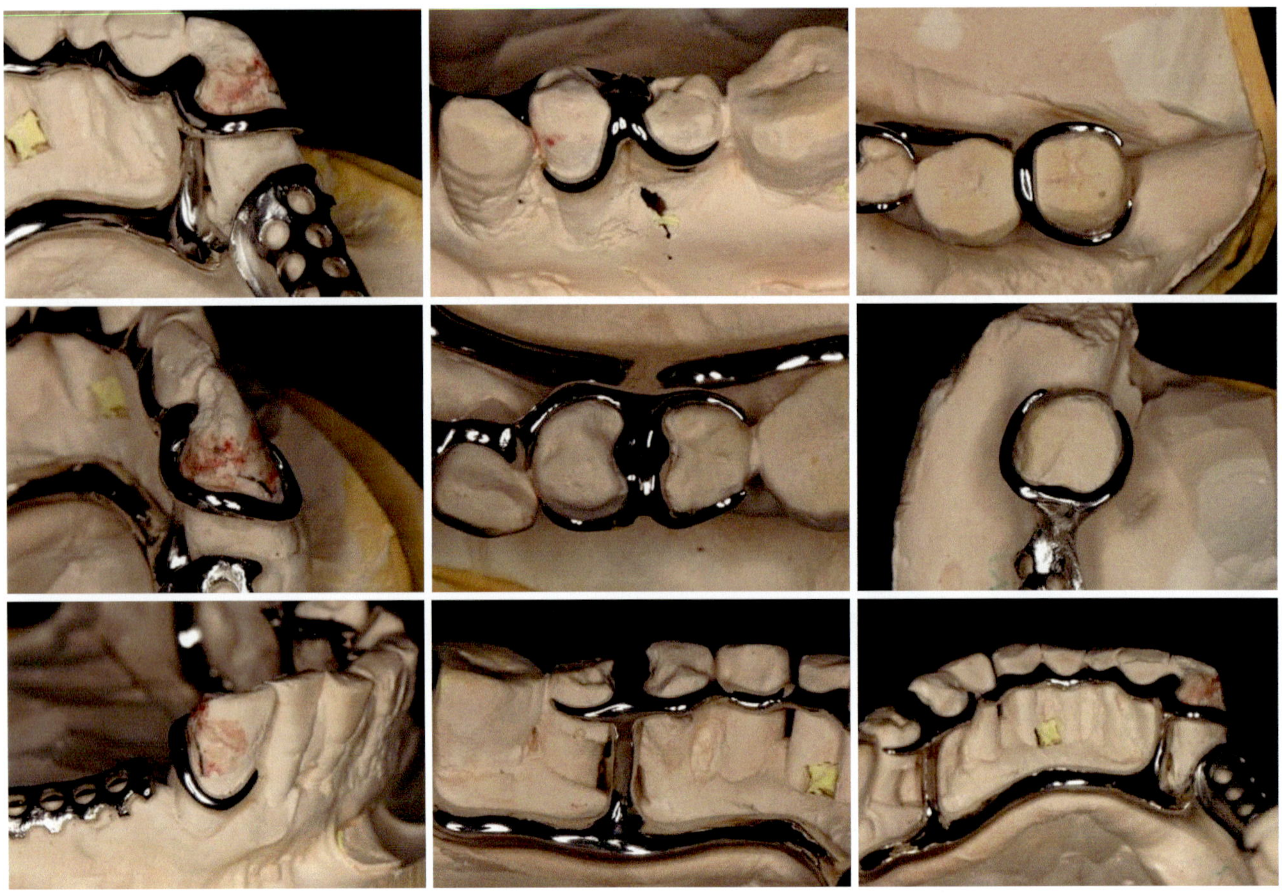

Fig. 6.185 Mandibular stent details

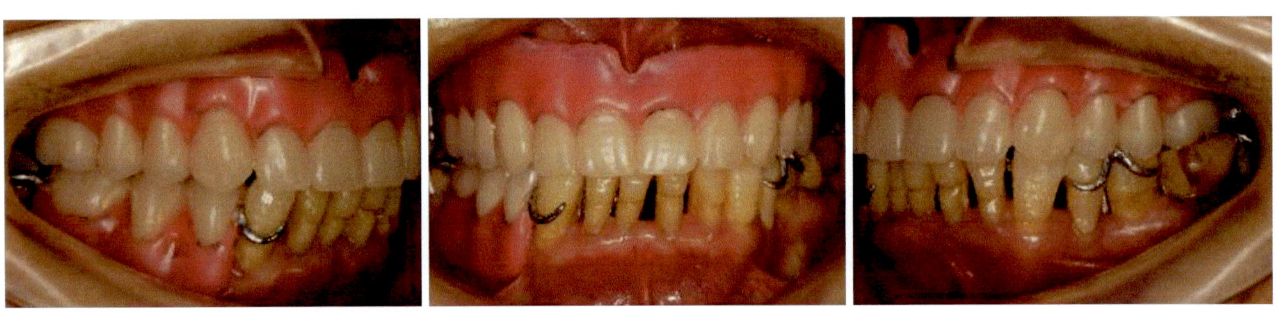

Fig. 6.186 Trying in of the wax pattern

3. *After restoration*

The final effect of wearing denture is shown in Fig. 6.187, the upper and lower jaws are well occluded (Fig. 6.188), there is no metal clasp exposure when smiling (Fig. 6.189), and the effect comparison before and after the main medical history is shown in Fig. 6.190.

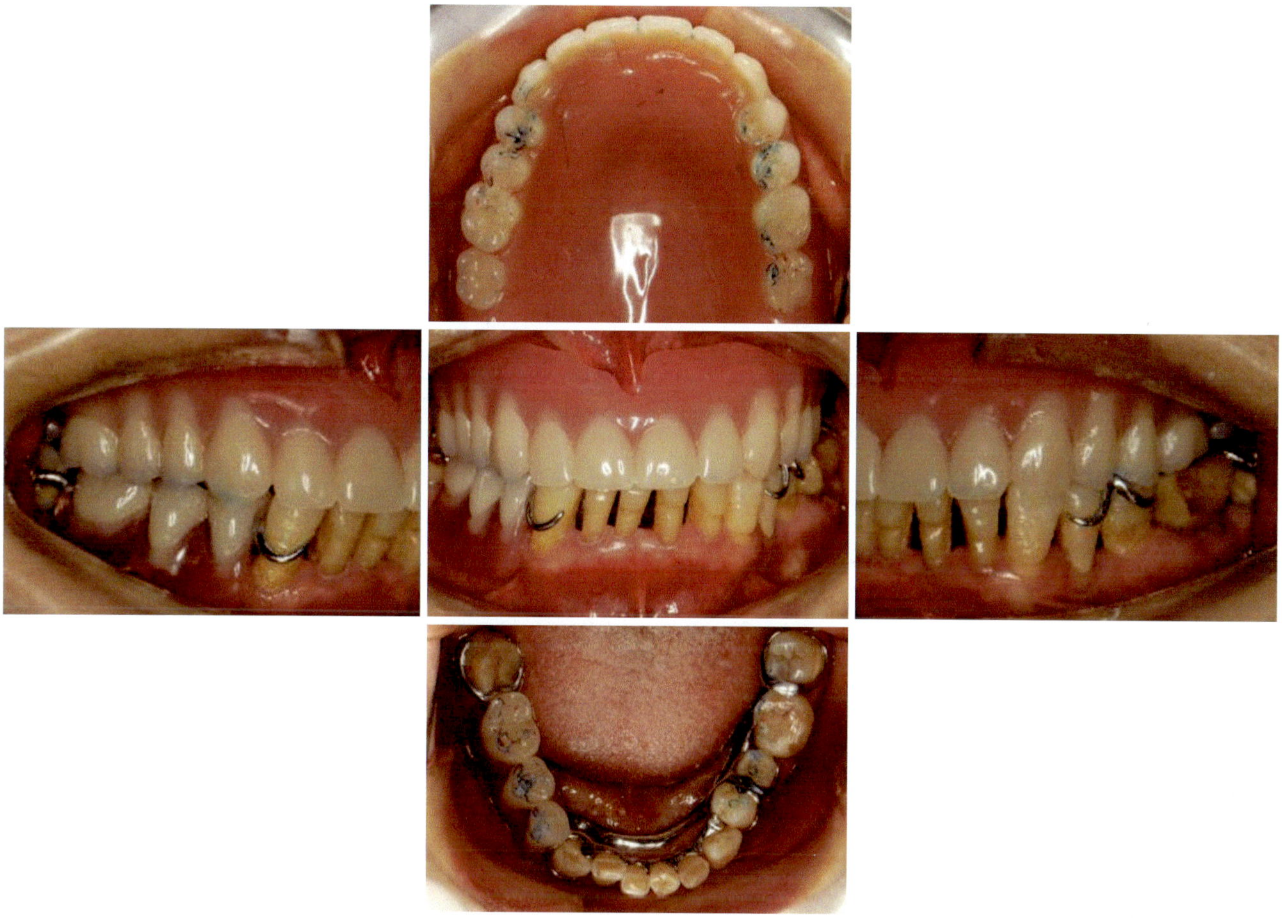

Fig. 6.187 The intraoral renderings

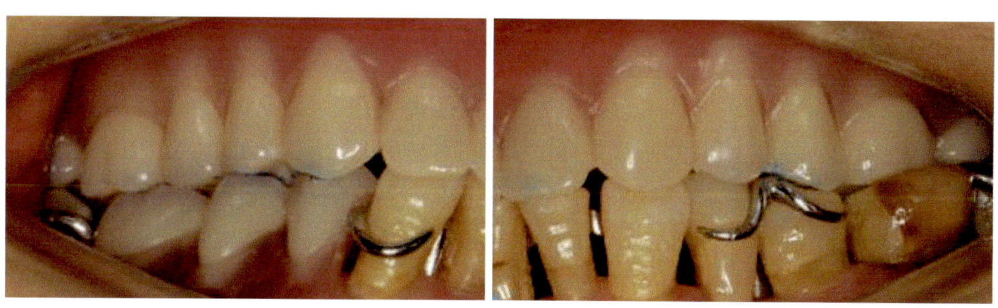

Fig. 6.188 Great occlusion of the upper and lower jaw

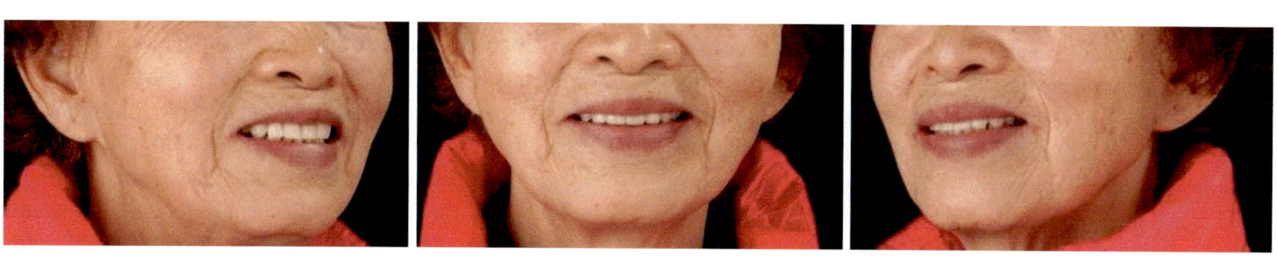

Fig. 6.189 Lower third of facial view

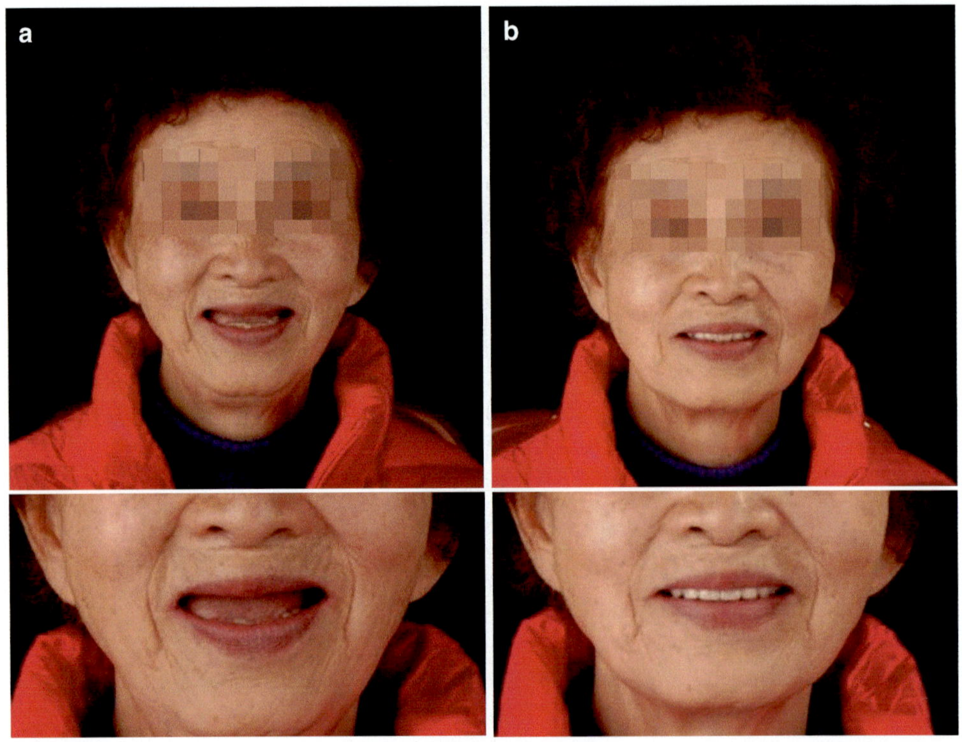

Fig. 6.190 Comparison before and after wearing denture. (**a**) Smile before wearing denture. (**b**) Smile after wearing denture

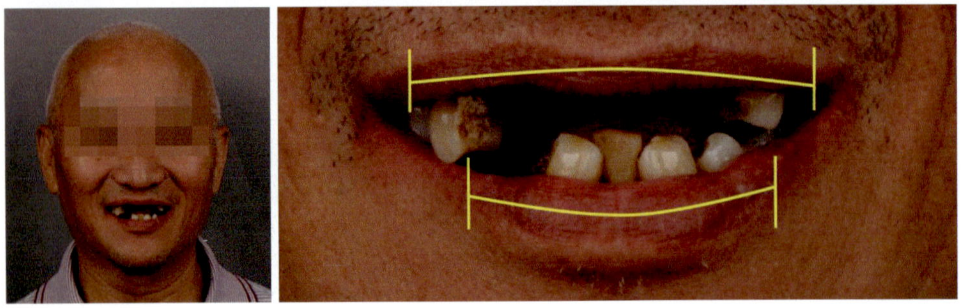

Fig. 6.191 Facial analysis

6.24 Case 24

A Case of Dentition Defect Repaired by E-Clasp Digital Stent Combined with Implant

1. *Before restoration*

   A man, 72 years old. In order to solve the problems of mastication and esthetics, he came to our department for treatment.

   Observing the exposed space of Gao's smile can be judged as the middle smile line (Fig. 6.191). Oral hygiene is poor. The alveolar bone is absorbed to 1/3 of the middle root; 16, 17, 13–24, 26, 27, 32, 41, 42, and 44–46 teeth were missing; 14, 15, 25, 35, and 36 teeth are loose for 1°; the mandibular anterior teeth are not arranged in an orderly manner. The color of oral mucosa is normal, and the size of tongue is normal (Fig. 6.192). Diagnosis: (1) maxillary and mandibular dentition defects, maxillary Kennedy class I, and mandibular Kennedy class III and (2) chronic periodontitis.

2. *RPD design and manufacturing*

   In Kennedy I and Kennedy II defects, the traditional removable partial denture design is difficult to provide enough retention and stability for dentures. In order to improve the retention of the denture, we often implant implants in the distal space of missing posterior teeth [1], change the type of the defect, and reduce the instability of the denture, so that the denture can play a better role.

   In this case, RPD is design and manufactured. The patients underwent implant surgery first, and two implants were implanted at the sites of 17 and 27 teeth in the upper jaw, and one implant was implanted at the right premolar area of the lower jaw. In the second stage, the healing cap was exposed, and the locator abutment was connected (Fig. 6.193). Considering that the patient has implant retention, the e-clasp is mainly used as an auxiliary retention function.

   In this case, the hollow design is used to reduce the foreign body sensation in the upper jaw, the buccally retentive clasps are designed on A5 and B4, and the mesh structure of the edentulous area is used to avoid the implant. In the case of sufficient retention, unilateral design is adopted to reduce the denture area, and combined clasp is designed between C6 and C7 (Fig. 6.194).

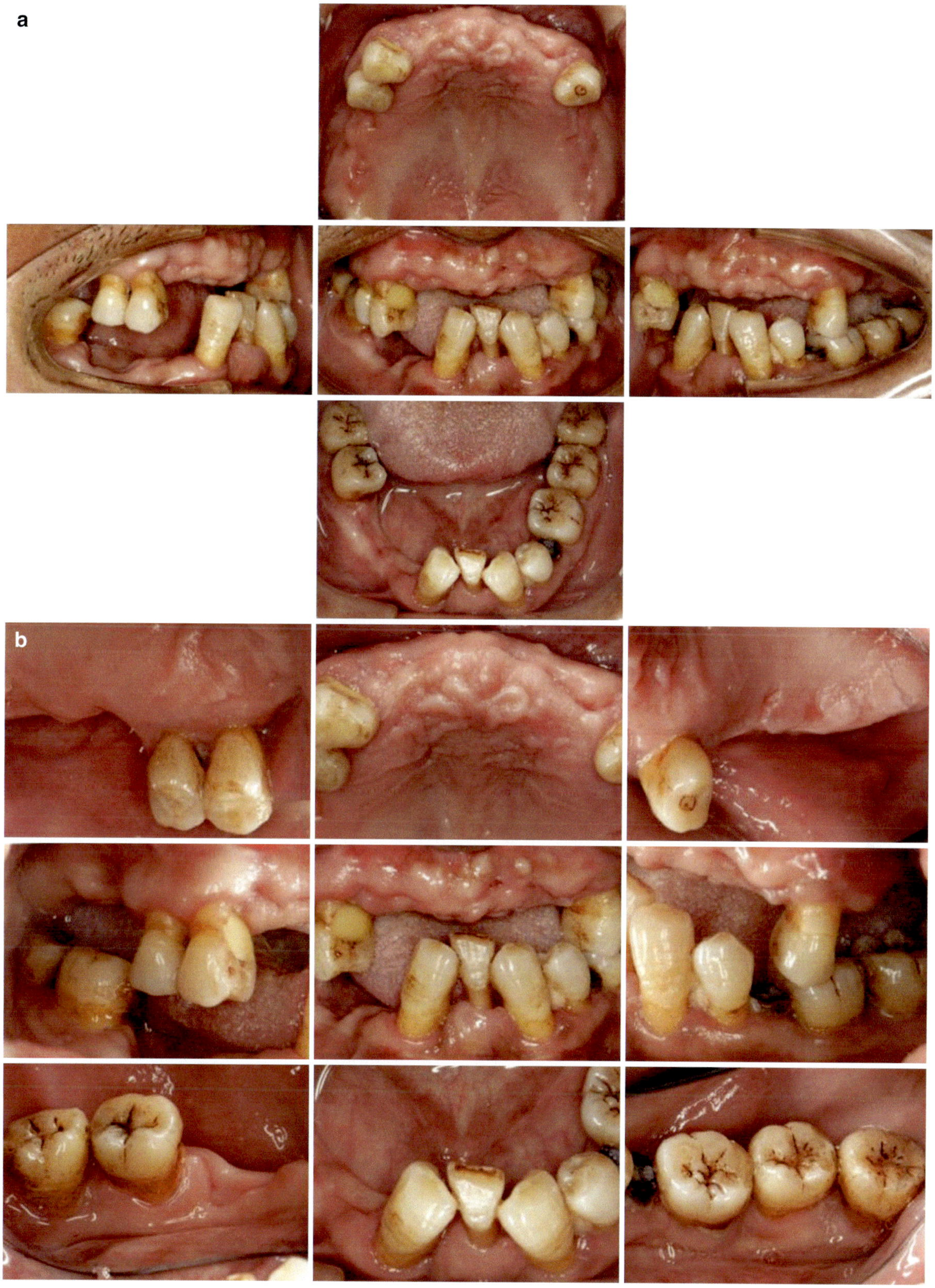

Fig. 6.192 Intraoral condition. (**a**) Intraoral condition. (**b**) Intraoral Local analysis

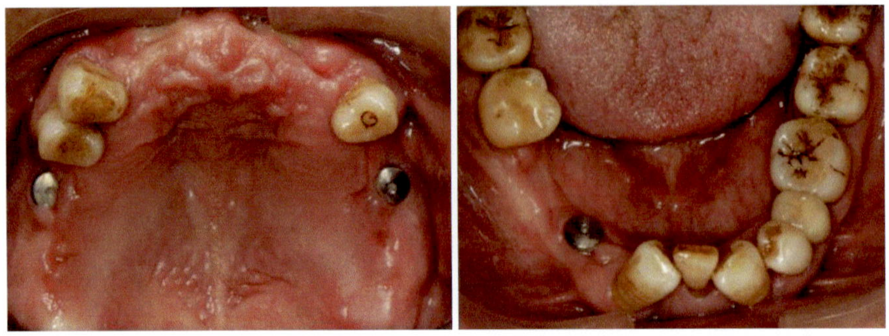

Fig. 6.193 Two implants were implanted at the sites of 17 and 27 teeth, respectively, and one implant was implanted at the right premolar area of the mandible

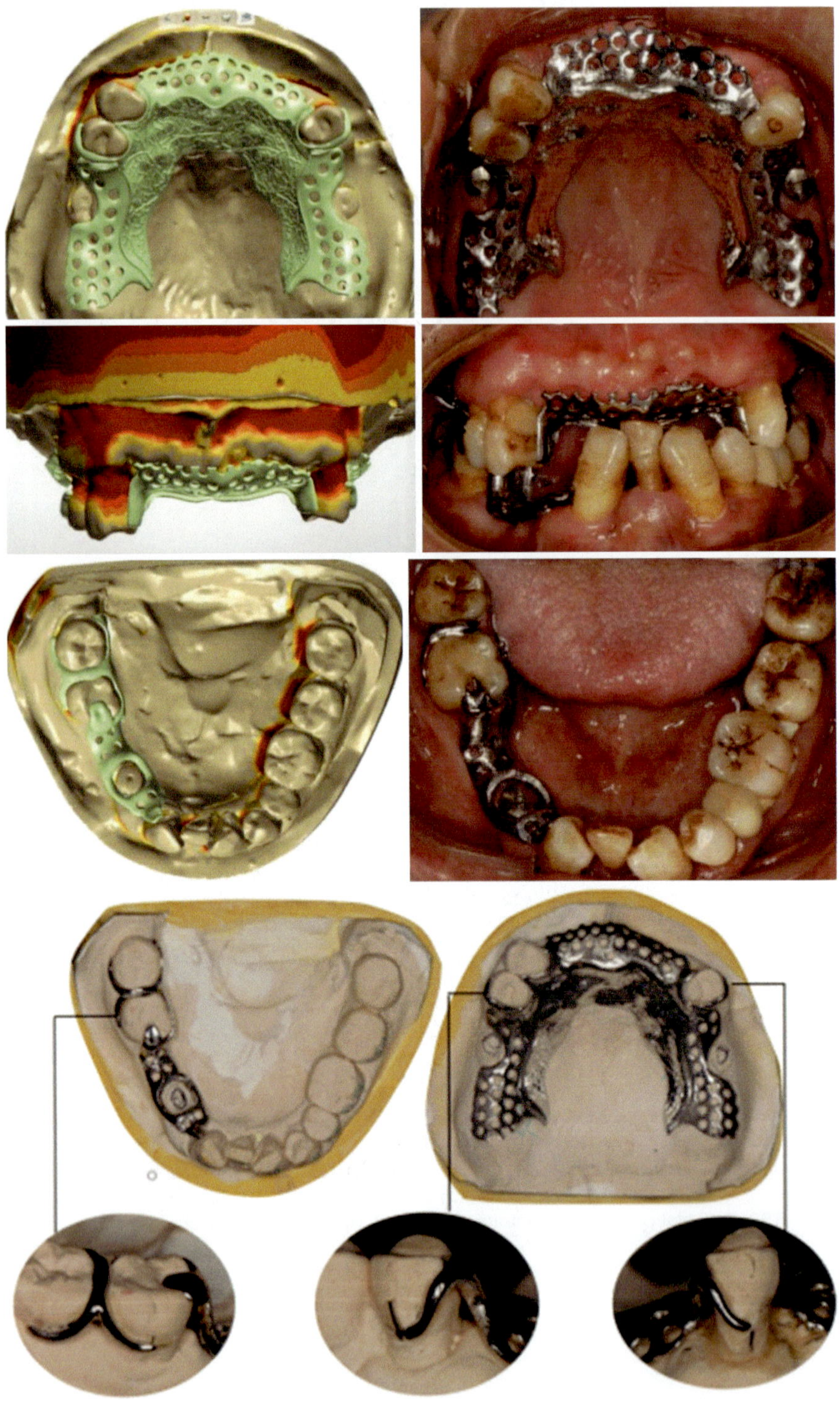

Fig. 6.194 Design of upper and lower jaw framework

3. *After restoration*

The final effect with denture is satisfactory (Figs. 6.195 and 6.196).

The combination of RPD analysis, design, and manufacture not only includes the advantages of wide indications and relatively low requirements for abutment teeth but also includes the natural esthetic effect of fixed dentures. The following case is a combined repair of mobile and fixation [2].

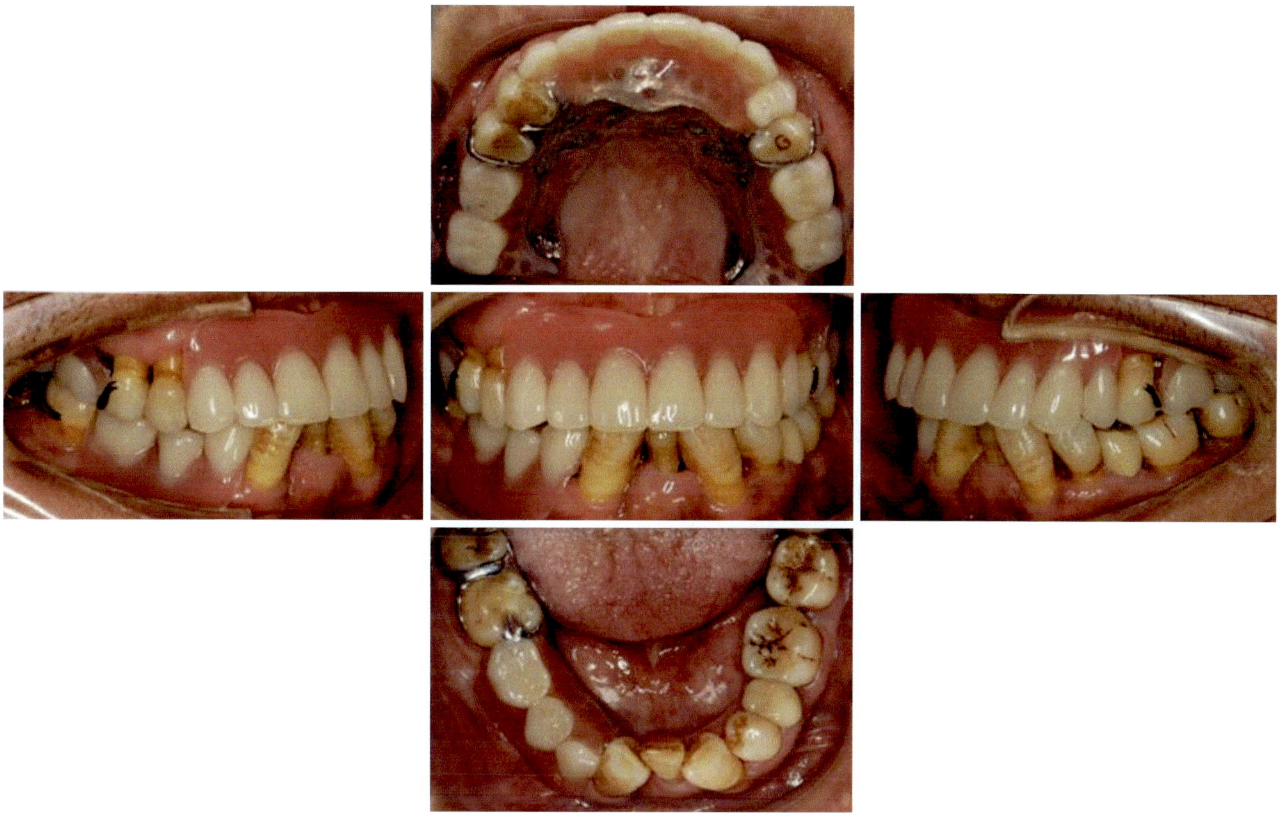

Fig. 6.195 The intraoral renderings

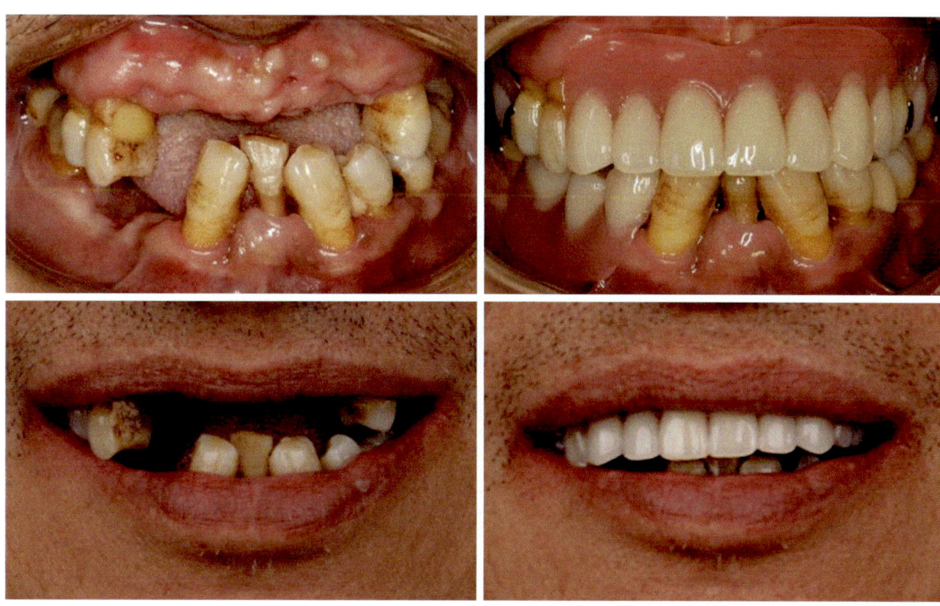

Fig. 6.196 Comparison before and after wearing denture

6.25 Case 25

A Case of Fixed-Removable Prostheses with Digital E-Clasp Bracket Based on the Simulate Production of Personalized Artificial Teeth

1. *Before restoration*

   A woman, 82 years old. On the front view, the distance between the lower facial 1/3 is slightly short, and the nasolabial groove is obvious, and on the side view, the protrusion of the mandible and the upper and lower lips are all over the esthetic line (Fig. 6.197). When smiling, the protrusion of the upper anterior teeth is serious, showing "bucktooth" shape. Observing Cao's smiling exposed zone, it can be judged as the middle high smile line (Fig. 6.198).

   The patient complained of slight protrusion of the upper anterior teeth when he was young. After the accident, the anterior teeth were missing due to trauma, and the protrusion was more and more serious year by year. The anterior teeth has deeply overbite and overjet, and the mandibular anterior teeth are directly bitten on the palatal neck of the anterior teeth of the upper jaw. The cusps of A3 and B3 teeth are ground and dentin is exposed obviously. The maxillary premolars are also worn to different degrees. The sites of maxillary edentulous teeth are area A1, A6, A7 and area B2. The location of mandibular edentulous teeth is 1, 4, and 5 in area C and 4 and 6 in area D (Fig. 6.199).

   Due to the longtime of missing teeth on the right side of the jaw, the extension of the remaining teeth in the upper and lower jaw interferes occlusion, and the lower jaw can't move forward. No abnormal symptoms are found in the joint consultation. It is very difficult to adjust and grind. In order to avoid further damage and deepening of the root fossa on the palatal side, it is necessary to improve the occlusal position by 1–2 mm.

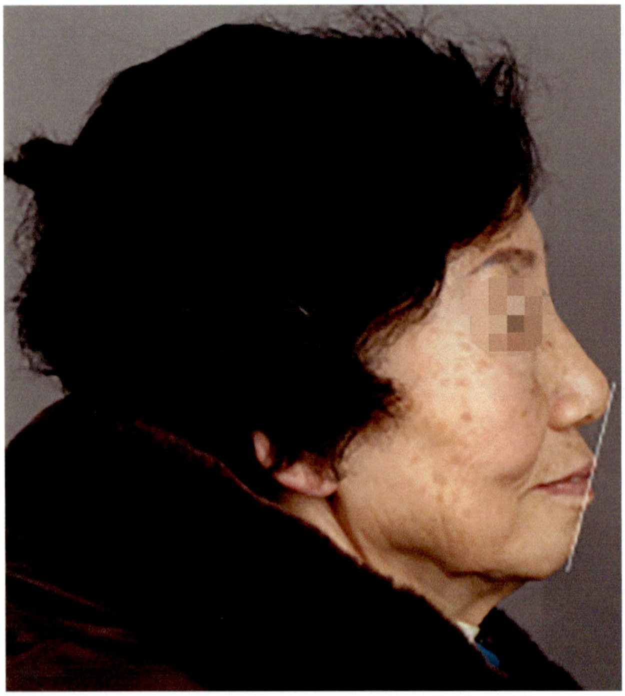

Fig. 6.197 Facial analysis

2. *RPD design and manufacturing*

   Because of the special shape, color, and arrangement of the anterior teeth, the arrangement of the artificial teeth cannot achieve a better esthetic effect. With the consent of the patients, the metal abutment teeth were designed at the missing teeth of the esthetic stent, and then the porcelain crown was used for bonding.

   First, make esthetic wax pattern on the model, and try to wear it in the mouth of the patient. After the patient is satisfied, determine the shape of the porcelain teeth (Fig. 6.200). The upper jaw is designed with three-arm clasps on A5 and B4. Because the missing teeth are located in the front, the clasps of the anterior teeth adjacent plate bar are placed on B3 to assist the retention. Design metal prefabricated abutment teeth in the position of missing teeth. The esthetic wax pattern can be used as a preparation to scan together and guide the preparation of abutment teeth. We designed lingual plate in mandible, three-arm clasp on C6 and D6, and design C clasp on D5. The location of missing teeth is also designed with prefabricated metal abutments (Fig. 6.201). After the occlusal relationship is recorded during the trial wearing of the stent, the porcelain fused to metal crown is made on the maxillary stent (Fig. 6.202).

Fig. 6.198 Smile analysis

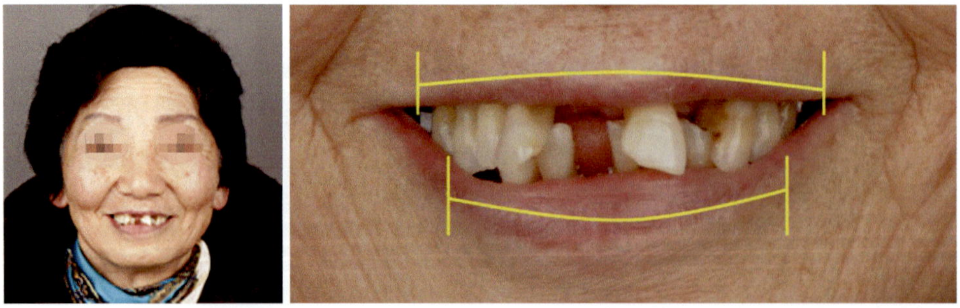

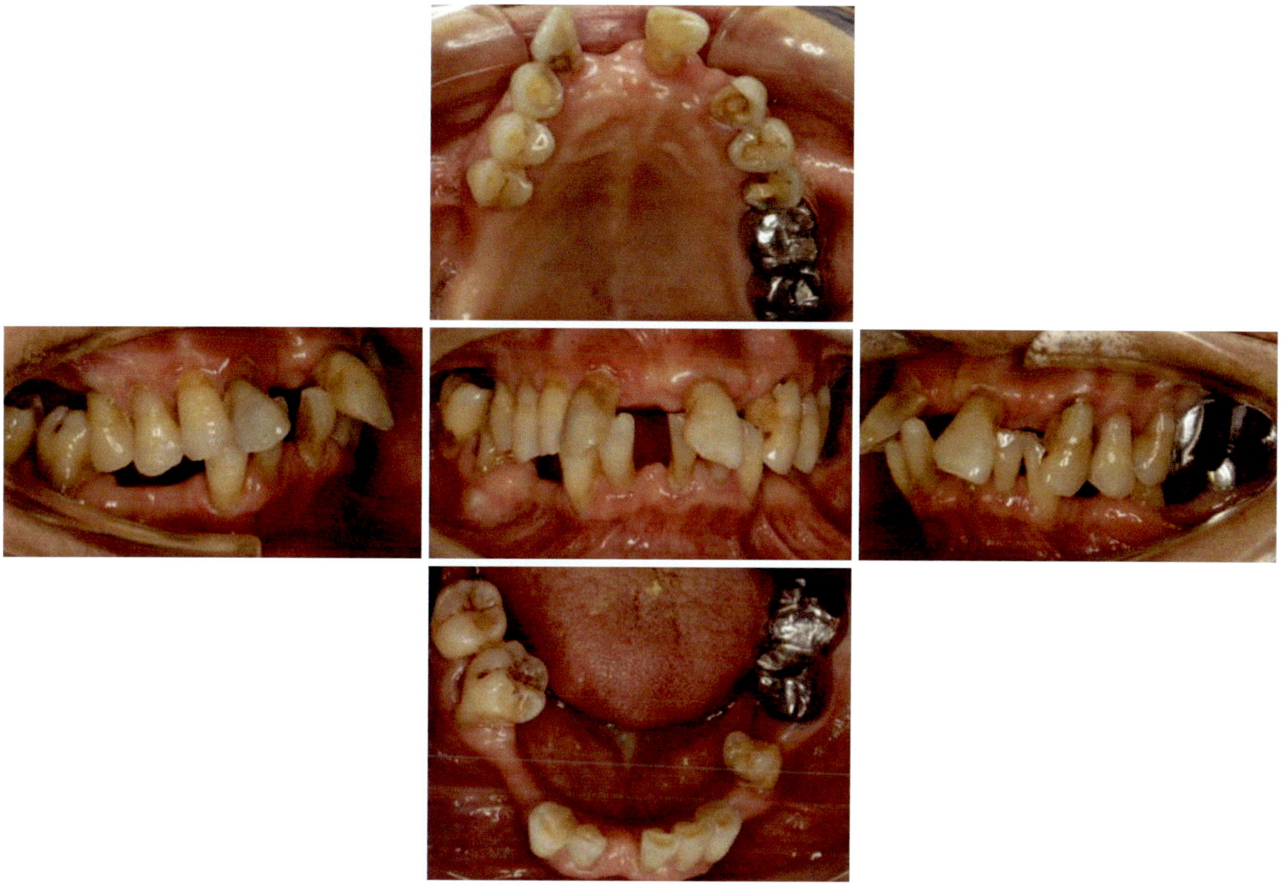

Fig. 6.199 Intraoral condition

Fig. 6.200 Production of wax pattern

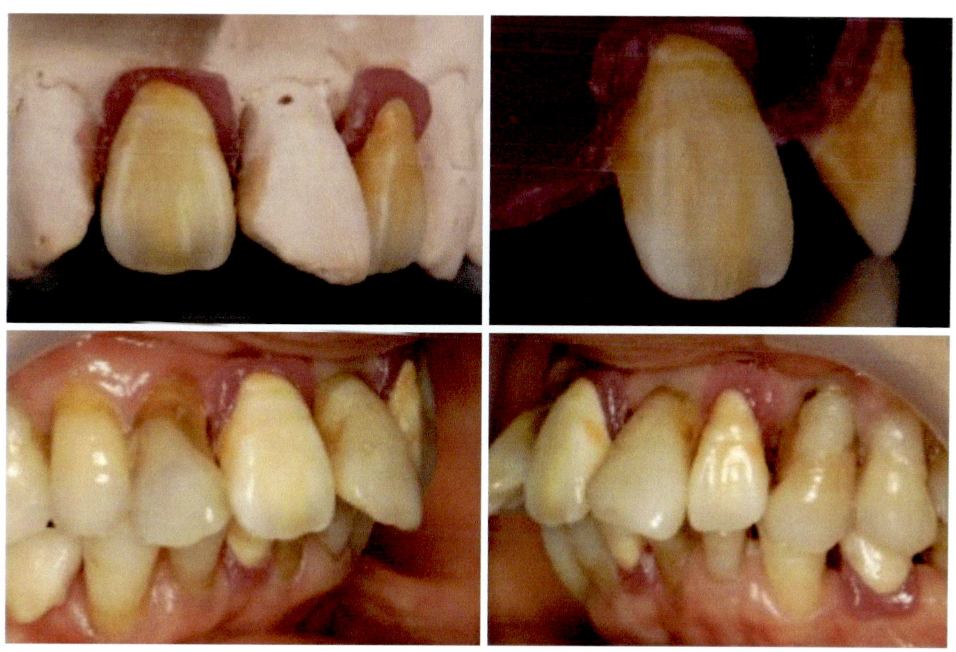

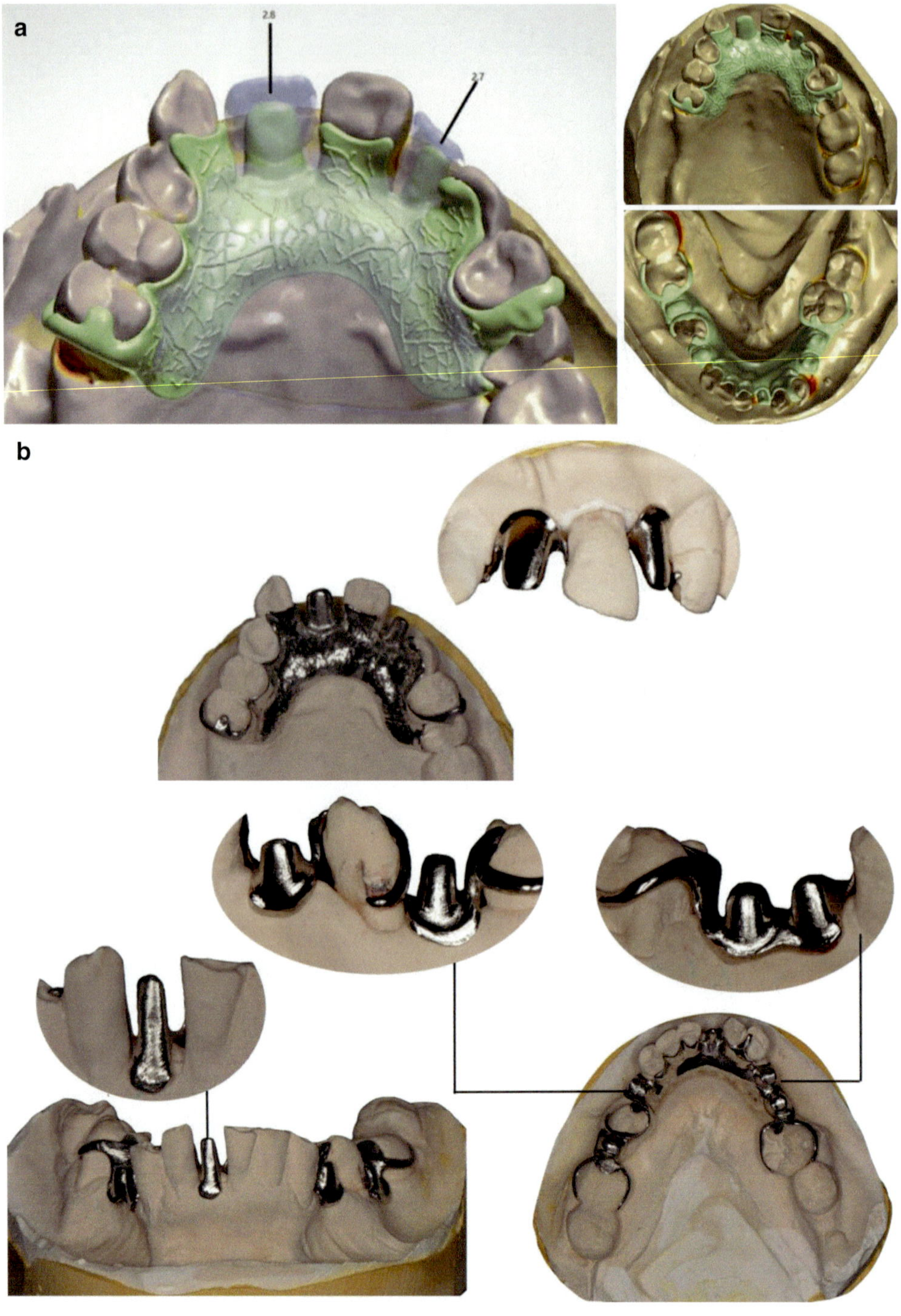

Fig. 6.201 The mandible and maxillary stents fit well in the model and mouth. (**a**) Match the model with the wax pattern, and design the abutment part of the stent according to the final shape of the prosthesis. (**b**) Fabrication of framework

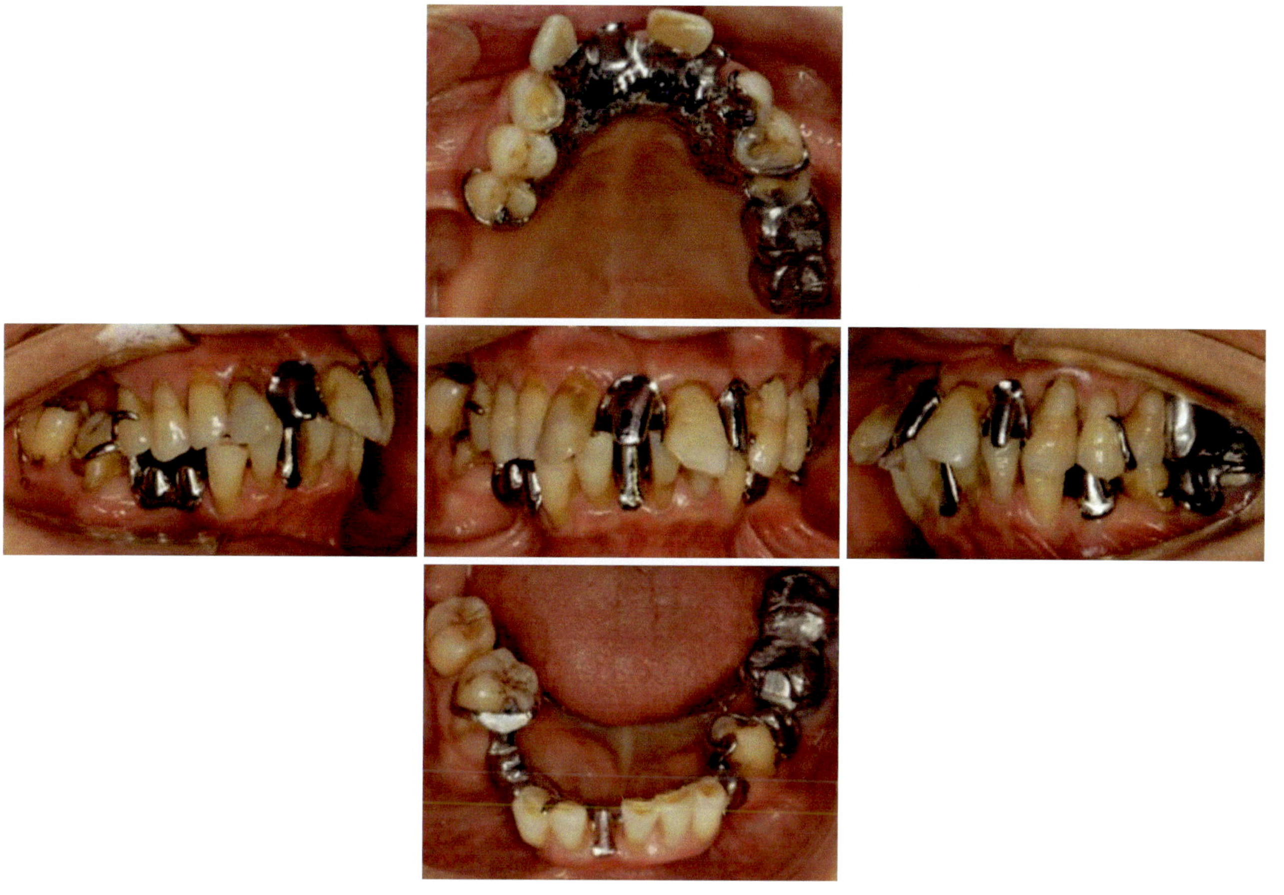

Fig. 6.201 (continued)

3. *After restoration*

The final result is shown in Figs. 6.203 and 6.204.

The above cases adopt the comprehensive repair method, which not only achieves the esthetic effect of fixed repair but also widens its scope of application, reduces the attrition of natural teeth, and reduces the cost of the whole repair. It is a multi-win repair method.

The intraoral prediction technique is an esthetic analysis plan for the main medical history of esthetic fixed restoration of anterior teeth. It is a new method of visualizing tooth esthetic design with the help of computer before creative operation. In the case of no need to grind and prepare teeth, the treatment plan is designed by software, which is not only intuitive but also noninvasive.

In the mouth, prediction technology can also be used in comprehensive RPD analysis, design, and manufacturing. In the following cases, multiple factors such as fixed-removable repair, intraoral prediction technology, simulated resin base, and simulated porcelain teeth were used.

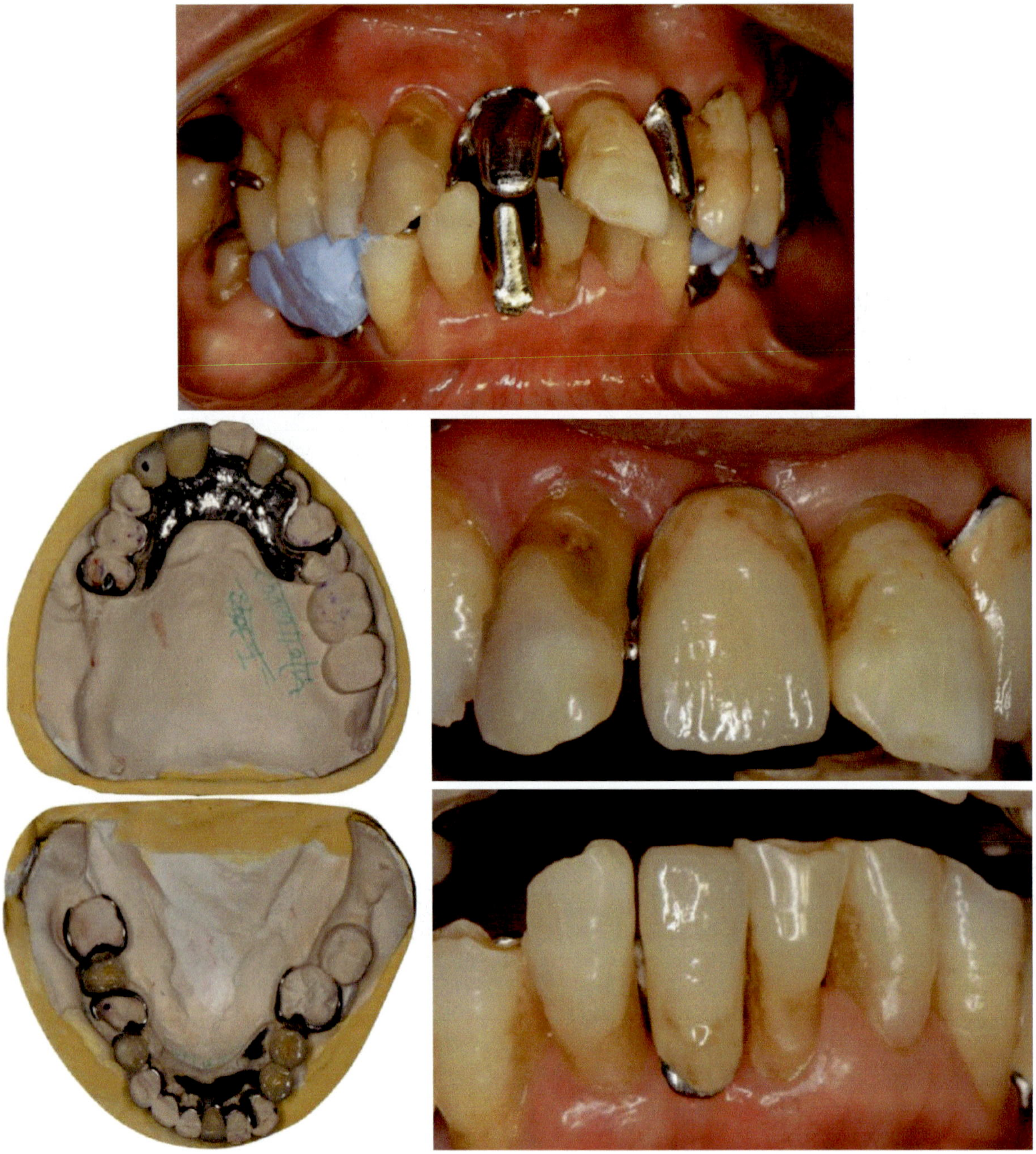

Fig. 6.202 Porcelain crown making

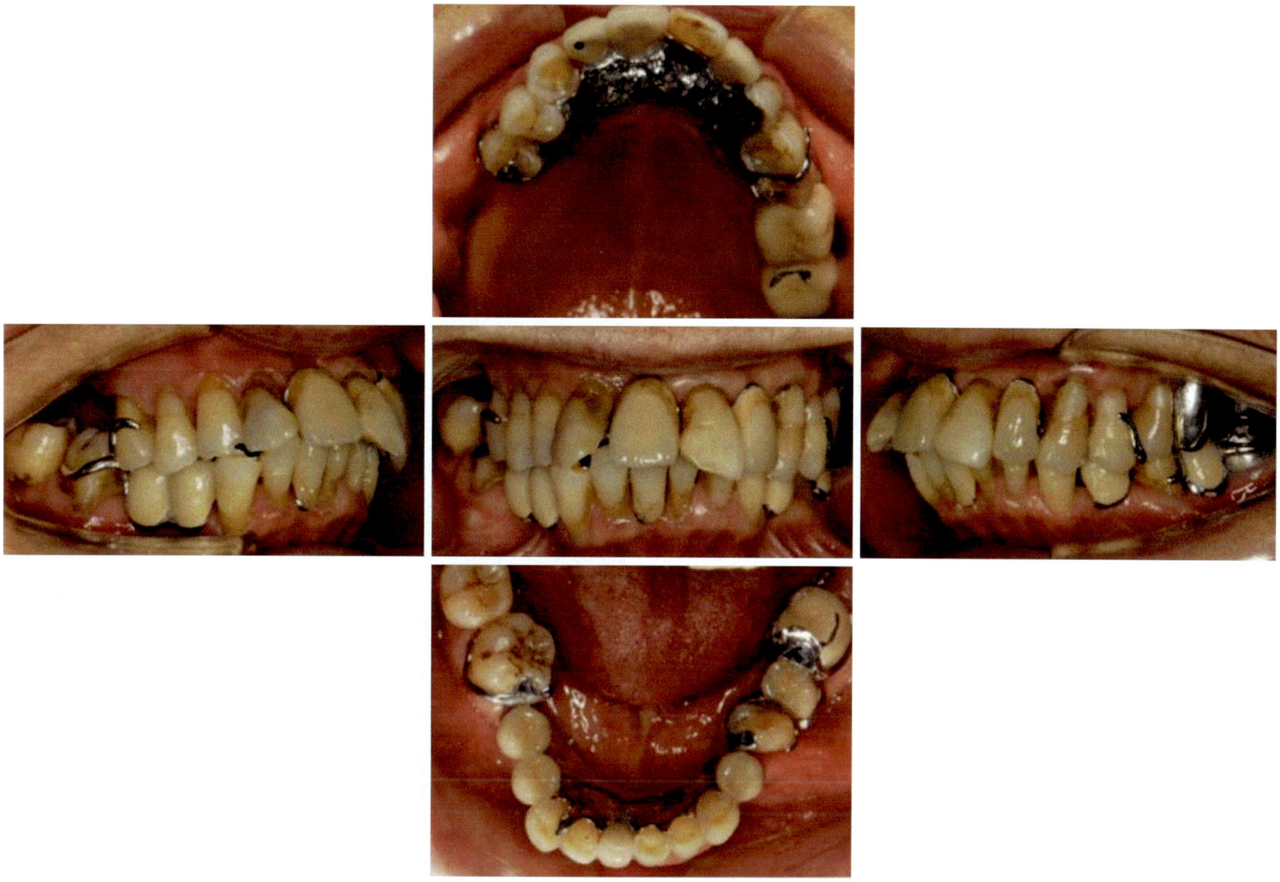

Fig. 6.203 The intraoral renderings

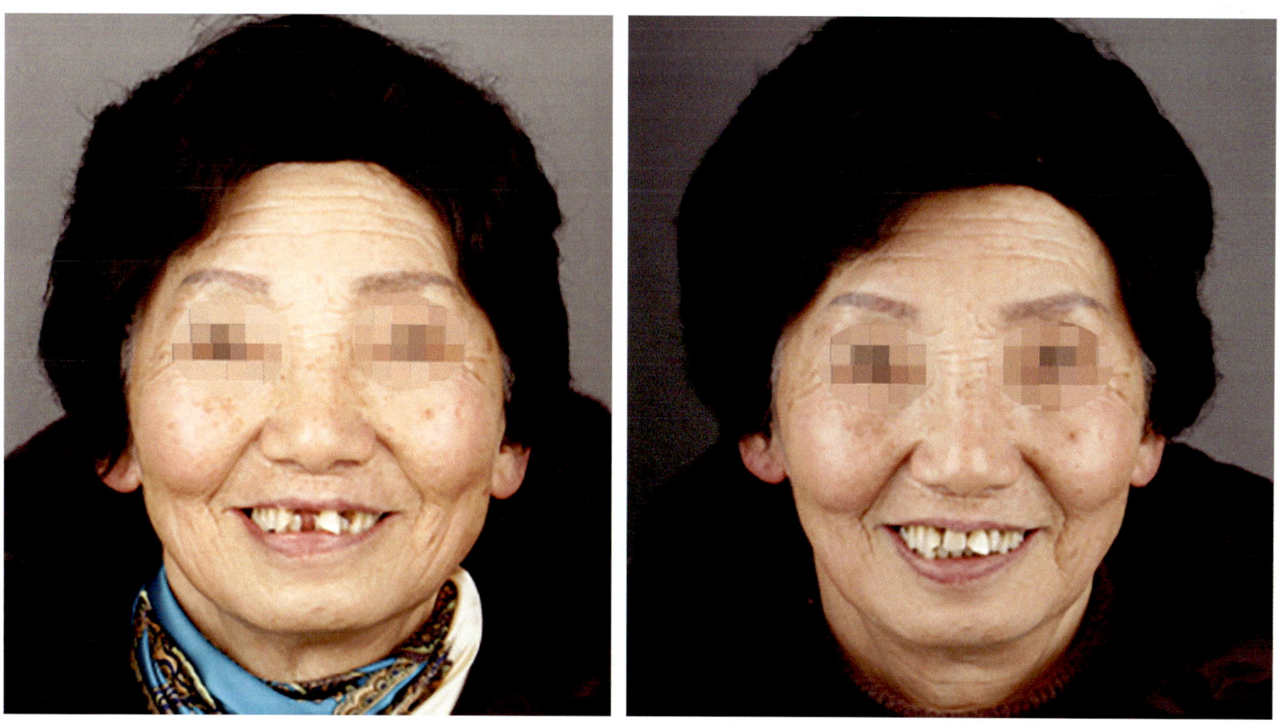

Fig. 6.204 Comparison before and after wearing denture

6.26 Case 26

A Case of Fixed-Removable Denture with E-Clasp Digital Stent Based on the Simulated Production of Multiple Anterior Teeth

A woman, 68 years old. The fullness of the lower facial 1/3 is normal (Fig. 6.205). The absence of upper and lower anterior teeth has a great influence on esthetics. Observing Cao's smiling exposed zone, it can be judged as a high smile line (Fig. 6.206).

1. *Before restoration*

   Patient has higher requirements for esthetics and hopes to achieve real and natural repair effect. The teeth in the esthetic area are A5–B5 and C4–D4. The missing teeth on maxilla are 1, 2, 3, 6, and 7 in area A and 1 in area B, while the missing teeth on mandible are area C1–2 and area D1–2. The remaining teeth are in good condition, and the buccal inverted concave of area B6 is smaller (Fig. 6.207).

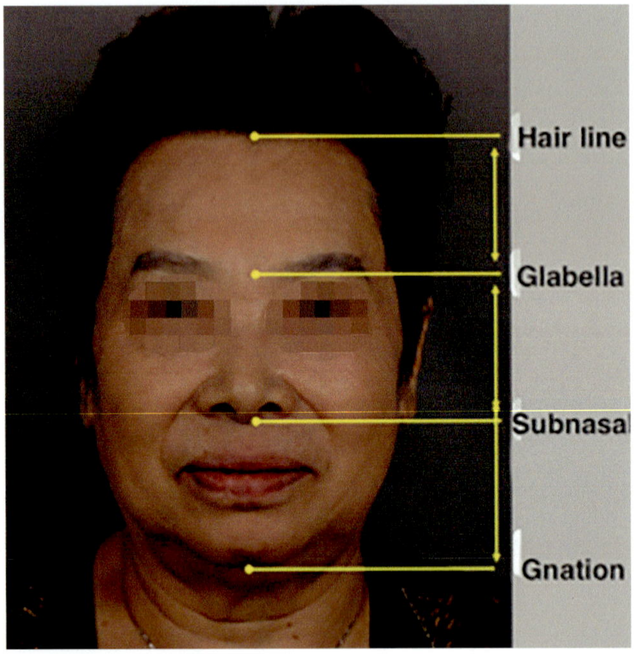

Fig. 6.205 Facial analysis

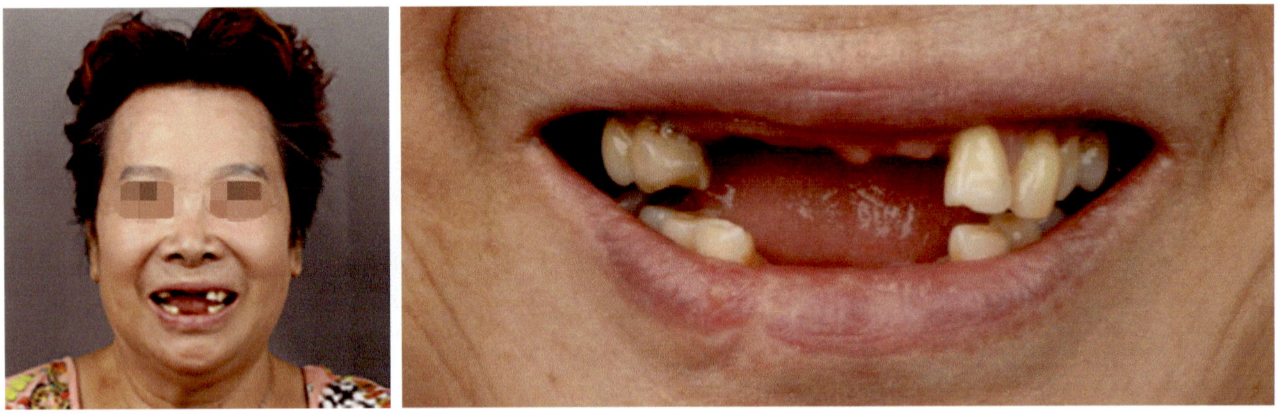

Fig. 6.206 Smile analysis

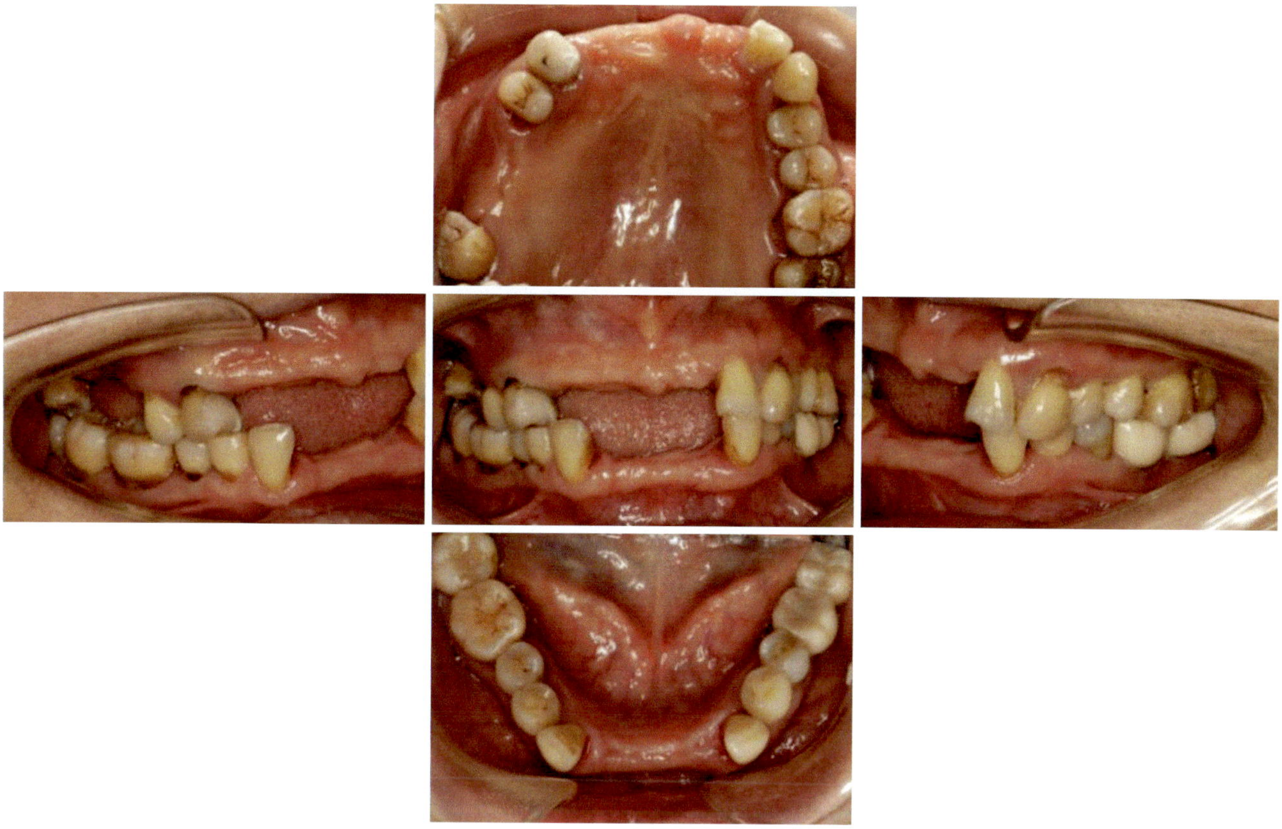

Fig. 6.207 Intraoral condition

2. *RPD design and manufacturing*

Intraoral prediction technology: The first step is software design. In order to compare the effect, we make two designs:

(a) Common design: Put C clasp of normal length on A5, and place embrasure clasps on B4 and B5. Place the circumferential clasp on A7.

(b) Esthetic design: Place the short buccally retentive clasp on A5, and place the traditional clasp on area B6. Because of the tight occlusion, we do not design the rest of B6. The buccal inclination of B6 is obvious, and the position of clasp is higher (Fig. 6.208).

The second step is to fit the photos in the mouth with the designed stent shape. Let's look at the results of the common design after fitting. The clasps in areas A and B are all at risk of exposure. Looking at the fitting results of the lower part, we can see that the clasps on B4 and B5 have been exposed, and the esthetic effect is not good. As for the effect map of esthetic design facial fitting, it can be seen that there is no clasp exposed in the range of A5–B5 and the normal shadow of the corner of the mouth should cover the part of clasp that B6 is exposed to (Fig. 6.209). Compared with the two schemes, the effect of esthetic design is better. After communicating with patients, patients chose to use the second esthetic design.

The third step is personalized dental preview, similar to DLD dental preview of fixed repair. Here, the tooth shape prediction can be realized with the tooth assistant software (Fig. 6.210). According to the patient's satisfied esthetic design tooth shape prediction, we make the esthetic wax pattern. The wax pattern needs to copy the original design parameters, and try wearing it in the mouth of the patient. After trial wearing, it can be modified again according to the actual situation. Finally, the wax pattern is used to guide the final repair system (Fig. 6.211).

We design e-clasp + porcelain-fused metal framework and simulate base for Miss Peng. At the position of the missing tooth, a metal pre-prepared abutment part must be designed to bond with the subsequent porcelain tooth. The design points are as follows (Figs. 6.212 and 6.213):

(a) Maxillary support design: most of the maxillary anterior teeth are missing. AB11 (C clasp) clasp is designed on A5, and three-arm clasp is designed on A8 and B6

(b) Major connector to avoid the gum, so that the gum can get sufficient food massage to ensure oral health.

(c) Labial retention bead design—to combine with the maximum area of the simulation base. For gingival tissue defect, it is suitable for patients with esthetic effects.

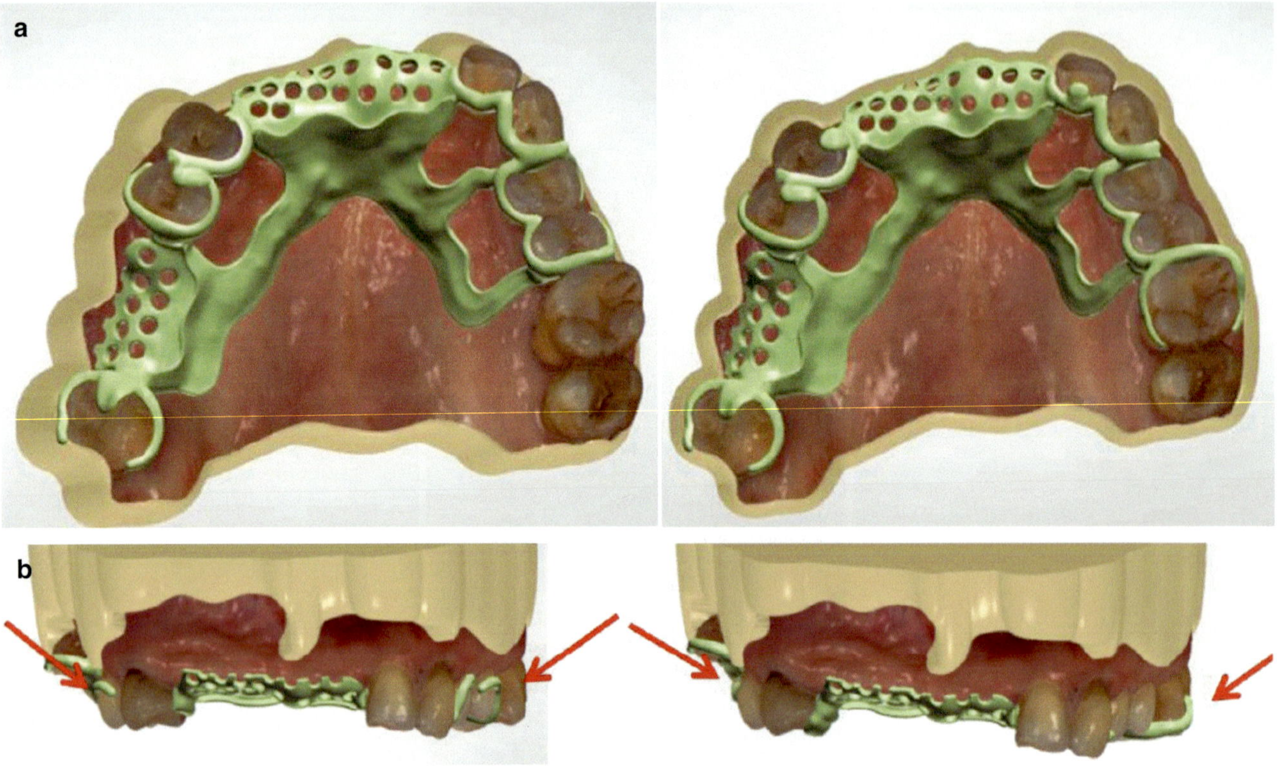

Fig. 6.208 Bracket design: complete the two designed bracket forms in the design software. Now, we can see the front view of the two designs. The common design is easy to expose the metal because the abutment tooth is located in the front and the clasp is long (half-page version). (**a**) Occlusal view of bracket design. (**b**) Front view of bracket design

(d) The best position of the cervical line is consistent with the esthetic wax pattern or more under the gum. The simulate base can slightly cover the neck of the teeth, and the esthetic effect is better.
(e) The design of shoulder is the same as that of abutment to ensure the color of porcelain layer.
(f) The junction line of the trailing edge is flushed with the cervical edge, which is equivalent to the effect of metal reinforcing belt.
(g) Fit esthetic wax pattern in three-dimensional directions, labial surface, incisal surface, and lingual surface, and reserve appropriate thickness of porcelain layer. It can be measured with the tool provided by the software and adjusted accordingly.

According to the results of color comparison, the porcelain teeth are made, and the esthetic wax pattern turns guide plate to guide the porcelain process (Fig. 6.214).

The patient is satisfied with the porcelain teeth made at present. The clinical bonding can be carried out in or out of the mouth. Figure 6.215 shows the bonding in the mouth. Layered stacking of gum resin: different colors of gum resin are used in different positions of the gum to achieve vivid simulate effect (Fig. 6.216). According to the patient's esthetic design tooth shape prediction, we make the esthetic wax pattern. The esthetic wax pattern need to copy the original design parameters, and try to wear it in the patient's mouth. After the trial wear, it can be modified again according to the actual situation. Finally, the wax pattern is used to guide the final repair system.

3. *After restoration*

The final result is shown in Figs. 6.217 and 6.218.

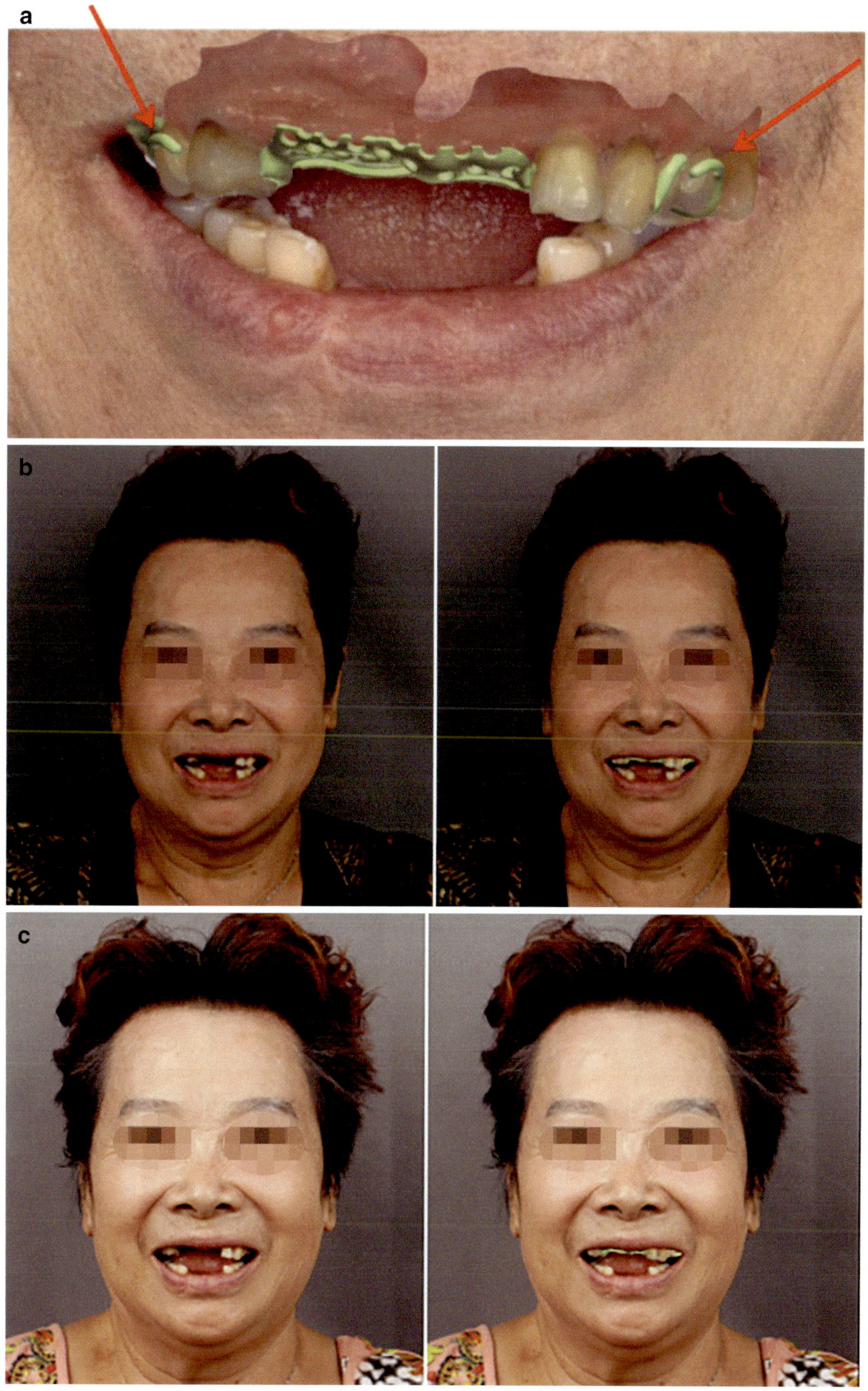

Fig. 6.209 Oral photos and shape fitting of designed bracket. (**b**) General Intraoral prediction. (**c**) Esthetic Intraoral prediction

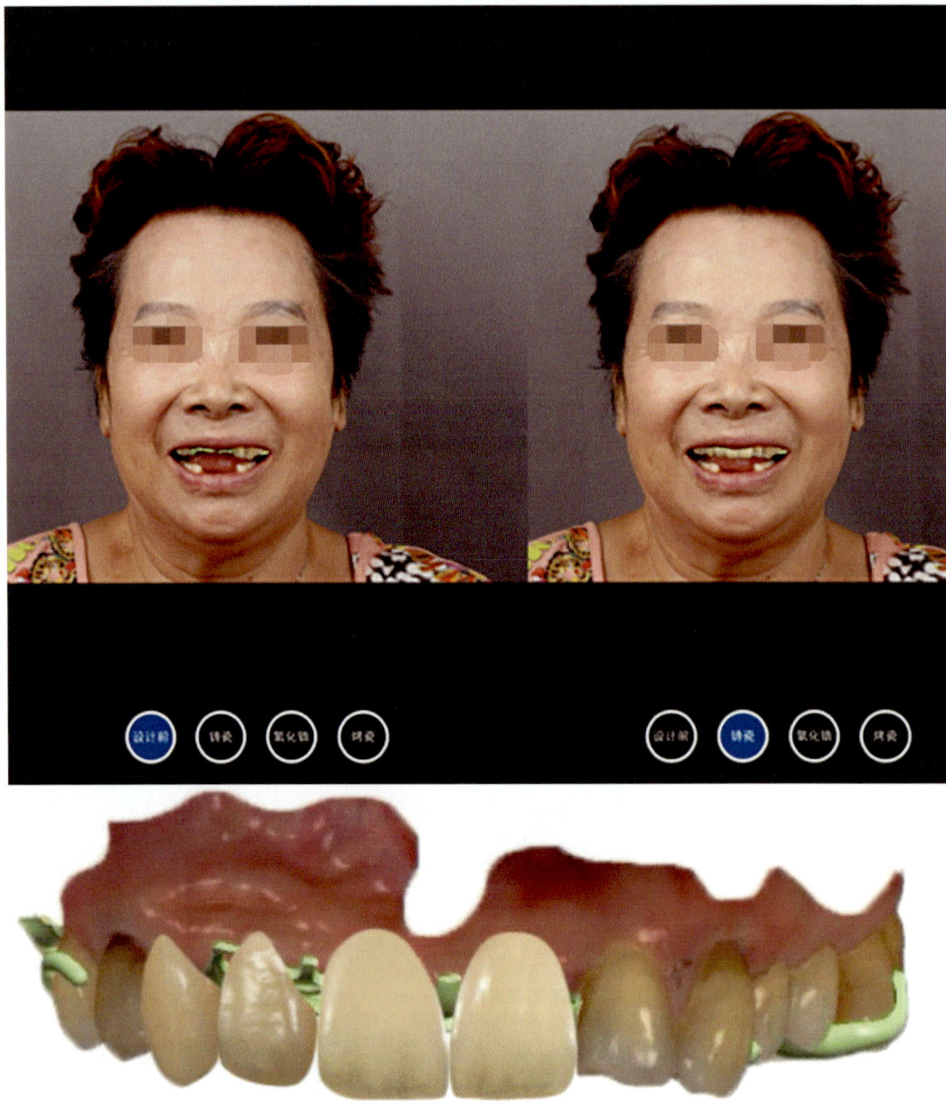

Fig. 6.210 Personalized tooth shape prediction

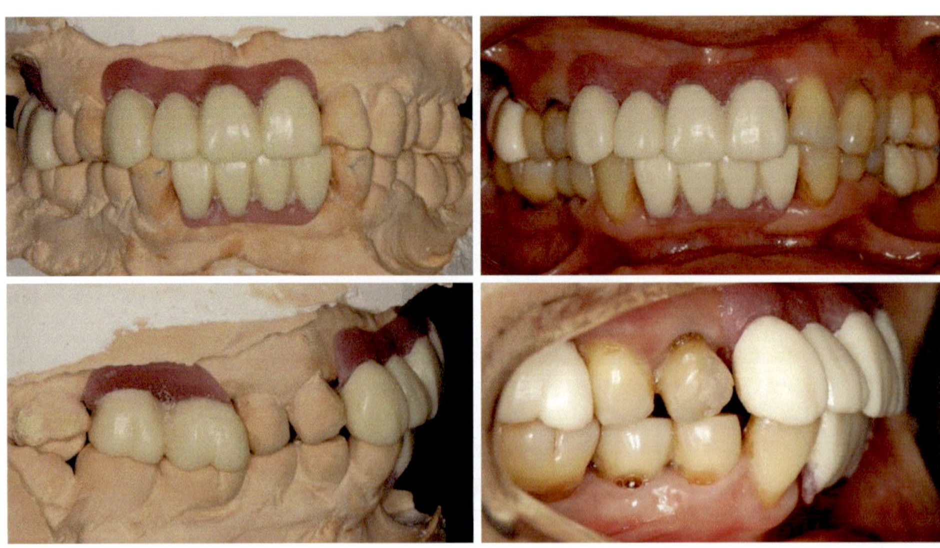

Fig. 6.211 The wax pattern is tried on in the mouth, and the shape is well coordinated with the adjacent teeth. Determine tooth shape

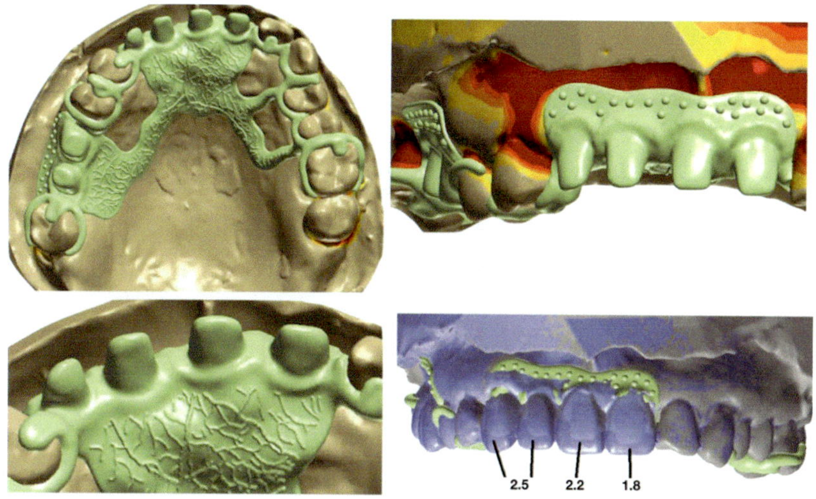

Fig. 6.212 Design of maxillary bracket

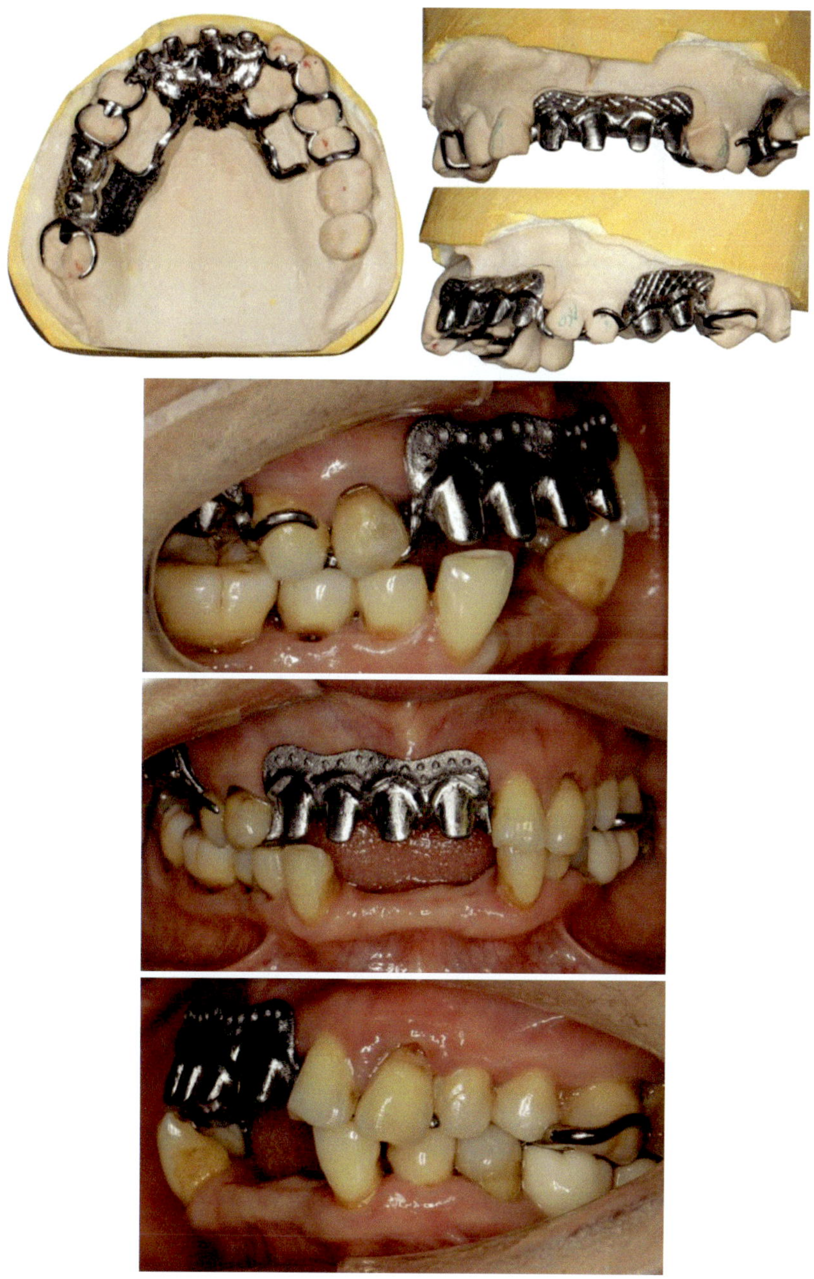

Fig. 6.213 Trial wearing of bracket in mouth

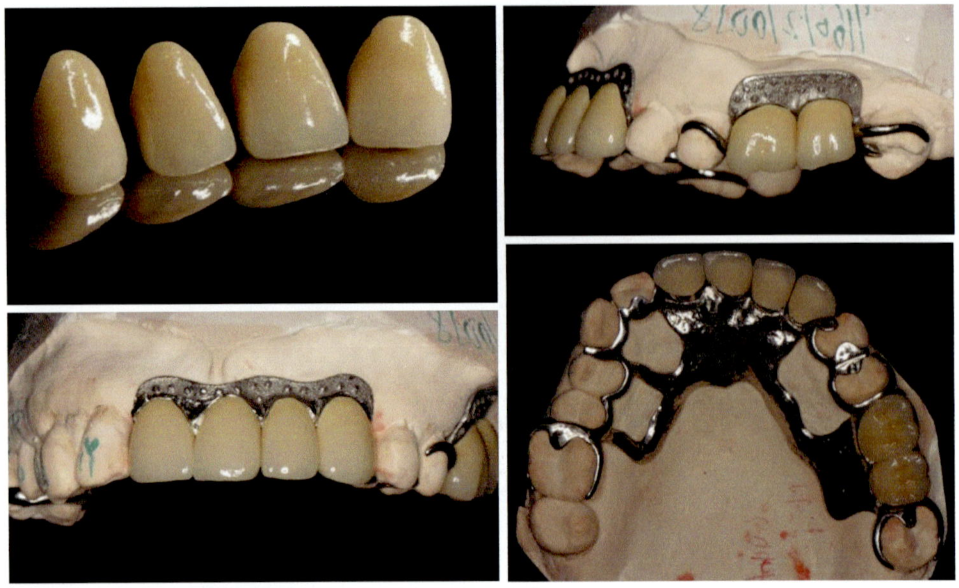

Fig. 6.214 Trying to wear the porcelain teeth on the bracket

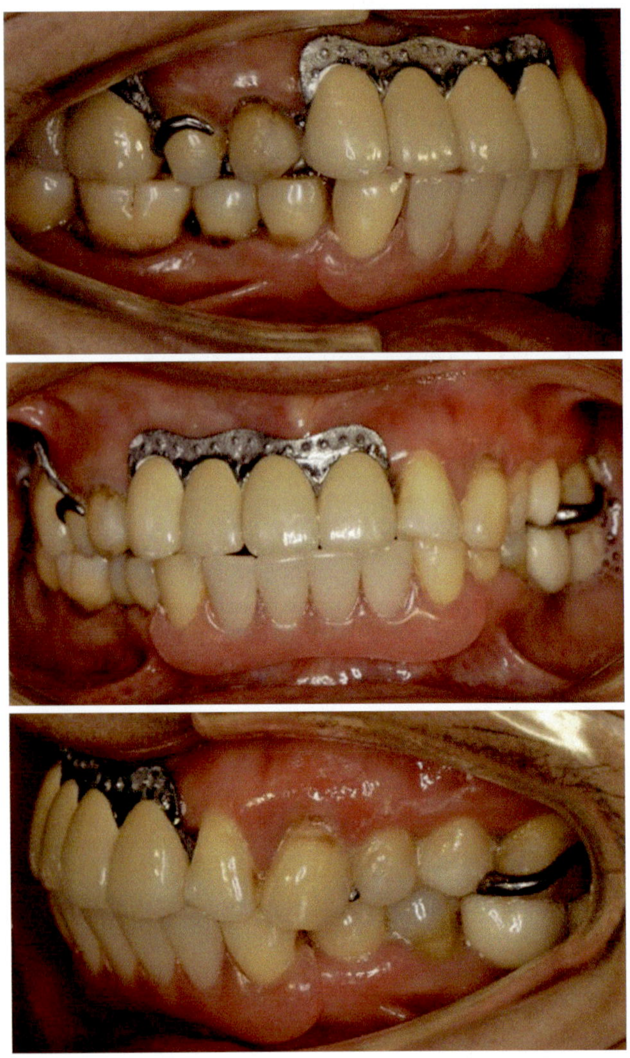

Fig. 6.215 Bonding of the porcelain teeth with the brackets in the mouth

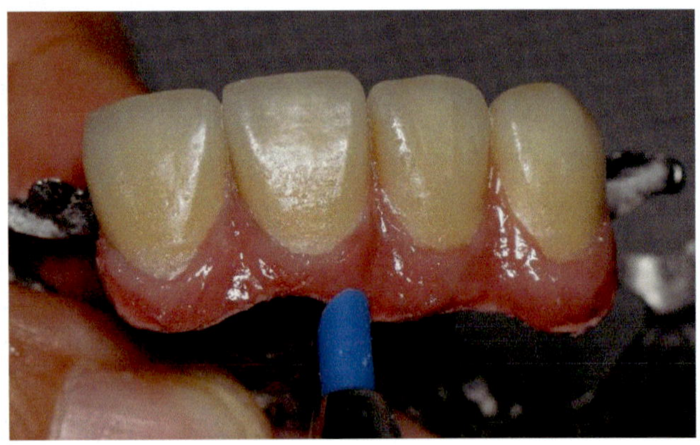

Fig. 6.216 Layered stacking of gum resin

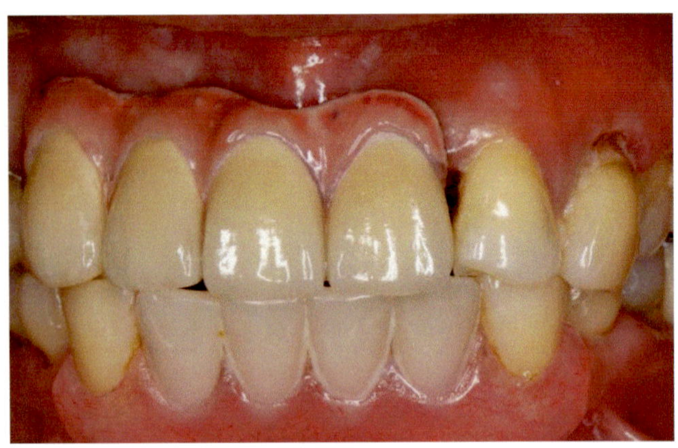

Fig. 6.217 The intraoral renderings

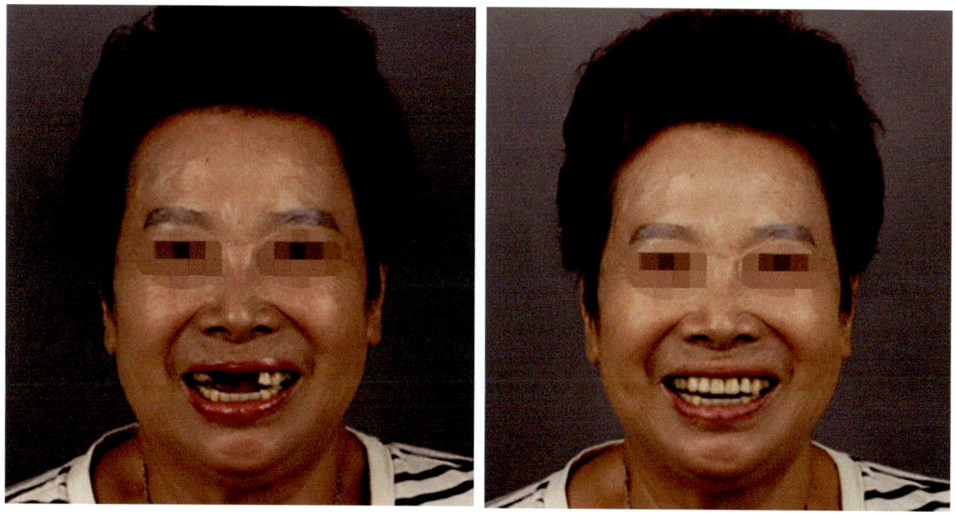

Fig. 6.218 Comparison before and after wearing teeth

6.27 Case 27

A Case of Esthetic Restoration of Porcelain Teeth with RPD

A woman, 43 years old. As a professional teacher, she have had severe attrition and masticatory weakness of complete dentition for 20 years. After the joint treatment in the joint department, the occlusal reconstruction and the restoration of the remaining teeth with porcelain crowns were completed in the repair department, the patients felt that the removable dentures were not esthetic (Fig. 6.219), and the retention stability was poor, so the restoration was required.

1. *Before restoration*

   The patient's face proportion is normal and the face is symmetrical (Fig. 6.220). The upper and lower jaws were all Kennedy II deletions. A12367 and B126 of the upper jaw are missing, and A1 and B12 are residual root, and A45 and B345 porcelain crowns were used for restoration. C567 and D67 of mandible were missing, and C1234 and D1234 porcelain crowns were used for restoration (Fig. 6.221). The patients had normal occlusion, normal overbite, normal overjet, normal joints, and good oral health. Due to the high esthetic requirements of patients, we should consider the e-clasp restoration of personalized artificial teeth.
2. *RPD design and manufacturing*

   The remaining teeth in the mouth of the patient are all porcelain teeth. The design of the scaffold should be on the premise of ensuring the stability and esthetics of the fixation, and try to disperse the force as much as possible to avoid the stress concentration leading to porcelain fracture of the porcelain teeth. See Fig. 6.222 for the prediction of diagnosis wax pattern in the mouth.

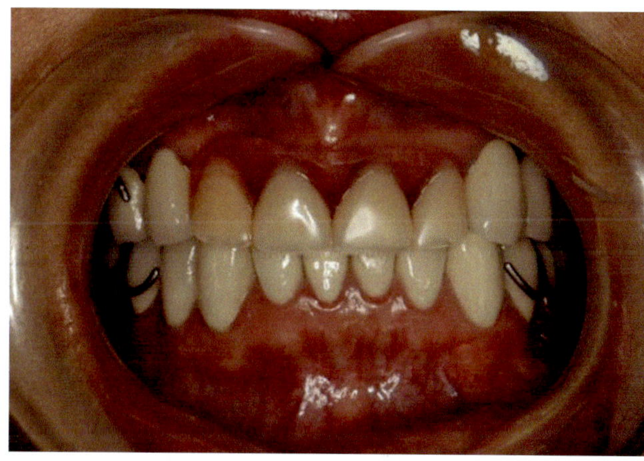

Fig. 6.219 Old denture in the mouth

Place C clasp and distal adjacent plate on the A5, combined with A4 distal occlusal rest and lingual reciprocal arm. When the free end of area A is under the dislocation force, because the point of C clasp is adjacent to the artificial teeth, the rest is located in the mesial, which is more likely to form the locking effect, effectively preventing the free end of the saddle base from warping toward the occlusal direction; when the free end of area A is under the chewing force, the base and the clasp arm sank at the same time, and the mucosa and A4A5 jointly disperse bite force, which can reduce the burden of porcelain teeth.

We place the short buccally retentive clasp on B5 and extend the lingual antergic arm to B3 to disperse the force and enhance the stability (Fig. 6.223).

We design I bar on buccal side of C5 and distal plate. Because the frenum linguae is too high, the variant "human"-shaped double lingual bar is used. When the free end of area C is under the dislocation force, the I bar can effectively prevent the free saddle base from rising to

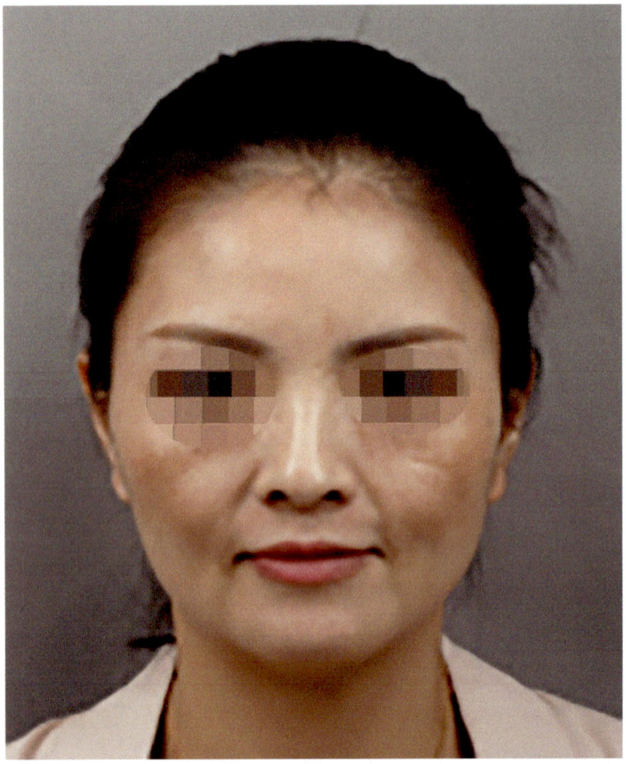

Fig. 6.220 Full-face view

the occlusal direction; when the free end of area C is under the mastication force, the I bar is out of contact with the abutment teeth, avoiding the torque exerted by the clasp on the porcelain teeth and dispersing the bite force to the mucosa.

We design half-and-half clasp without occlusal rest on D4. When the saddle base in D area is chewed, the base and the clasp arm sank simultaneously, dispersing the bite force to the mucous membrane and reducing the burden of porcelain teeth (Fig. 6.224).

After the stent is completed (Fig. 6.225), try it in the mouth (Fig. 6.226).

Due to the high esthetic requirements of patients, personalized artificial teeth are customized through wax pattern production (Fig. 6.227), and the wax pattern is used to complete tooth arrangement, and the we try it in the mouth (Fig. 6.228). The posterior teeth are filled with glue (Fig. 6.229), and the anterior teeth are made of metal substrate and then porcelain on them (Fig. 6.230). Because there are five missing teeth in the anterior tooth area, the actual space is only allowed to repair four teeth, and the space was too large for the target repair space of four teeth, so it is necessary to reduce the distance between mesial and distal line angles and deepen the

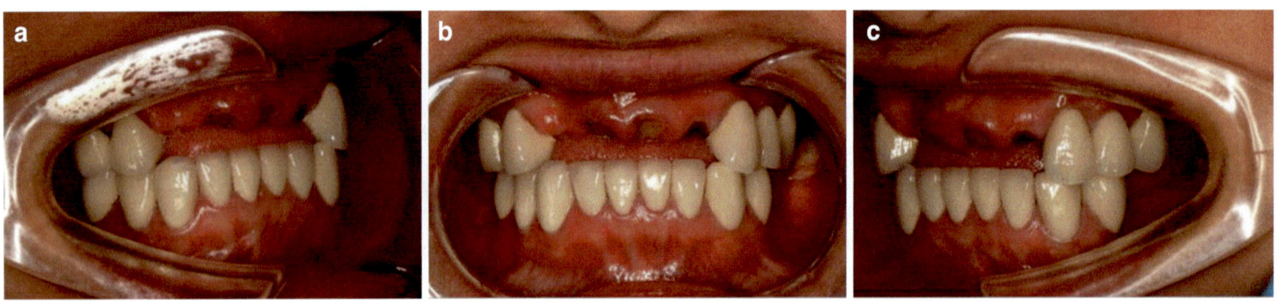

Fig. 6.221 Intraoral condition. (**a**) Right view of occlusion. (**b**) Positive view of occlusion. (**c**) Left view of occlusion

Fig. 6.222 Intraoral prediction

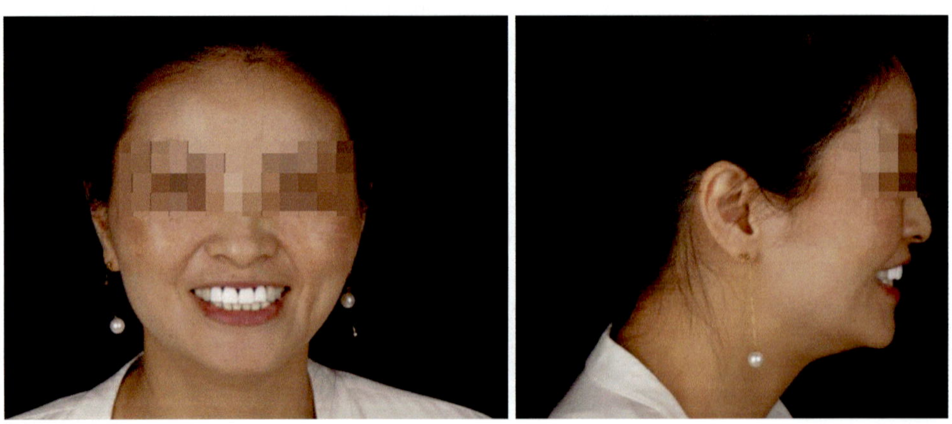

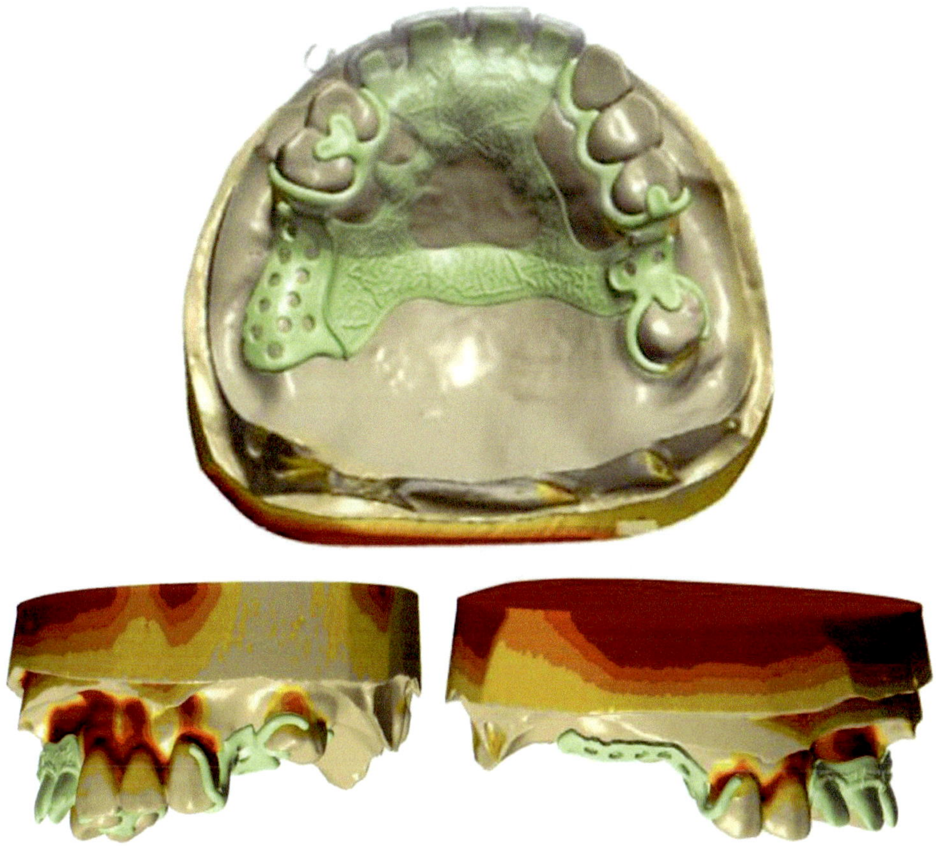

Fig. 6.223 Design of maxillary bracket

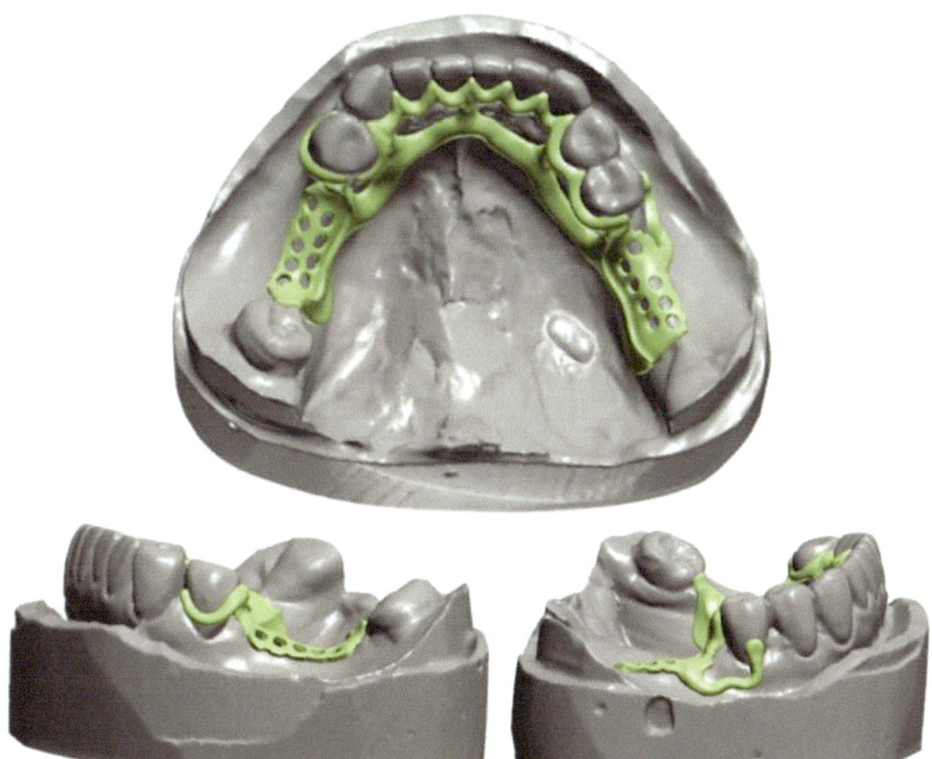

Fig. 6.224 Design of mandible bracket

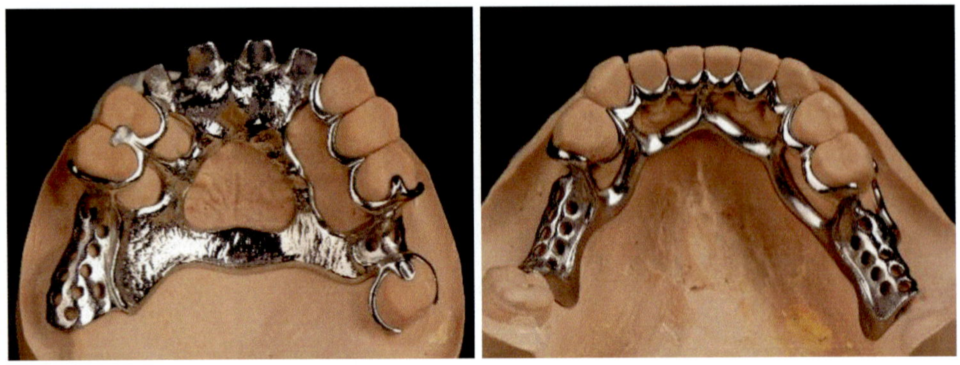

Fig. 6.225 Bracket completion

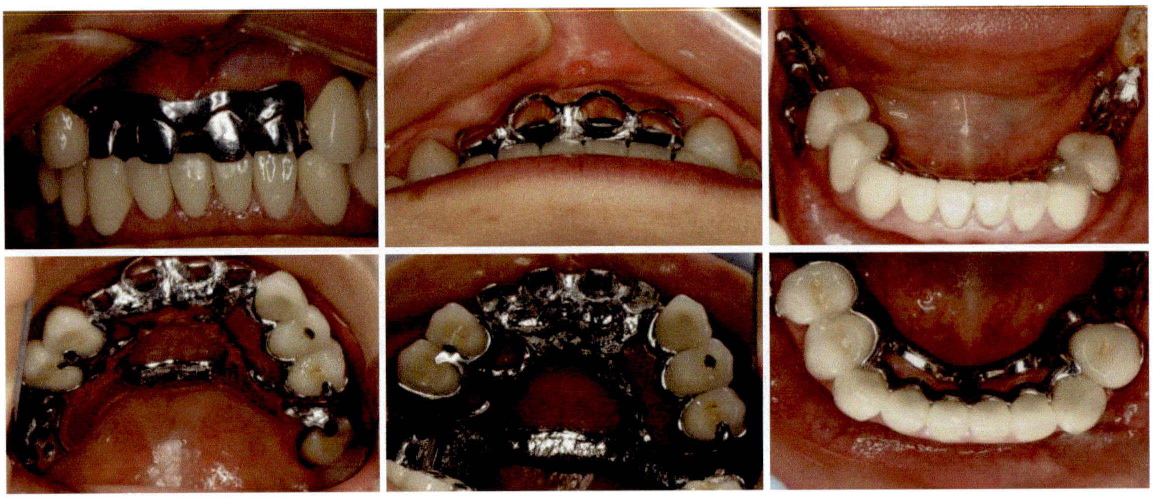

Fig. 6.226 The fitting of the stent in the mouth is great

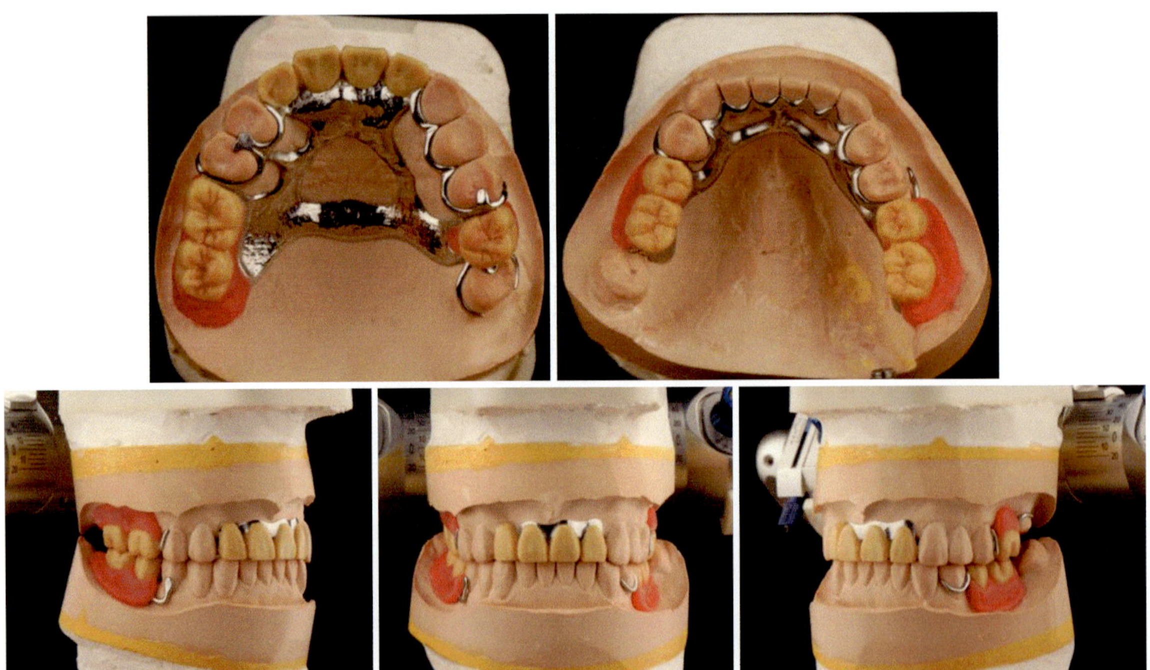

Fig. 6.227 Personalized artificial wax teeth

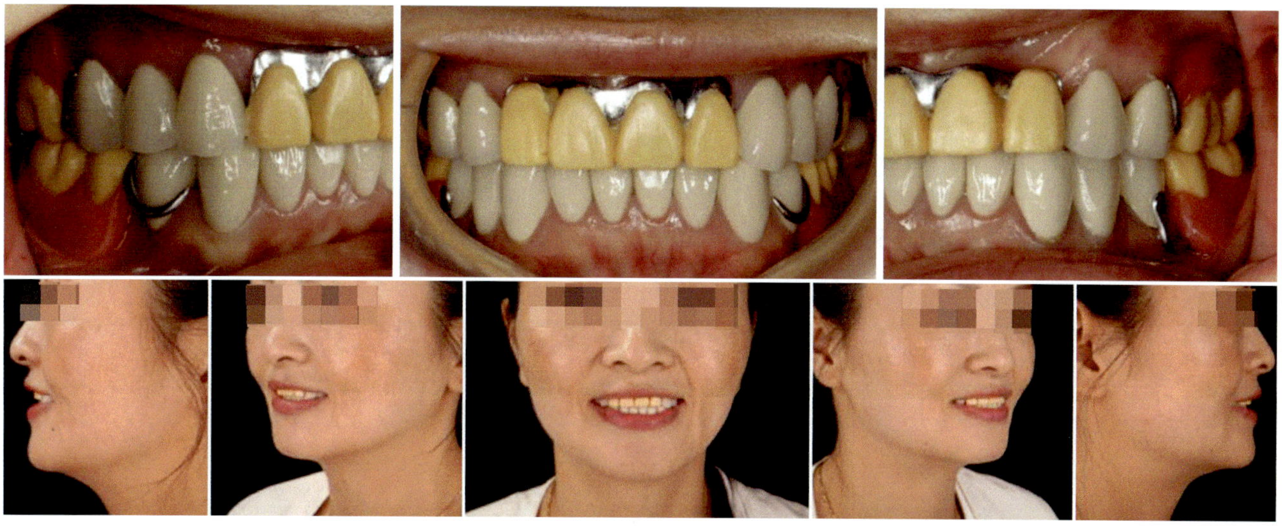

Fig. 6.228 Try wearing after tooth arrangement

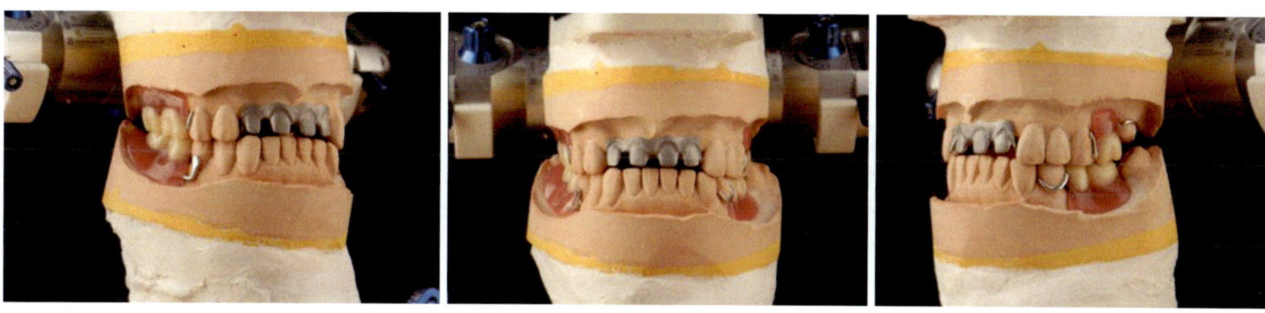

Fig. 6.229 In order to avoid overweight of the stent, the posterior are made of resin teeth

Fig. 6.230 Porcelain after making substrate of anterior teeth

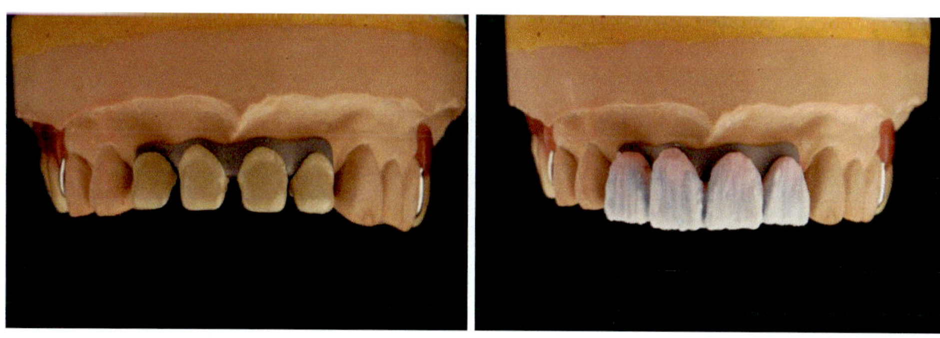

color of the adjacent surface, so as to achieve the effect of crown narrowing visually while retaining the adjacent contact (Fig. 6.231). After the porcelain teeth are bonded, the gingival porcelain is porcelained, and the restorations are finally completed (Fig. 6.232).

3. *After restoration*

Denture retention stability is good, and the production of personalized artificial teeth and the design of e-clasp met the patients' higher esthetic expectations. The patient is very satisfied (Figs. 6.233, 6.234, and 6.235).

PEEK (polyether ether ketone) is a kind of special engineering plastics with high performance. Since it was developed, it has been used as an important strategic military material. Due to its excellent chemical stability, good biological properties, and mechanical properties close to

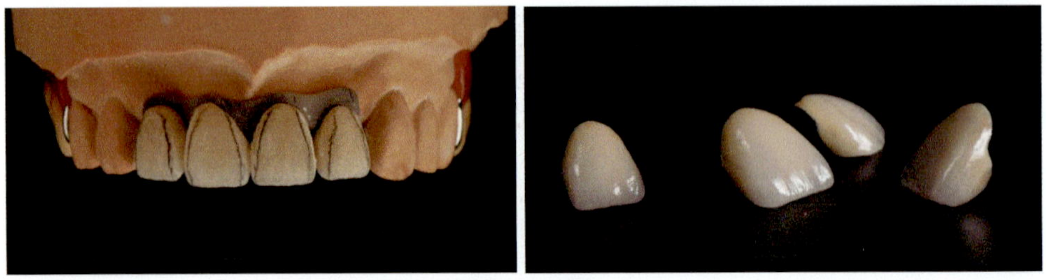

Fig. 6.231 Porcelain teeth completion

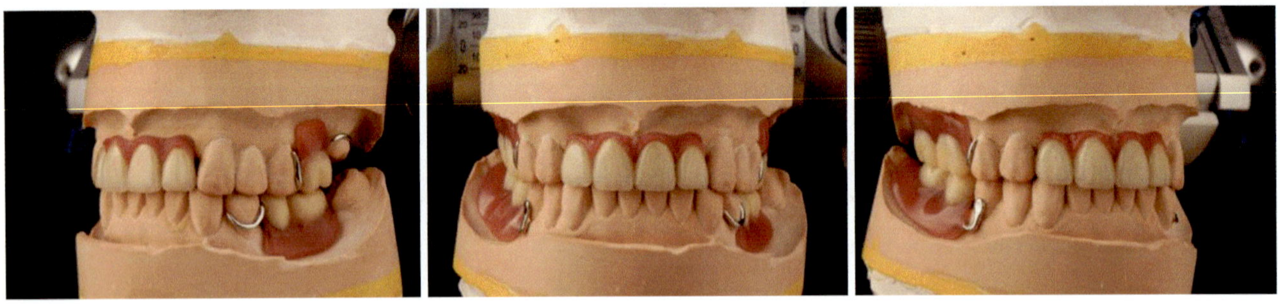

Fig. 6.232 After the porcelain teeth are bonded, gingival porcelain is porcelained; the restorations are finally completed

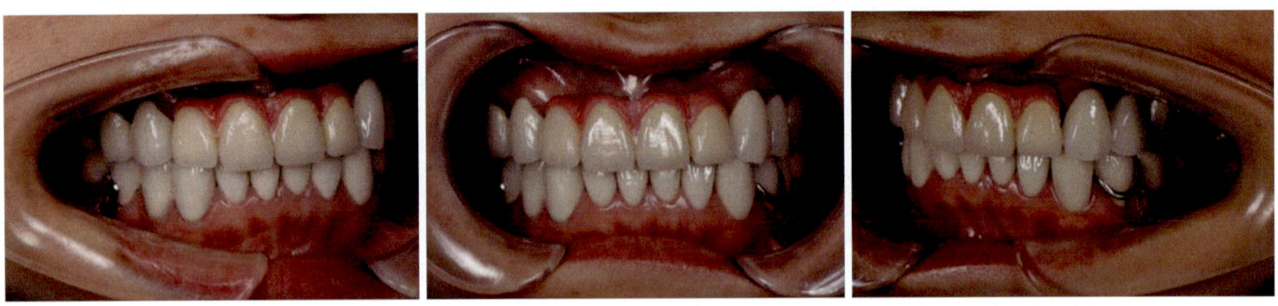

Fig. 6.233 The intraoral renderings

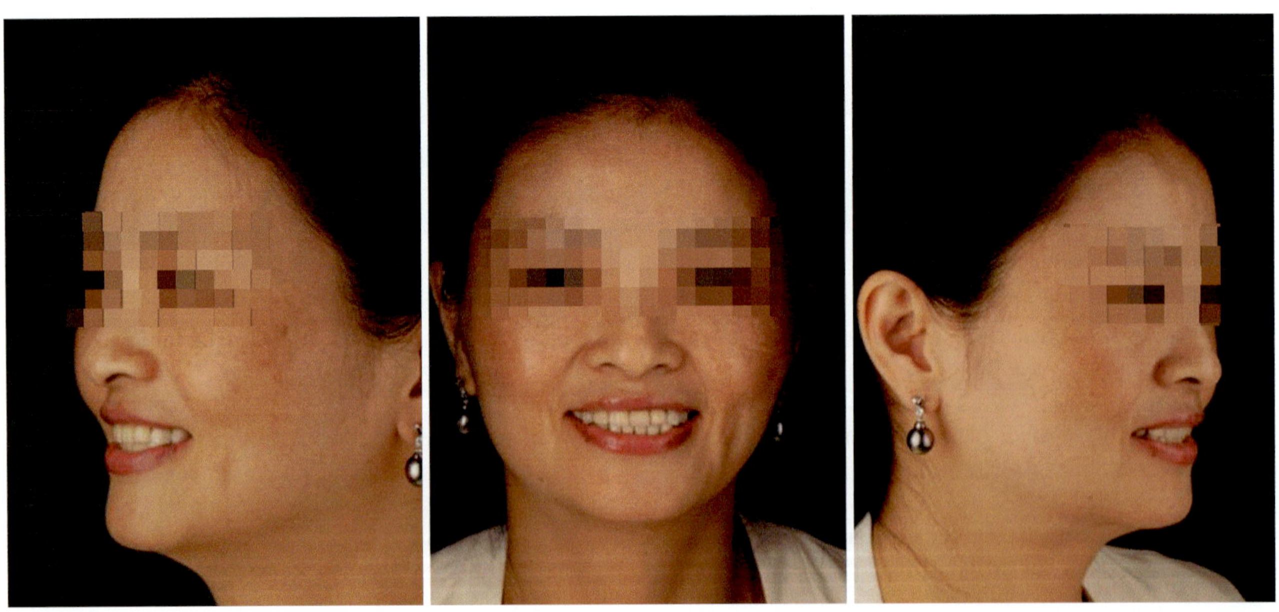

Fig. 6.234 Full-face view

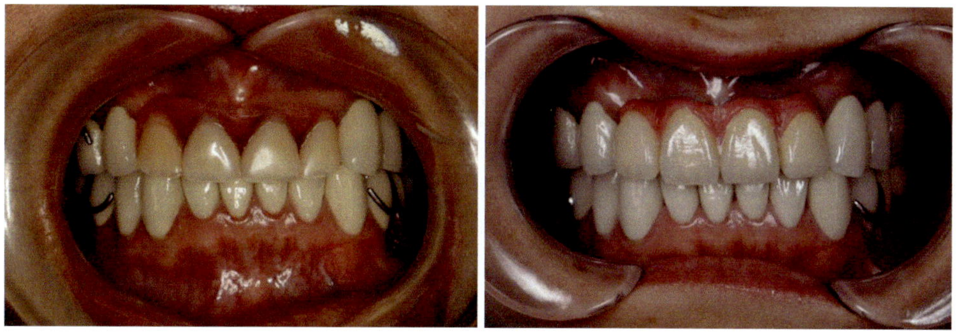

Fig. 6.235 Comparison before and after wearing teeth

natural teeth and dense bone, PEEK and its composite materials have attracted attention in the field of stomatology. At present, PEEK and its composite materials have been used in fixed repair, removable partial denture repair, and implant repair.

In the field of removable restoration, PEEK shows many advantages: because PEEK has high elasticity, it can reduce the torque on the distal and mesial abutment teeth and is especially suitable for the cases of free-end loss; PEEK has no metal color and peculiar smell, and the taste of patients is better, and compared with the traditional metal stent, PEEK stent has no metal color and is more esthetic; PEEK is lighter than metal, and patients wear better. It is also reported that PEEK material has low plaque adhesion, which is helpful for periodontal health. However, PEEK is not a perfect material. Although its elasticity is high, its relative strength is insufficient, and it may not be suitable for some delicate structures. Therefore, PEEK tends to make relatively simple stent, especially plate structures. However, due to the limited scientific evidence and the lack of generally accepted stent design rules, it is less used in clinical final repair and is more commonly seen in temporary repair.

In the next four cases, we used PEEK as the stent material for repair and achieved good results.

6.28 Case 28

A Case of Non-free-End Mandibular Loss Repaired by PEEK Bracket RPD

1. *Before restoration*

   A woman, 65 years old. There are fixed restoration on A4–A7 and B5–B7, and C126 and D126 are missing. The anterior teeth have tight occlusion with deep overbite and normal overjet, and pigmentation is visible on the tooth surface. C4 is I°loose, and the remaining teeth are not loose (Fig. 6.236).

2. *RPD design and manufacturing*

   In this case, cobalt chromium alloy [3] and PEEK are used to make stent respectively. The mandible is Kennedy III dentition defection, and the remaining teeth are not loose, so it is considered to select the teeth on both sides of the missing space as the abutment and use the mesial rest to reduce the lateral force on the abutment. Consider placing combined clasps between C45 and D45, respectively, and ring clasp on C7. Double lingual bar is used in major connector. Due to the low strength of PEEK, it is necessary to thicken the metal stent structure properly and then cut it to get PEEK framework (Fig. 6.237).

3. *After restoration*

   The final result is shown in Figs. 6.238 and 6.239. The patient is much satisfied.

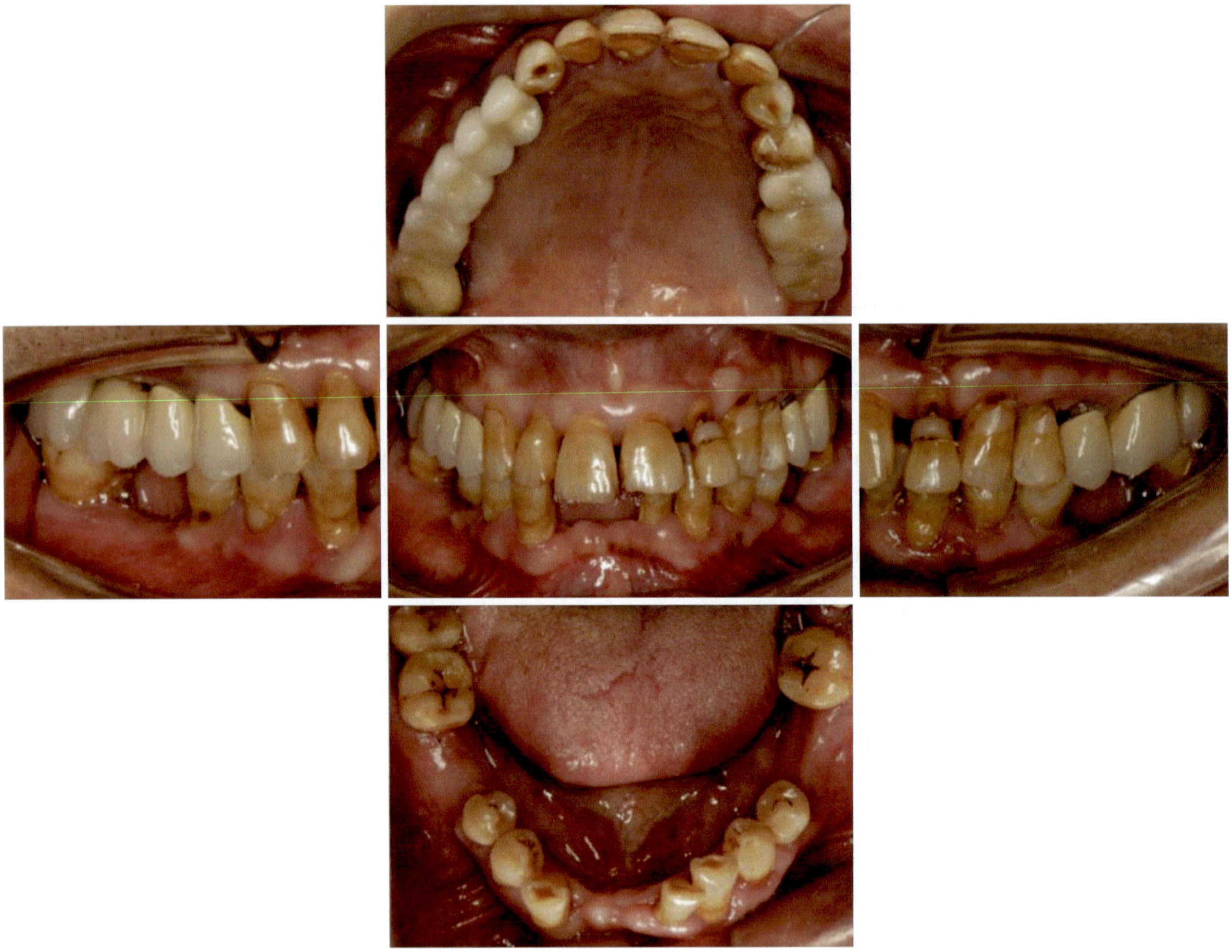

Fig. 6.236 Intraoral condition

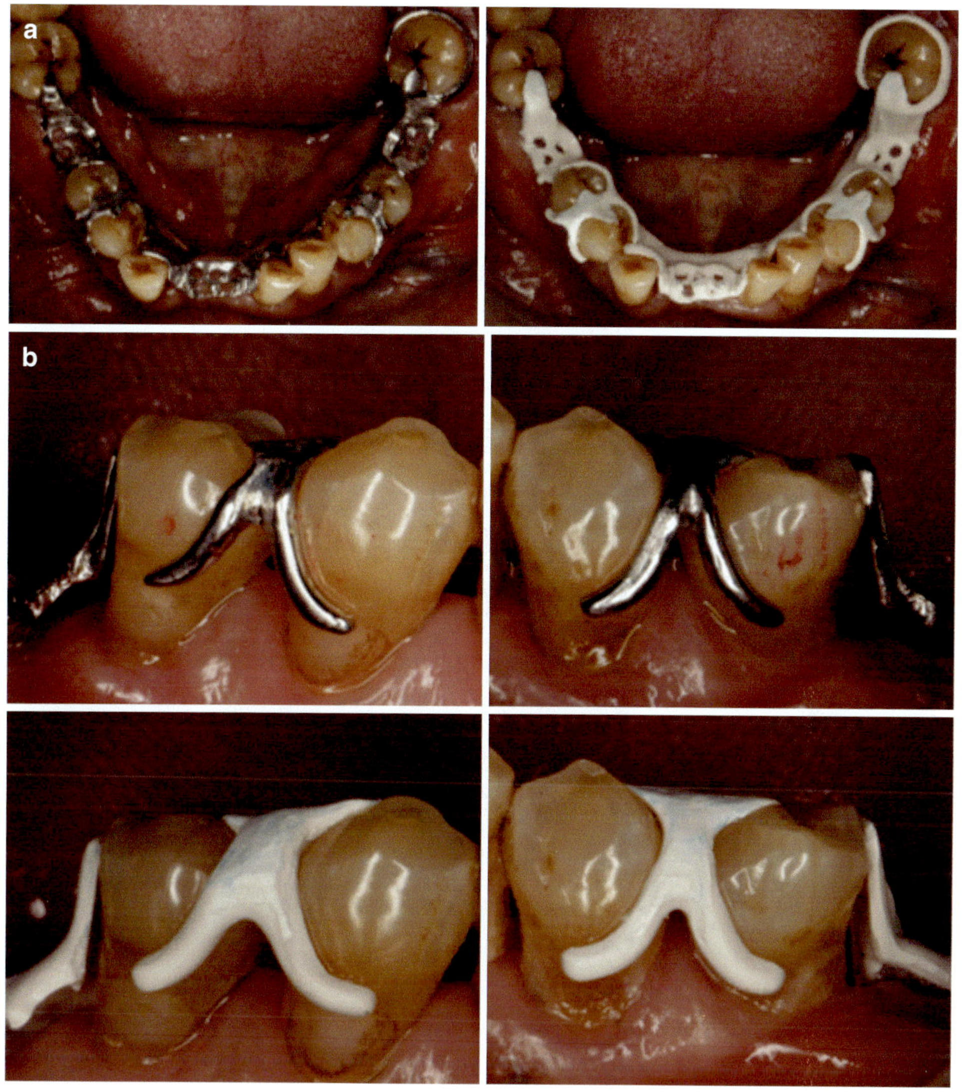

Fig. 6.237 Bracket design. (**a**) Machining of two kinds of stent materials (cobalt chromium alloy on the left and peek on the right). (**b**) Proper thickening of PEEK clasps

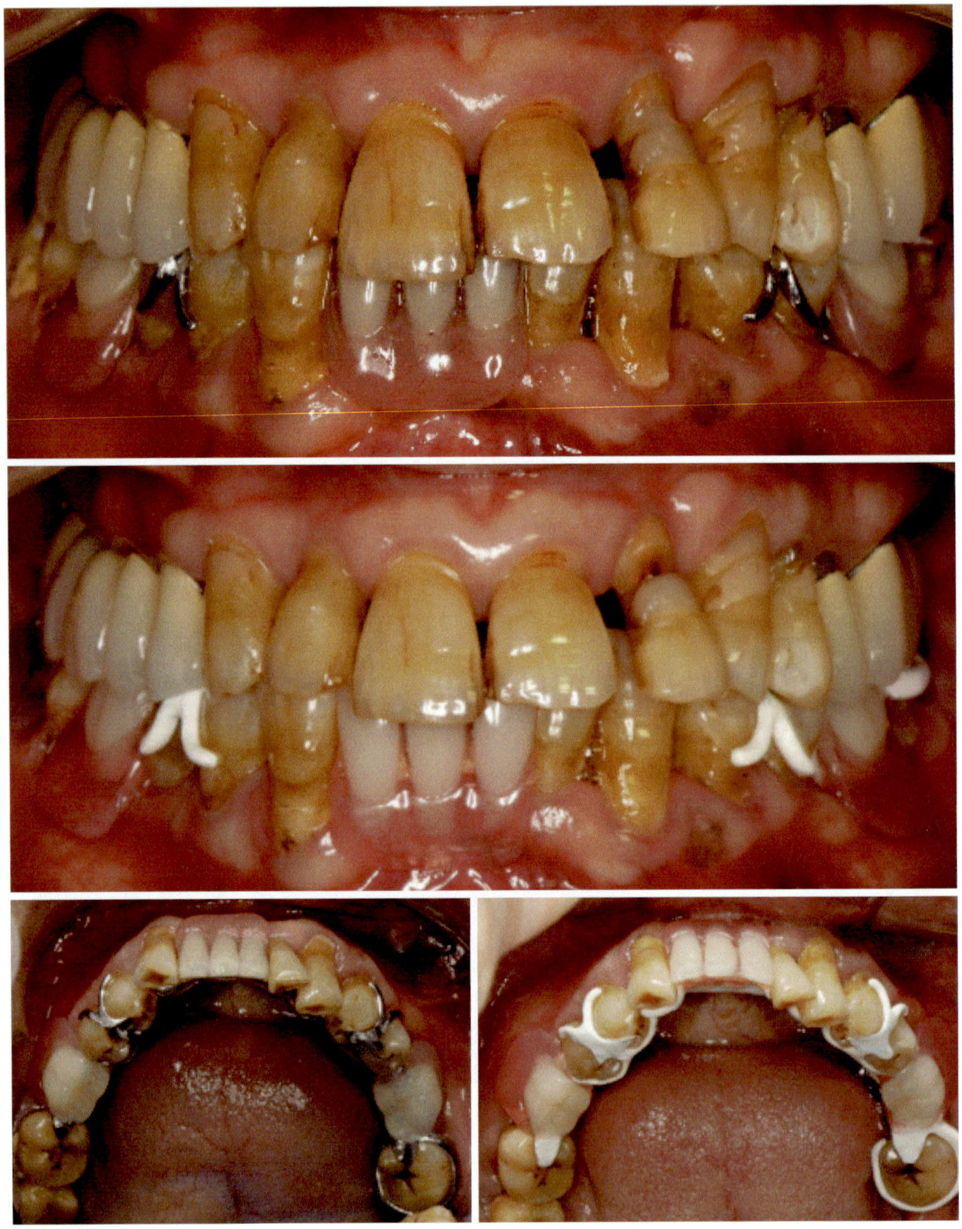

Fig. 6.238 The intraoral renderings

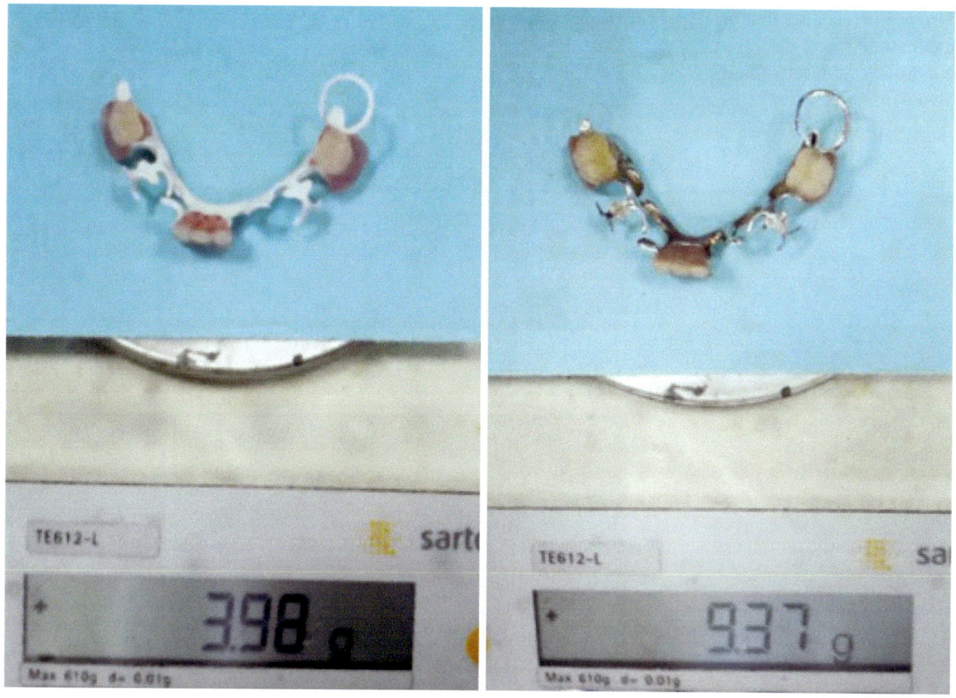

Fig. 6.239 The weight of PEEK bracket is 58% lighter than that of CO-Cr alloy bracket

6.29 Case 29

One Case of Dentition Defect Repaired with PEEK Stent Combined with RPD

1. *Before restoration*

   A woman, 66 years old. The upper jaw is Kennedy III dentition defect, the remaining teeth in the upper jaw are A3–B3, and only C3 is left in the lower jaw; C3 is once loose. It can be seen that alveolar bone resorption is serious, especially that the mandibular alveolar bone is in poor condition (Fig. 6.240).

2. *RPD design and manufacturing*

   For the patients with few remaining teeth, the main support mode of removable denture is mucous membrane support, and when using the remaining teeth for retention, it needs to use the base for retention, which requires that the base has a certain range, and the edge of the base is well sealed. Therefore, this case combines two techniques of esthetic clasp with absorbable denture to obtain good retention and esthetic effect. First, make the primary impression (Fig. 6.241), obtain the primary model (Fig. 6.242), make individual trays (Fig. 6.243), make the final impression (Fig. 6.244), obtain the final model (Fig. 6.245), design the bracket on the final model (Fig. 6.246), and make the wax pattern (Fig. 6.247) after the bracket is completed.

3. *After restoration*

   After the repair, the facial pattern is good without clasp exposure. The patient feels comfortable and satisfied (Figs. 6.248 and 6.249).

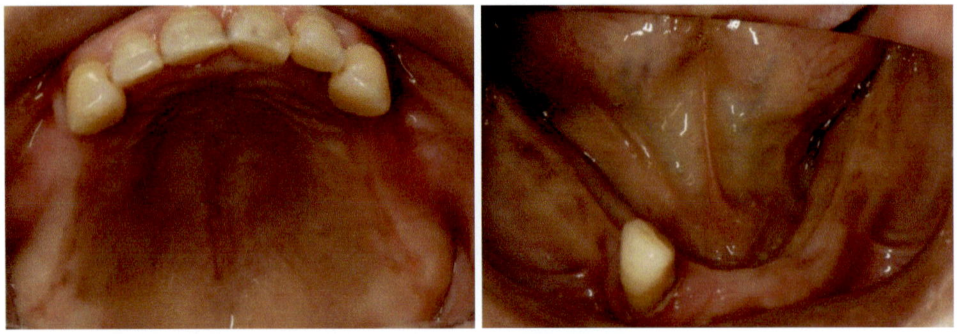

Fig. 6.240 The remaining teeth are few, and the condition of the remaining alveolar bone is poor

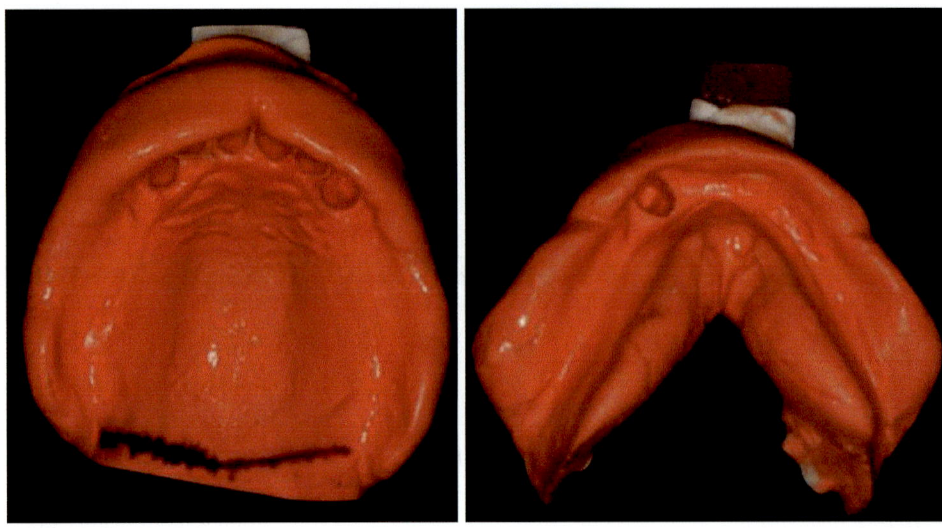

Fig. 6.241 Primary impression

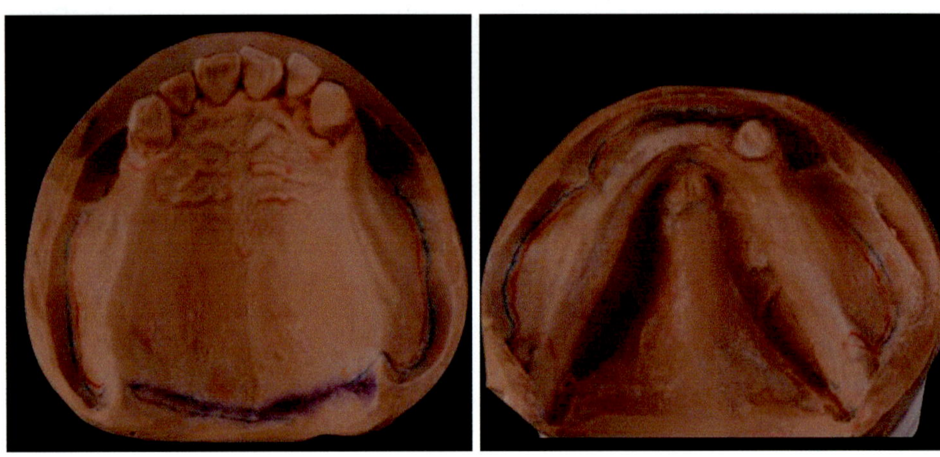

Fig. 6.242 Primary model

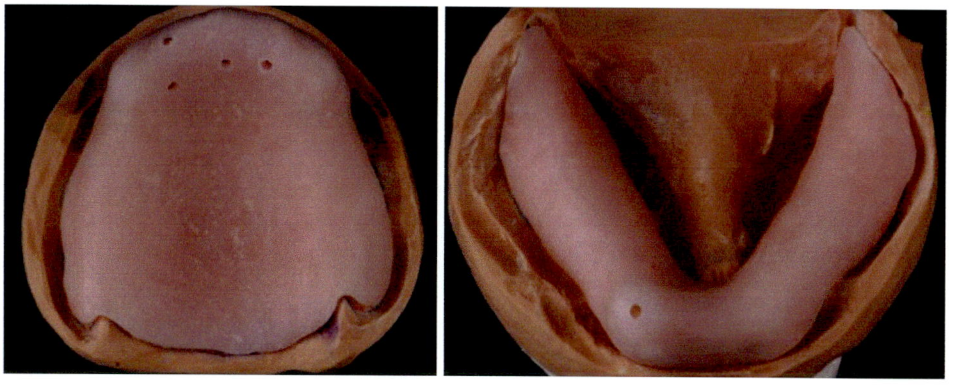

Fig. 6.243 Making individual trays

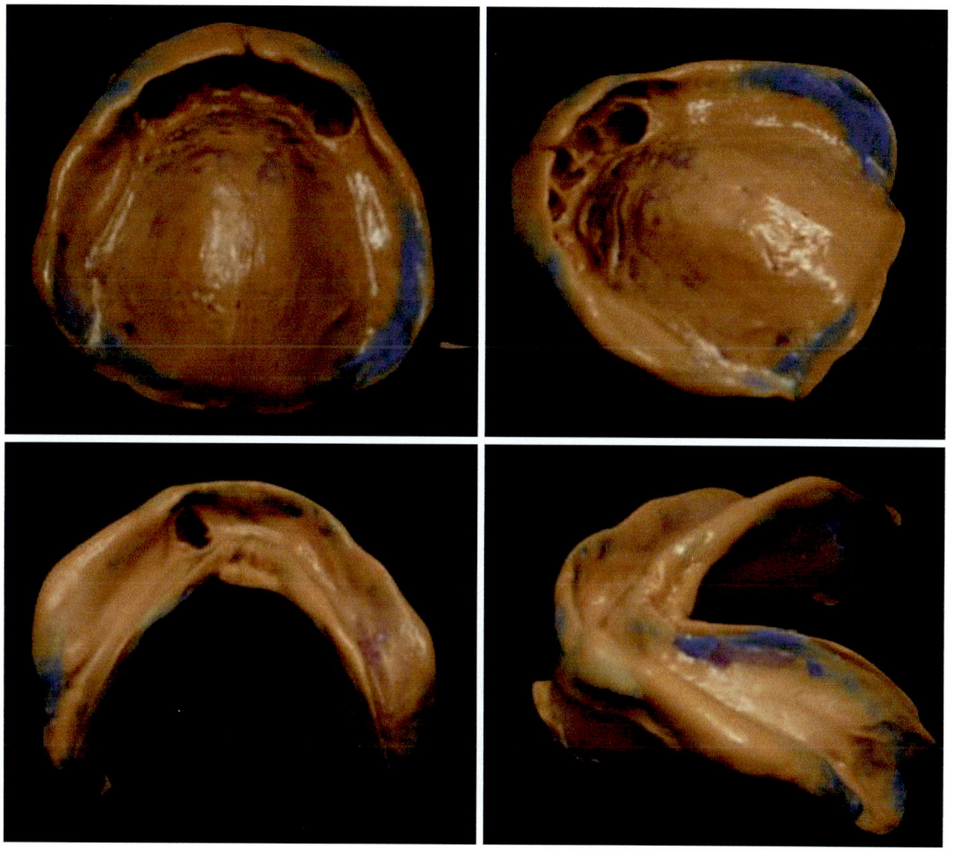

Fig. 6.244 Silicone rubber for final impression

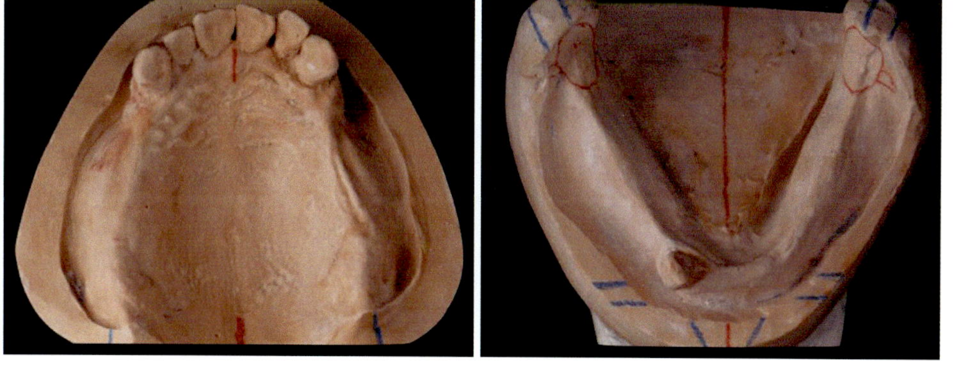

Fig. 6.245 Final model

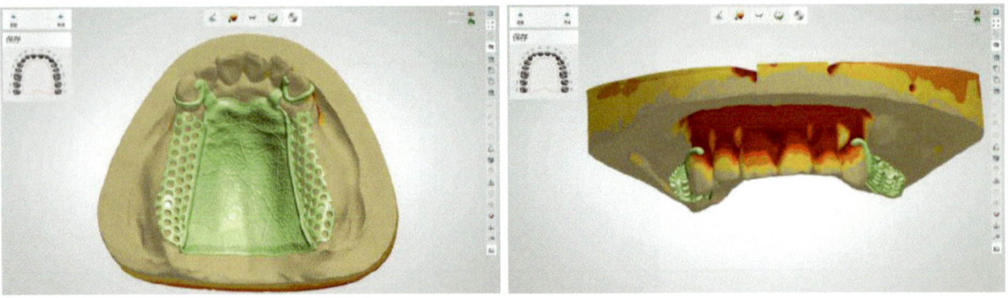

Fig. 6.246 Design of maxillary bracket

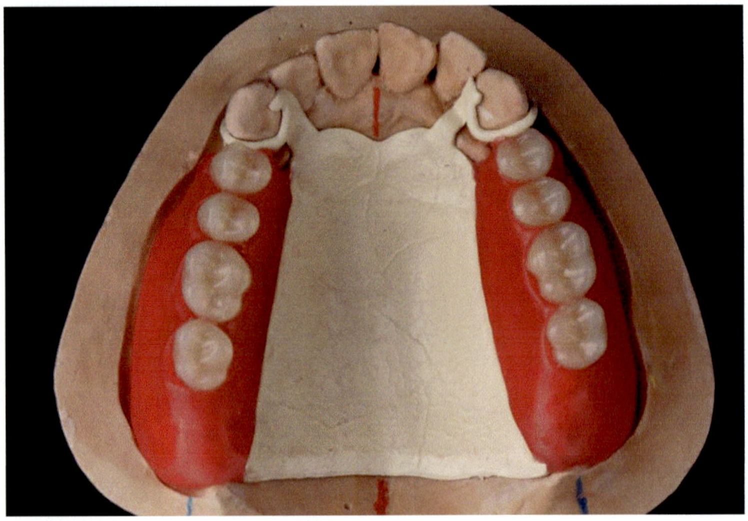

Fig. 6.247 Bracket completion and wax pattern production

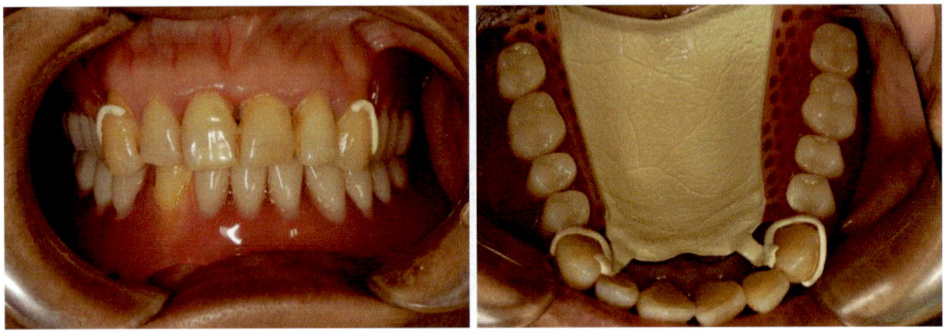

Fig. 6.248 The intraoral renderings

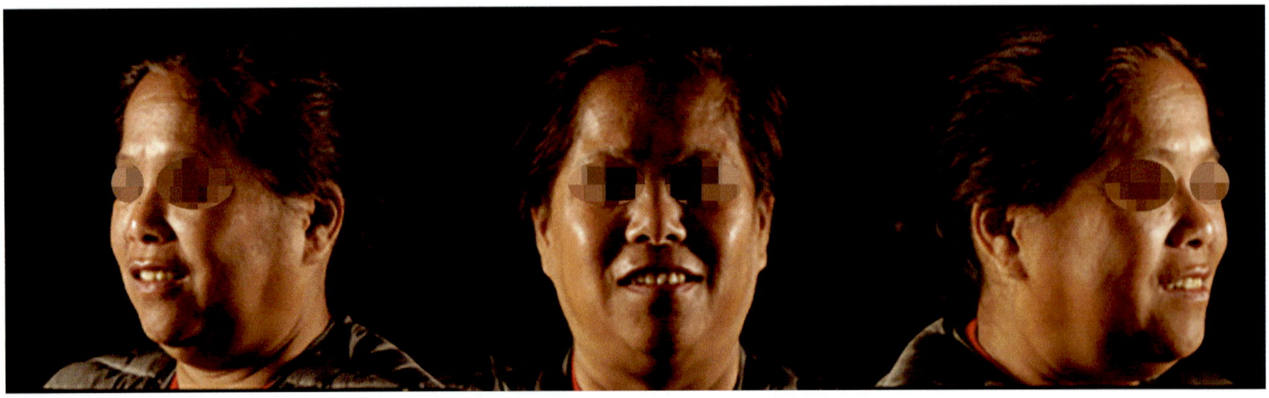

Fig. 6.249 Full-face view

6.30 Case 30

A Case of Upper and Lower Dentition Defect Repaired by PEEK Stent RPD

1. *Before restoration*

   The proportion of the patients' face is normal, but it is not symmetrical. The line between the pupil and the line between the mouth corner are not parallel. According to the main medical history before restoration, the smiling exposed zone of Zhang is observed, which could be judged as a low smile line, and the tooth position of the esthetic area of the upper jaw is A3–B3 (Fig. 6.250).

   The upper jaw are Kennedy I dentition defection, and the lower jaw are Kennedy III dentition defection. It can be seen that there is a black triangle between A1 and B1. The remaining teeth are not loose. The oral hygiene condition is general, and pigmentation can be seen on the tooth surface (Fig. 6.251).

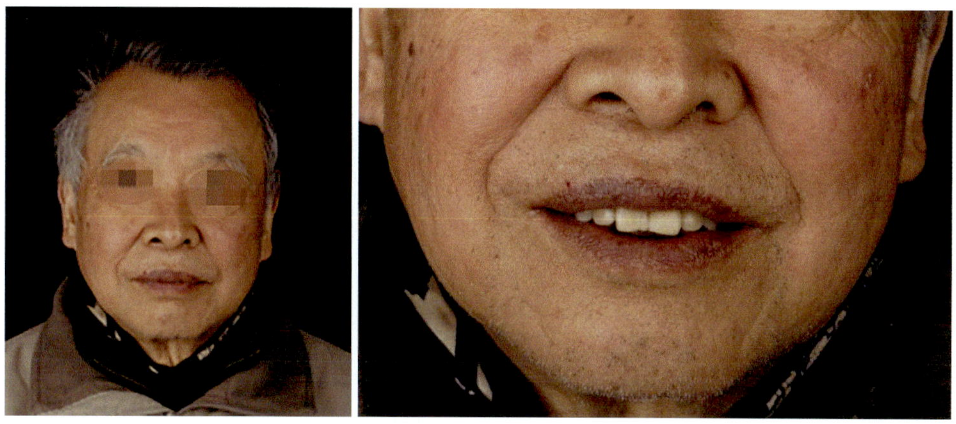

Fig. 6.250 Lower 1/3 facial view

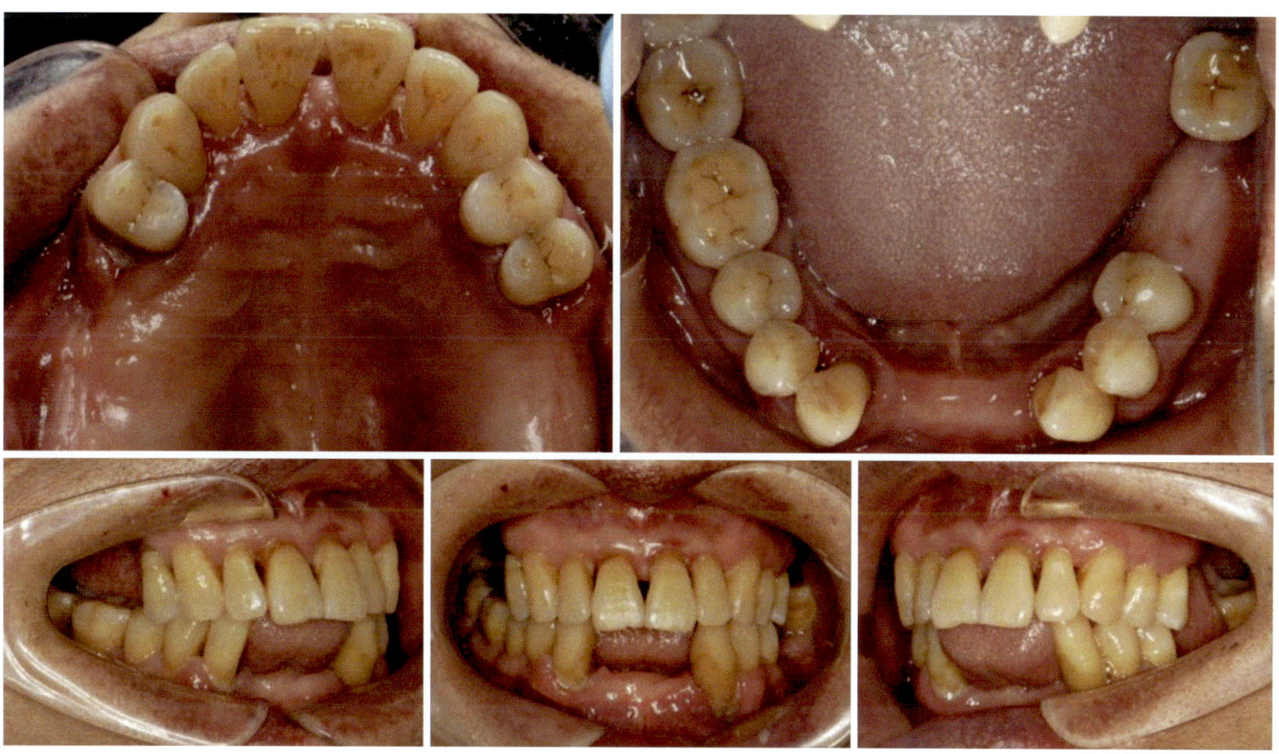

Fig. 6.251 The intraoral renderings

2. *RPD design and manufacturing*

Because the patients are not willing to receive too much attrition, we only prepare a small number of teeth in the mandible and use the existing conditions of the remaining teeth as much as possible to place the rest. The palatal plate was extended to the lingual side of A3B3, so as to achieve the purpose of both abutment teeth and mucosa support. A one-arm clasp is placed on A4. In order to make full use of tooth undercut to increase retention force, the clasp of B5 is extended to B4. The anterior teeth avoid the gums to ensure self-cleaning effect. There are Kennedy III mandibular defect. C4 and D5–D6 are selected as abutment teeth. We place a one-arm clasp on C4 and three-arm clasps on D5D6 to ensure the mandibular retention. Lingual plate is used for major connector (Fig. 6.252). After completing the bracket, arrange teeth and try wax patterns on (Fig. 6.253).

3. *After restoration*

The final result is shown in Figs. 6.254, 6.255, and 6.256.

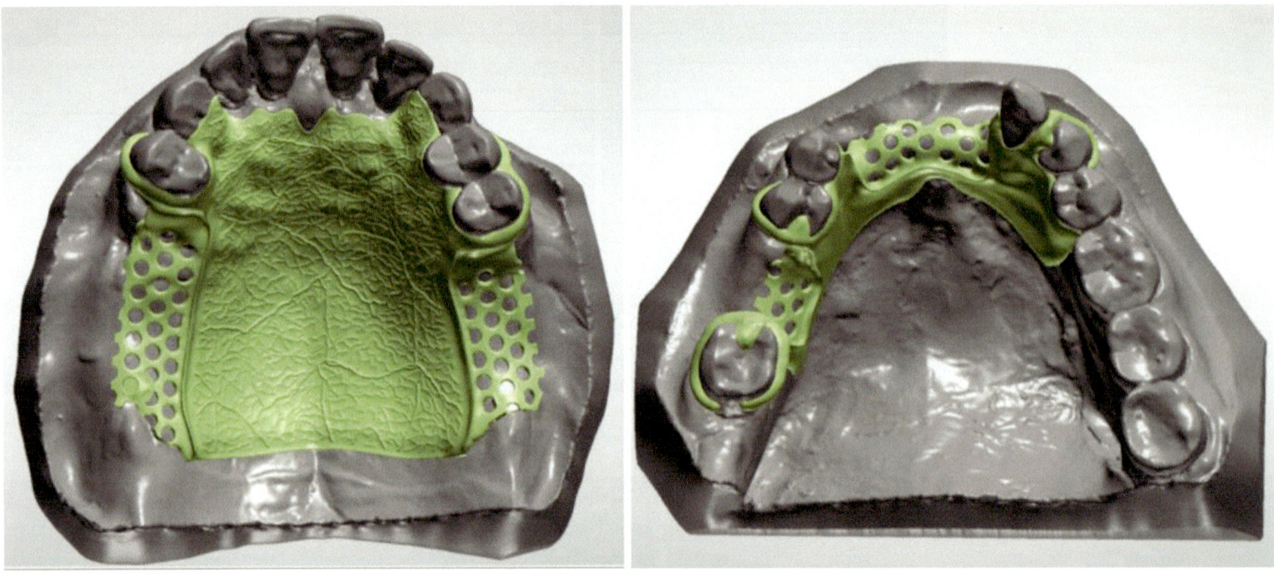

Fig. 6.252 Design of upper and lower jaw bracket

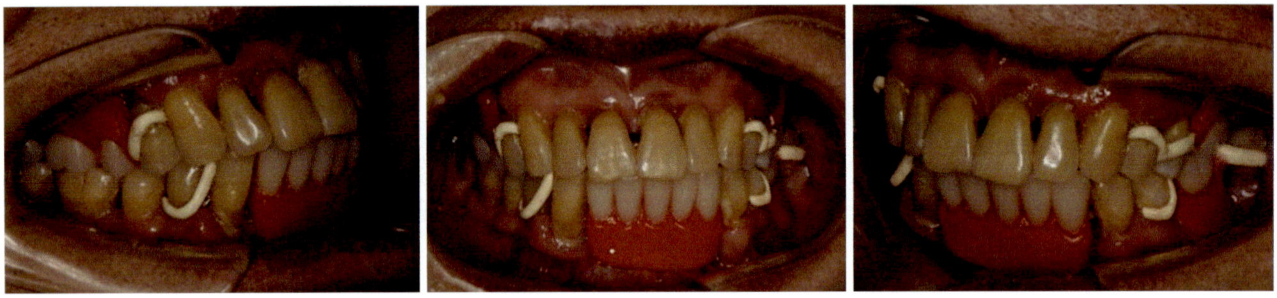

Fig. 6.253 After completing bracket, arrange teeth and try wax patterns on

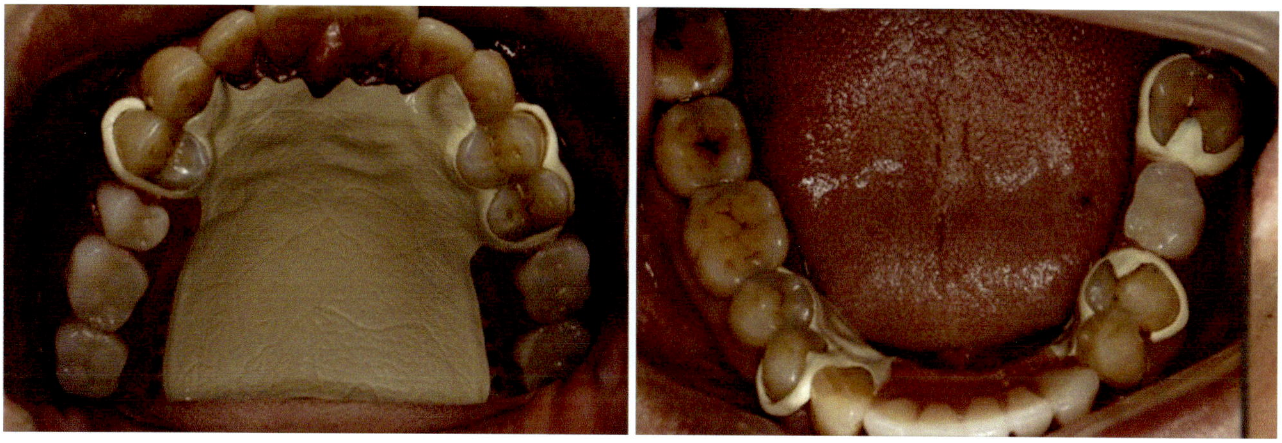

Fig. 6.254 The intraoral renderings

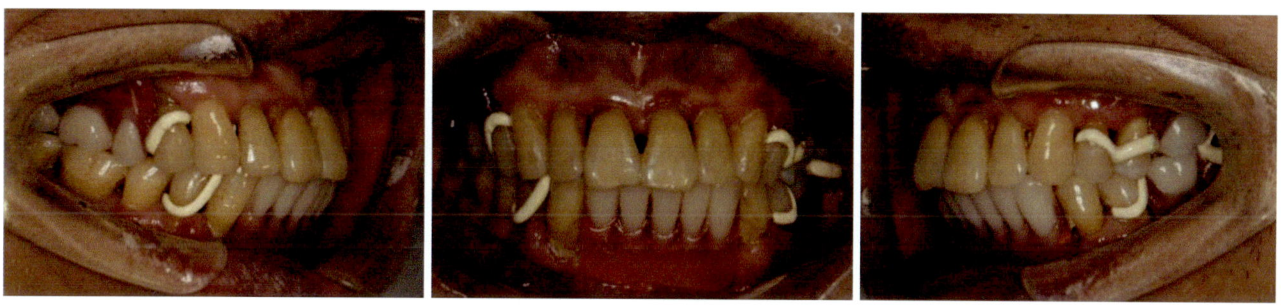

Fig. 6.255 Fitness and occlusion of denture are great

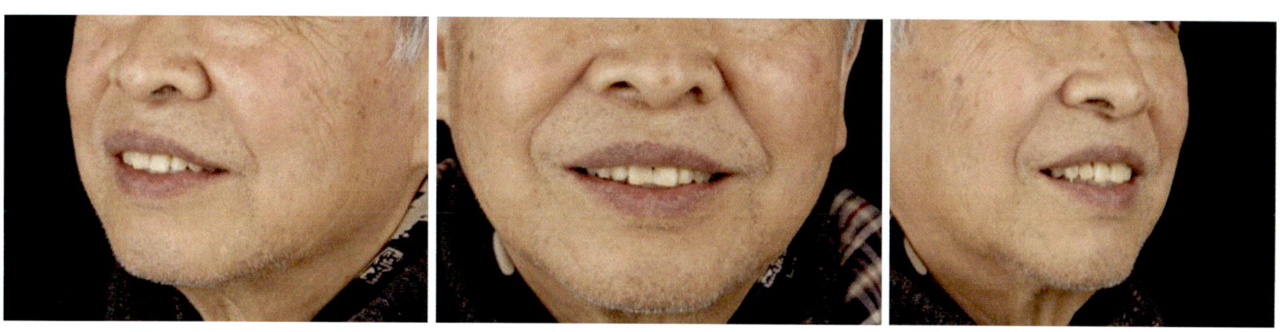

Fig. 6.256 Facial effects

6.31 Case 31

A Case Study on the Design of PEEK Stent and PEEK Integrated Removable Partial Denture

1. *Before restoration*

   A man, 86 years old. The facial asymmetry can be seen in the frontal view, but the middle line of dentition is in harmony with the middle line of the face. The esthetic tooth position which can be seen in the smile view of the face is 14–24 in the upper jaw (Fig. 6.257).

   In the oral examination, the upper jaw is Kennedy II dentition defect, and 25–27 are absent, 24 is residual root, 16 is I°loose, and 14 and 23 have wedge-shaped defects; the lower jaw is Kennedy II dentition defect, 37, 45–47 are absent, 36, 42, and 44 are I°loose. The oral health condition is poor, and there are many calculi (Fig. 6.258).
2. *RPD design and manufacturing*

   In this case, we have designed two schemes: one is traditional design, and the other is a combination of artificial teeth and stent to form integrated stent. Such stent will not form weak points because of the need to design

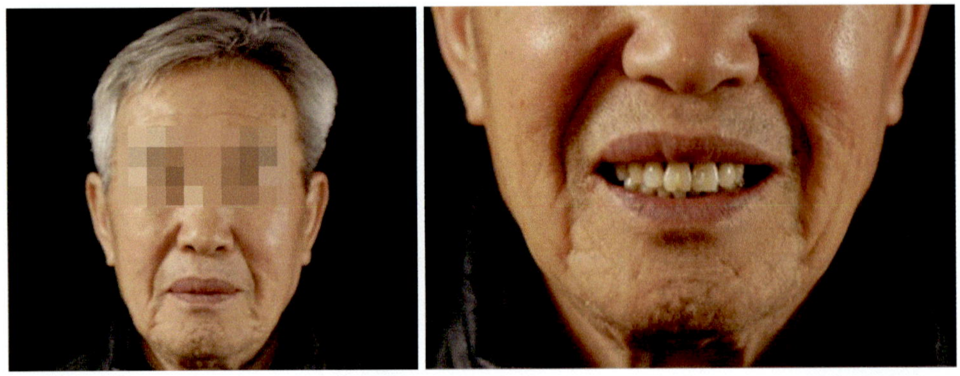

Fig. 6.257 Facial analysis

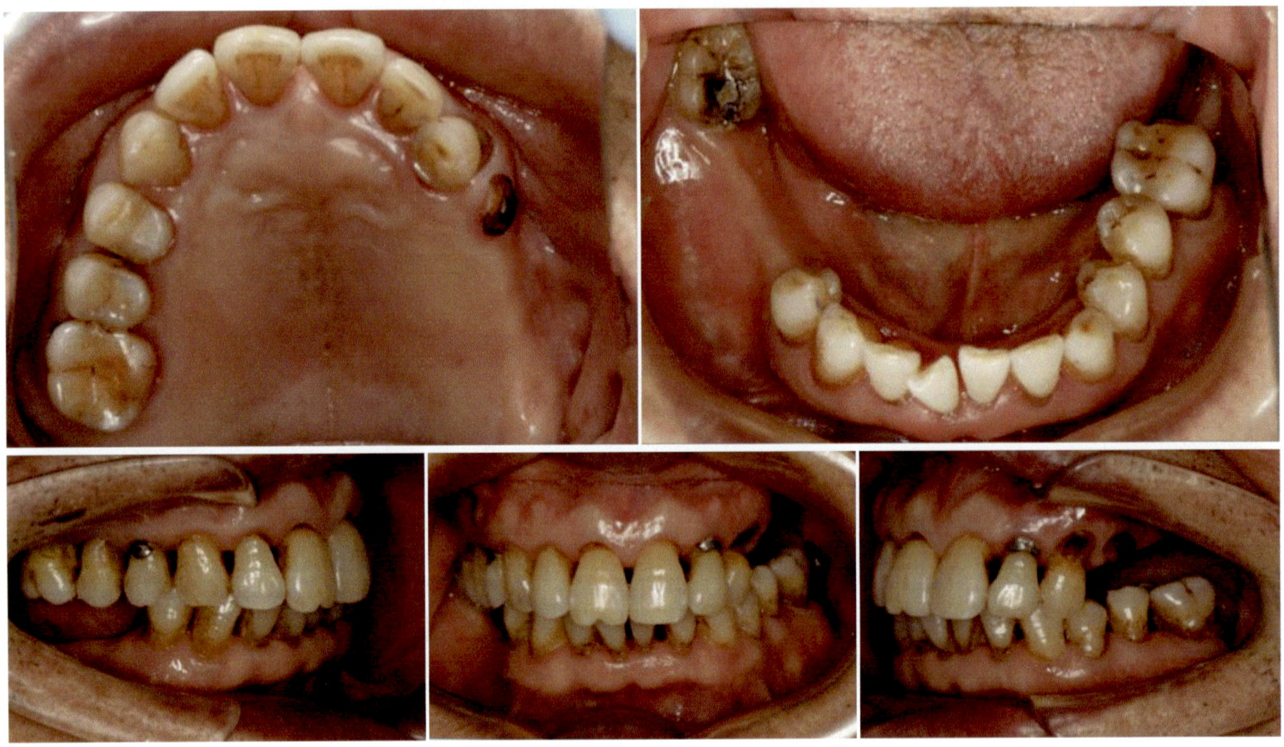

Fig. 6.258 Intraoral condition

the finish line. At the same time, due to the low density of PEEK, the weight of the whole stent is also very light.

(a) Scheme I

  (i) Conventional stent design: In this case, both upper and lower jaw major connectors were plate design, combined with the traditional one-arm clasp and three-arm clasp to sure the retention of the whole stent (Figs. 6.259, 6.260, 6.261, 6.262, and 6.263).

  (ii) Repair effect is in Fig. 6.264.

(b) Scheme II

  The design of rest and retainer in scheme I is not changed, and the artificial teeth and bracket are designed as a whole. Because the missing teeth are all posterior teeth, not in the esthetic area, so it will not affect the esthetics. In the second visit, alginate impression material was used to take impression, and the plaster model is filled, then temporary base and wax rim were made to obtain the occlusion relationship, and then the dental model scanner was used to scan to obtain the digital dentition model and occlusion relationship of patients.

  (i) Digital design of integrated bracket (Fig. 6.265)

  The dentition model and occlusion relationship of the patients were imported into the dental design software for the restoration design. The design of artificial teeth is carried out after confirming the path of inserting and automatically filling out the unwanted undercut. According to the shape of the remaining teeth, the suitable

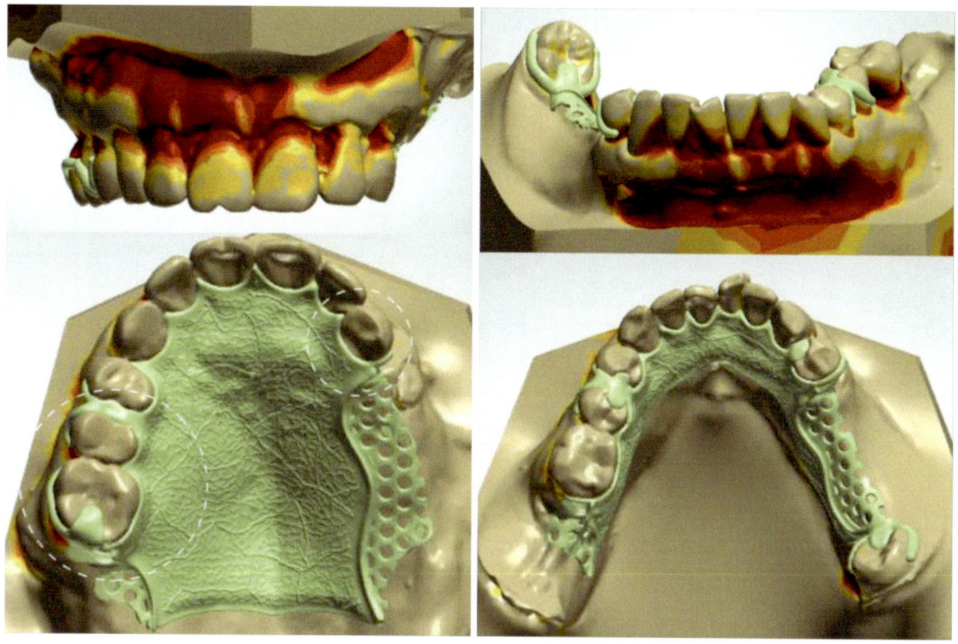

Fig. 6.259 The CAD design of PEEK bracket

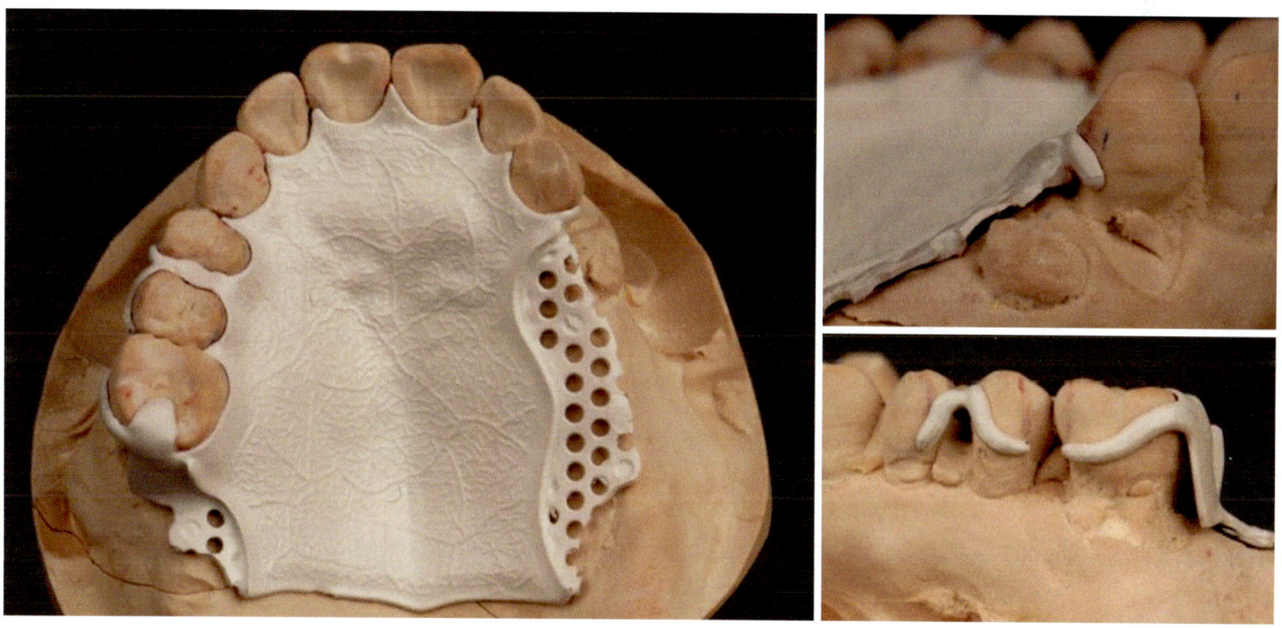

Fig. 6.260 Maxillary bracket completion

artificial teeth can be selected in the tooth shape database; and the size, axial direction, and shape of the teeth can be adjusted individually; and the teeth can be arranged according to the principle of alveolar crest.

After the tooth arrangement is completed, the bracket is designed. The palatal plate/lingual plate was chosen as the major connector to enlarge the stress area of the mucosa and avoid local pressure resulting in tenderness. The combined clasp was placed between 14 and 15, and the one-arm clasp was placed on 17 and 23. The combined clasp and the one-arm clasp were also used for retention of the mandible bracket. The clasp is semicircle, because PEEK elastic modulus is lower than that of metal clasp; in order to ensure the retentive force of clasp, set the depth of clasp tip into the undercut to 0.5 mm, the radius of clasp is 1 mm, the arm of snap ring is 1.3 mm, and the body of clasp is 1.5 mm. In addition, the net minor connector in the traditional bracket design is removed, and the plate-

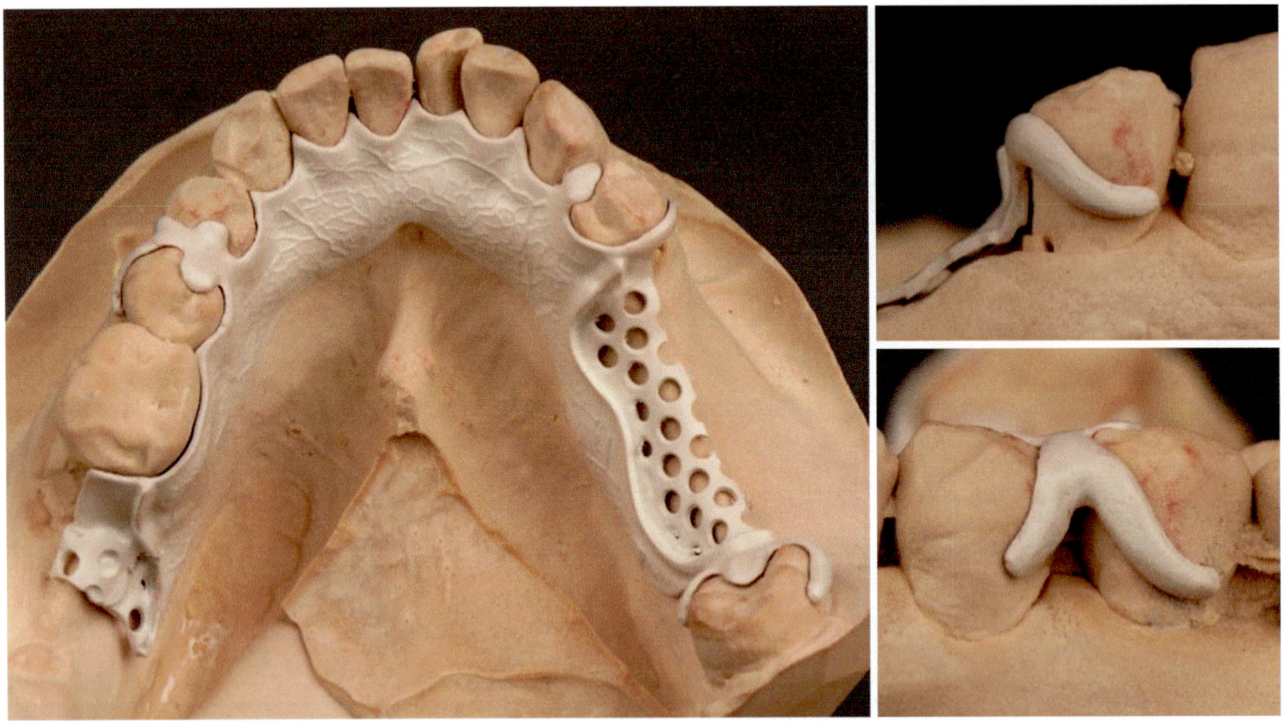

Fig. 6.261 Mandibular bracket complete

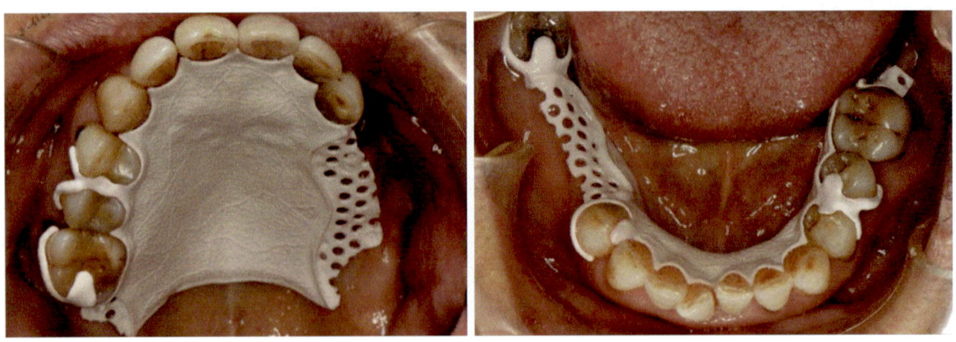

Fig. 6.262 It can be seen that the bracket is suitable for wearing

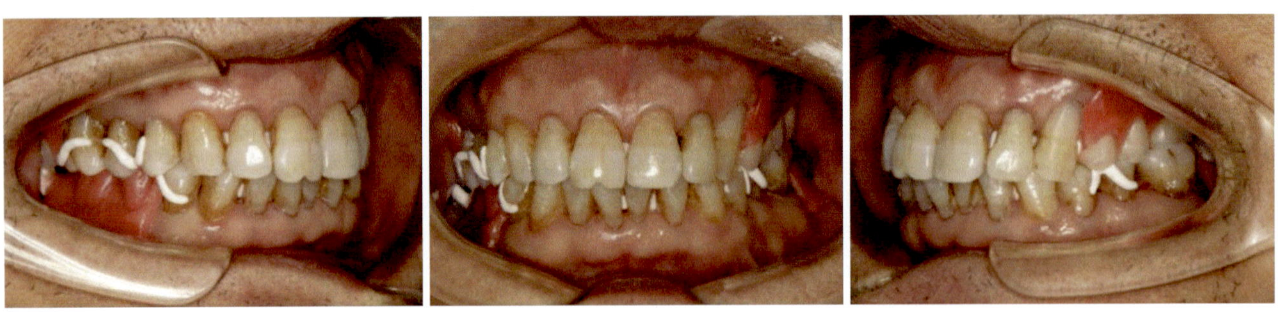

Fig. 6.263 Trying wax pattern on

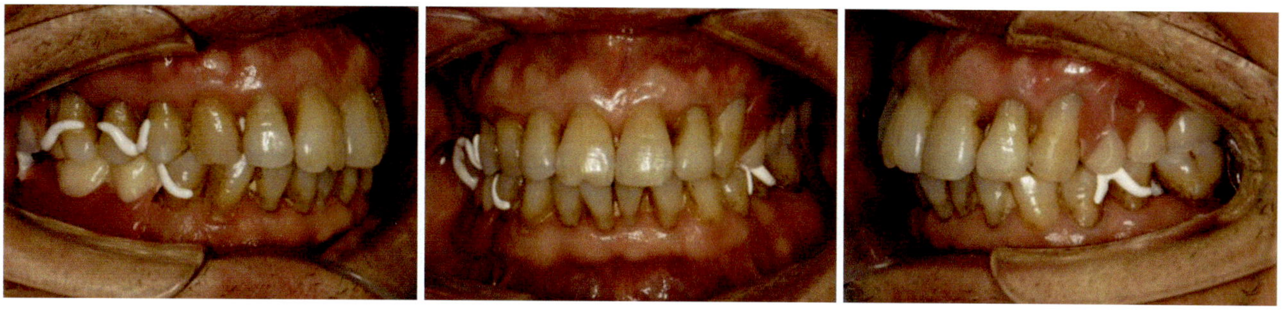

Fig. 6.264 The intraoral renderings

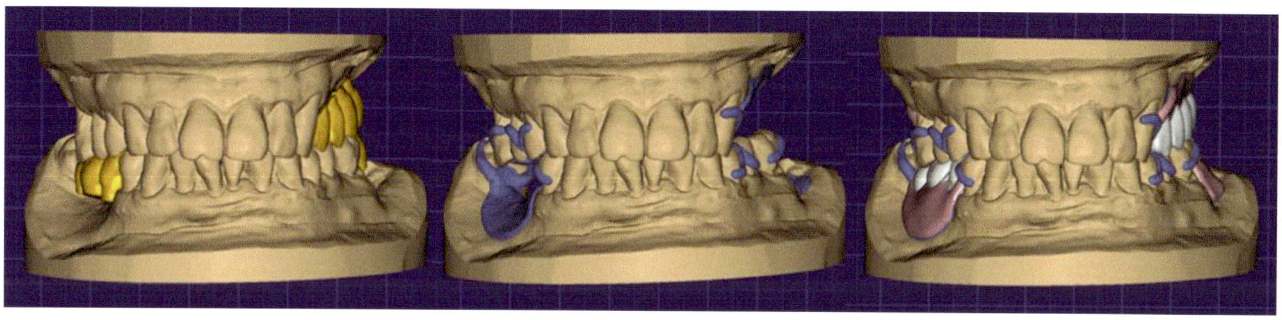

Fig. 6.265 Digital design of integrated bracket

Fig. 6.266 STL data export after bracket design

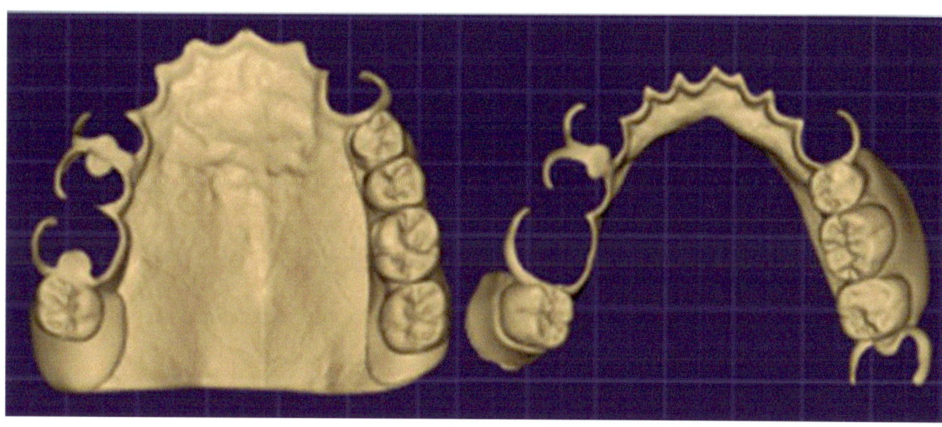

shape major connector is used to cover the extension range of the base in advance.

After the design of human teeth and brackets, the design of artificial gingiva was carried out. According to the shape of adjacent teeth, the natural cervical line, gingival papilla, and root protrusion are formed. Combine the STL data of the bracket, artificial teeth, and gingiva to obtain the designed data (Fig. 6.266).

(ii) Machining of integrated support

Use the CAD/CAM cutting machine to cut the PEEK disk, remove the support rod, and polish and finish the production of the integrated bracket (Fig. 6.267). The weight of maxillary stent is 8.2 g, while that of mandibular stent is only 6.9 g.

3. *After restoration*

Trying in of the denture shows that the stent is suitable, occluded well, and has good retention. The facial view shows part of the clasp entering the esthetic area (Fig. 6.268), but the patient indicates acceptance. The patient feels that the quality of the stent is very light, the self-report has no metal odor, and the comfort is better than the traditional metal removable partial denture. The patient was satisfied with the final results.

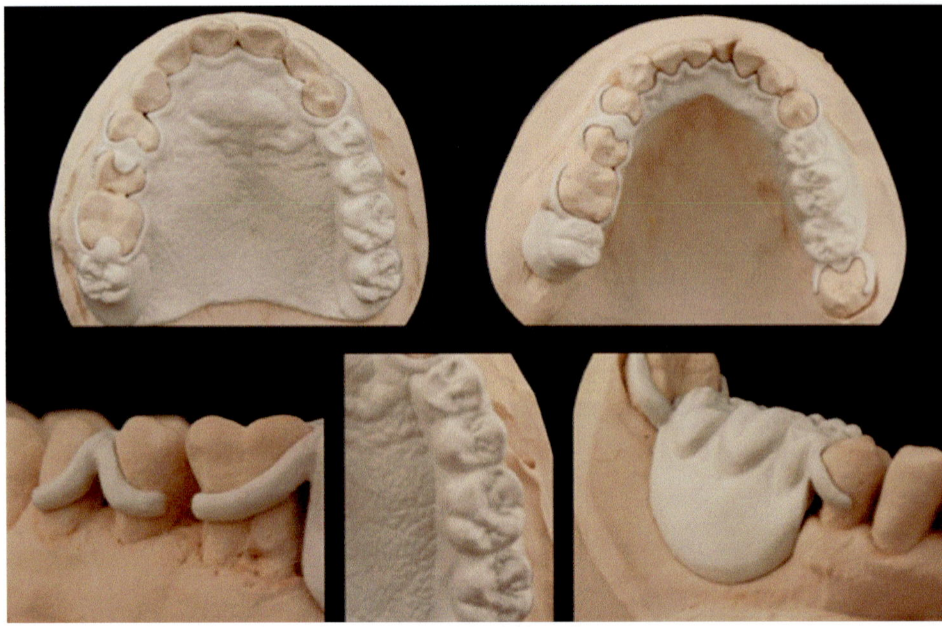

Fig. 6.267 Bracket fabrication completion

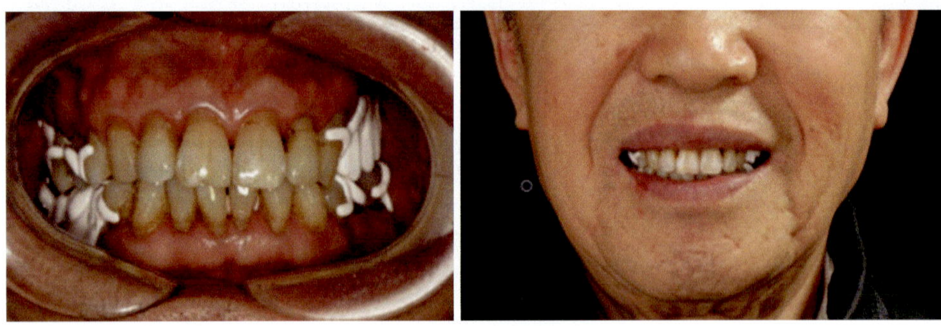

Fig. 6.268 Repair effect

6.32 Case 32

1. *Before restoration*

   A 58-year-old woman with severe dentition defection (Fig. 6.269), whose oral opening was limited to approximately 40 mm (width) and 25 mm (height) as the result of scleroderma. Oral examination showed a severely absorbed alveolar bone with 16, 17, 25–27, and 36–46 teeth missing. Mobility of 11, 12, 21, and 25 was degree III; mobility of 13–15 and 22–24 was degree I. Nonrestorable teeth (11, 12, 21, 25) were extracted.
2. *RPD analysis design and manufacturing*

   Record the maxillary and mandibular dentition size from CBCT data for tray design.

   Import digital files of another patient's casts with similar dentition scale. Adjust models to the same size of target dentition, and remove tooth dental crowns to simulate patient's dentition defect. Design and separate trays into two or three parts and 3D print them (Figs. 6.270 and 6.271). Insert CAD/CAM custom sectional trays into patient's mouth, and take each impression. Pour dental stone to make casts and then scan them after setting. Align sectional models to form final maxillary and mandibular models (Fig. 6.272).

   Embrasure clasps were planned bilaterally of the maxillary dentition (in 14–15 and 23–24 spaces) to further disperse occlusal forces to the abutment teeth. Also, the combined clasps can act as a periodontal splint to stabilize

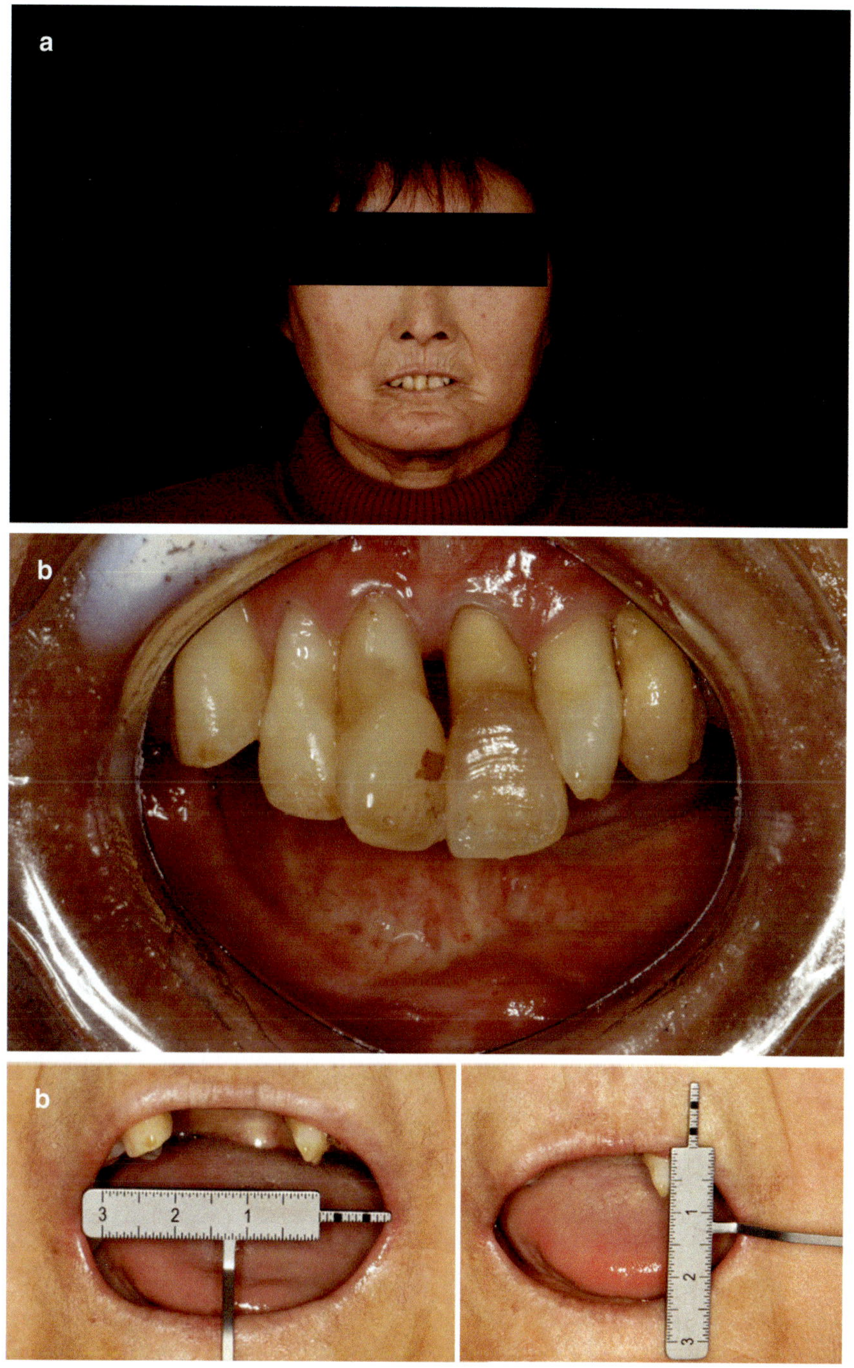

Fig. 6.269 Pretreatment condition. (**a**) Facial frontal view. (**b**) Oral condition. (**c**) Oral fissure evaluation

Fig. 6.270 Design process of custom trays. (**a**) Dentition size simulation. (**b**) Dentition defect simulation. (**c**) Models relief. (**d**) Custom trays design

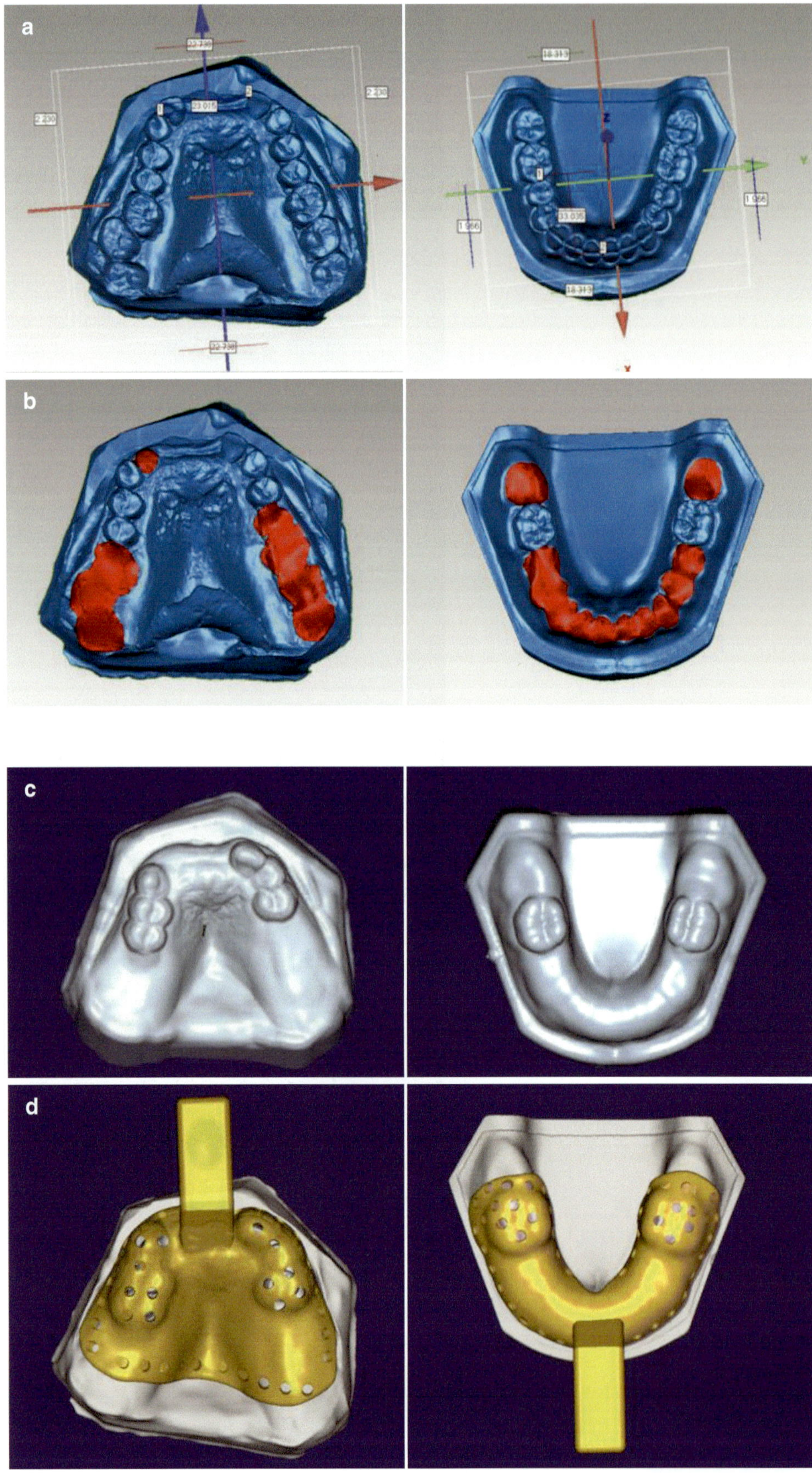

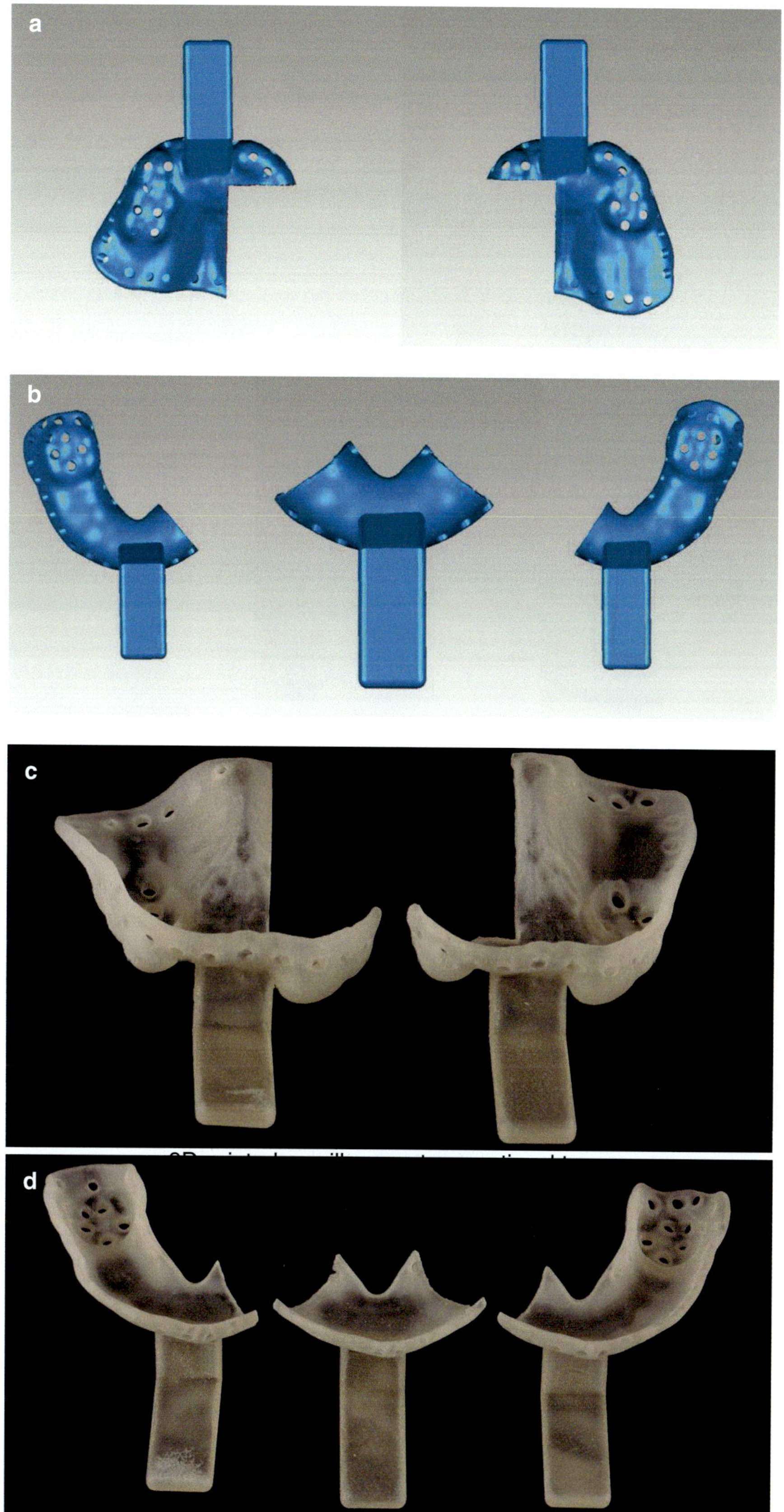

Fig. 6.271 CAD/CAM custom sectional trays. (**a**) Maxillary custom sectional trays. (**b**) Mandibular custom sectional trays. (**c**) 3D-printed maxillary custom sectional trays. (**d**) 3D-printed mandibular custom sectional trays

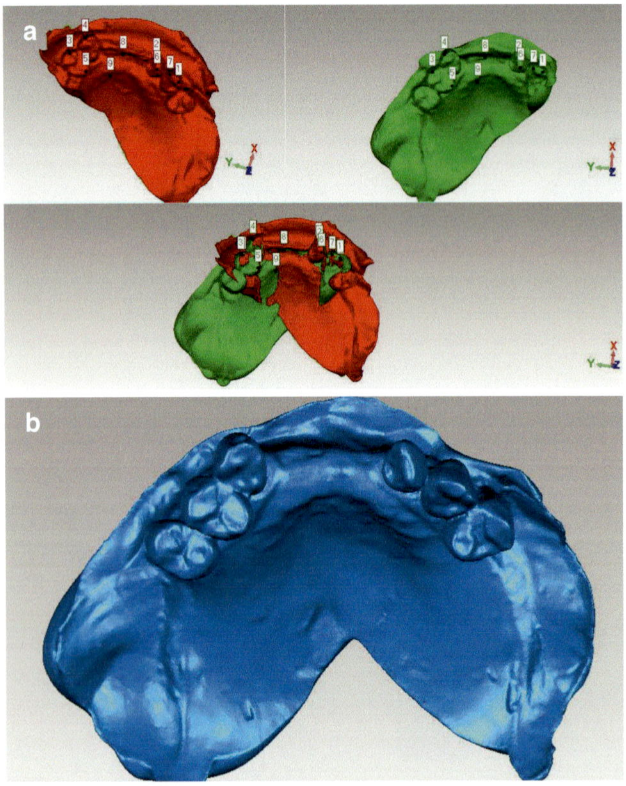

Fig. 6.272 Alignment of models. (**a**) Alignment of maxillary models. (**b**) Final maxillary model. (**c**) Alignment of mandibular models. (**d**) Final mandibular model

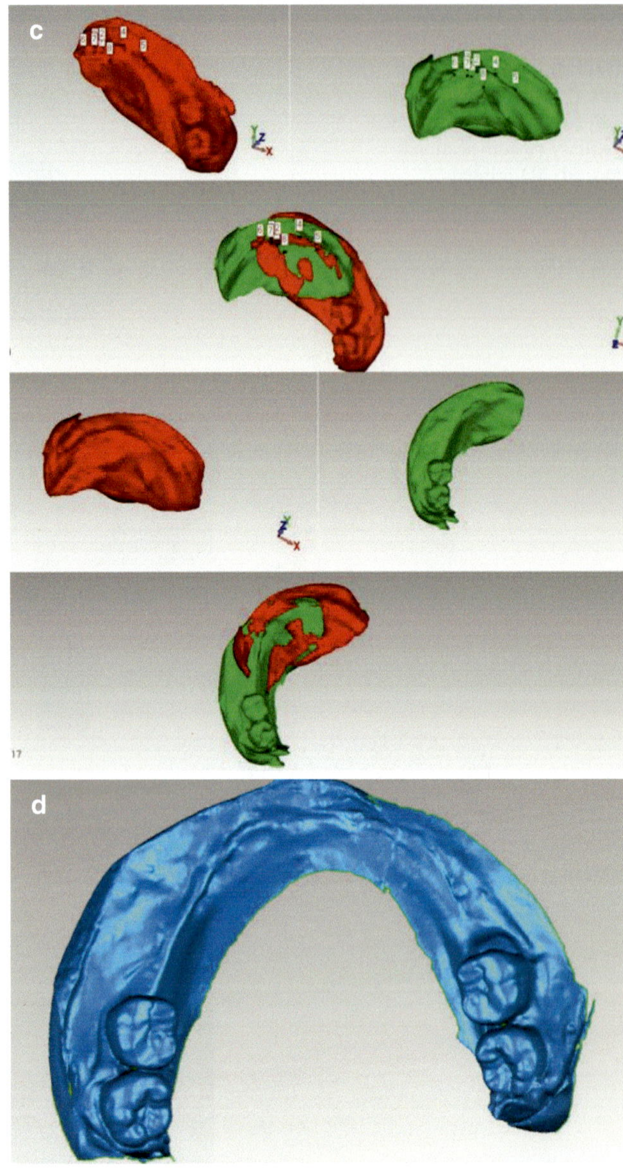

Fig. 6.272 (continued)

the remaining teeth, which had been influenced by severe alveolar absorption. Since the RPD is in one piece and not foldable, a shortened RPD design was adopted, which referred to the restoration of dentition only to the first molars instead of the second molars. As for the mandibular RPD, ring clasps with mesial rests were placed bilaterally on the second molars to provide more retention and stability. Due to the mesio-ligual inclination of the abutment teeth, the tips of clasps were placed at the lingual undercut area, and the rests were placed at the mesioocclusion surfaces. The third molars were excluded from the RPD design in order to reduce the RPD length (Fig. 6.273).

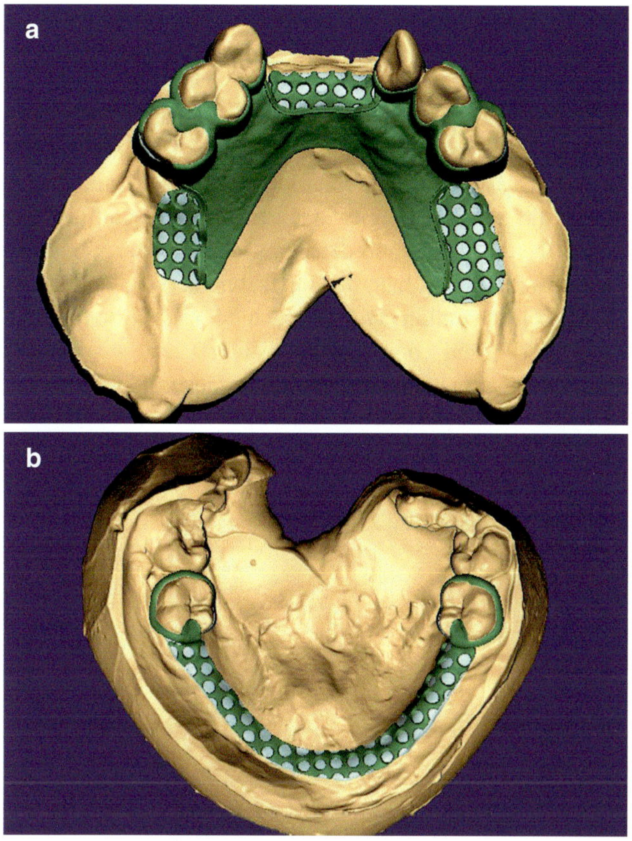

Fig. 6.273 Design of frameworks. (**a**) Design of maxillary framework. (**b**) Design of mandibular framework

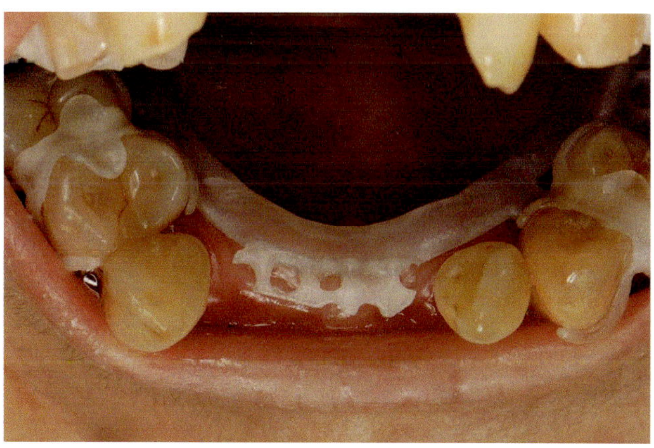

Fig. 6.274 Trying in of resin frameworks

The frameworks were 3D printed with Co-Cr alloy and were tried intraorally (Fig. 6.274); the maxillomandibular relationship in centric relation was recorded. The artificial teeth were arranged and were trimmed and polished (Fig. 6.275).

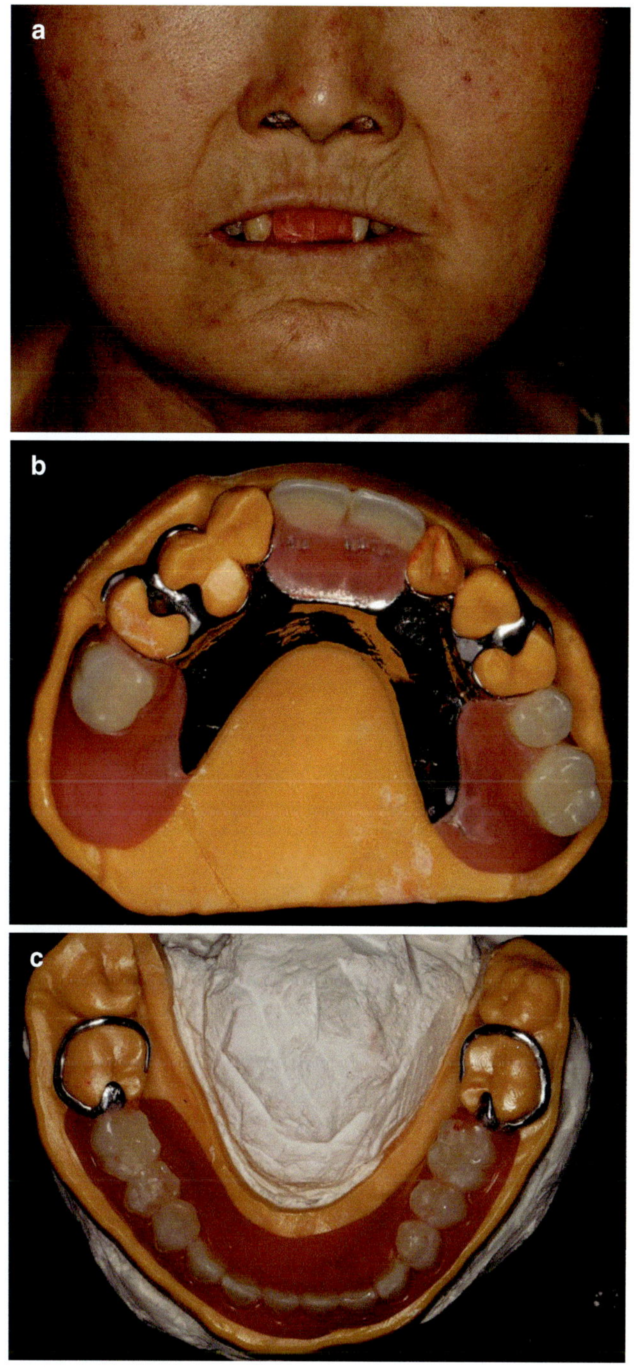

Fig. 6.275 Fabrication of RPD. (**a**) Record occlusal relationship. (**b**) Arrangement of maxillary dentition. (**c**) Arrangement of mandibular dentition

3. *After restoration*

It's the final effect of patient with denture (Fig. 6.276), reporting satisfaction with the treatment results.

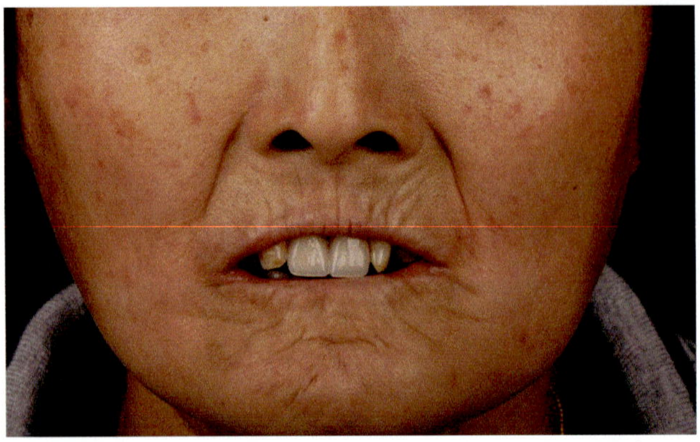

Fig. 6.276 Facial view with denture

6.33 Case 33

1. *Before restoration*

A 7-year-old kid diagnosed with ectodermal dysplasia (EDA) was referred for restoration treatment (Fig. 6.277).

EDA is a group of complex diseases with more than 200 different pathological damages, predominantly affecting the developmental defects of ectodermal tissues like the sweat glands, hair, nail, teeth, and nervous system. Its oral representation can be congenital missing tooth, tooth dysplasia, and conical tooth, which affect severely the chewing, pronunciation, and appearance of patients and will harm the physical and mental health of the patients.

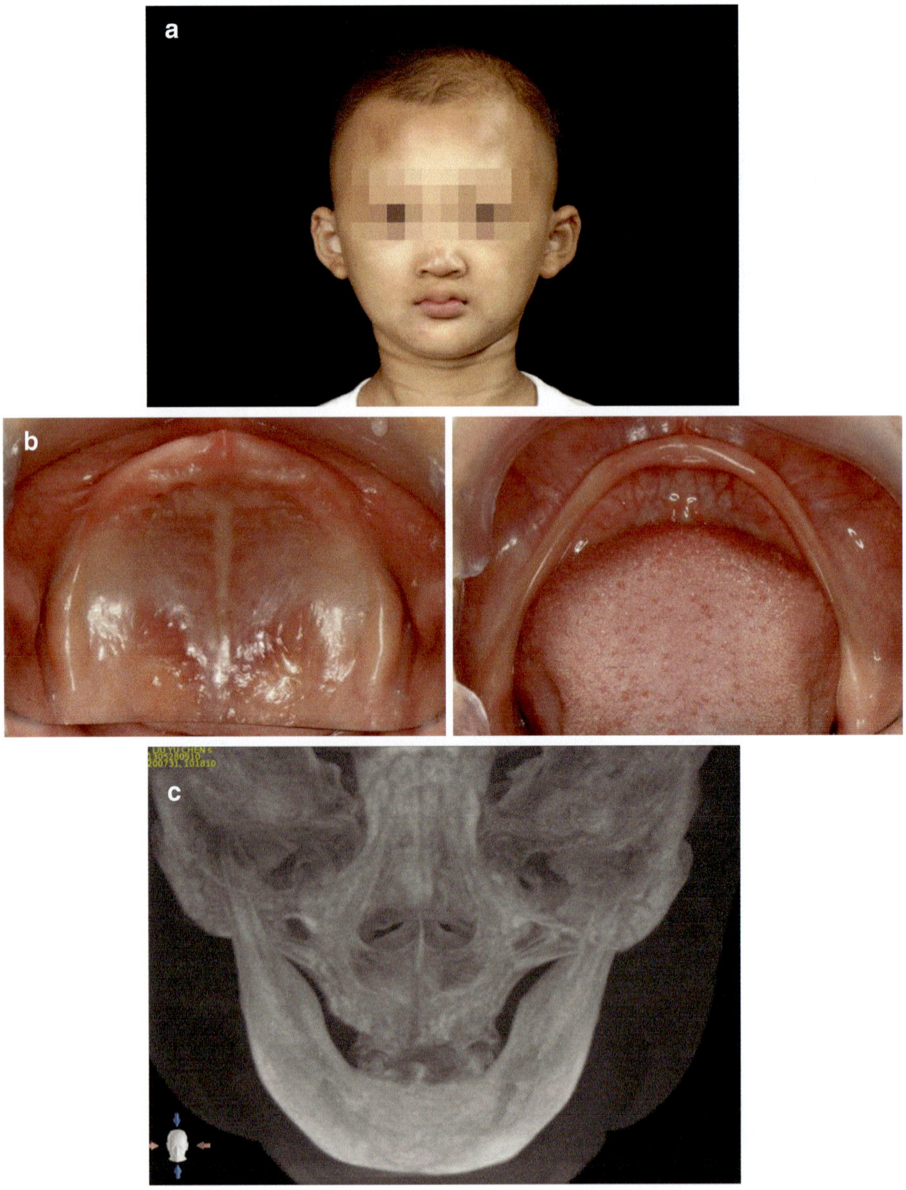

Fig. 6.277 Pretreatment condition. (**a**) Facial frontal view. (**b**) Oral condition. (**c**) CBCT

The patient's oral cavity was characterized by congenital missing teeth, and the patient is too young with active skeletal development to be repaired with implant denture. Early complete denture not only can restore the shape of teeth to reconstruct occlusion and the function of chewing and pronunciation but also can accelerate the development of jaw and temporomandibular joint, which can prevent malocclusion, improve patient's facial contour, establish good relations between the face and the skeleton, promote his physical and mental health, and raise the life quality.

2. *Treatment plan*

   Considering the particularity of the patient, we made a sequential treatment plan for him:

   (a) Stage I: Removable denture restoration immediately.

   Make the final impression with a two-step impression; after that, make the complete denture on the final model (Fig. 6.278). The treatment of the patient will be throughout the whole life cycle, so we record the change of the jaw position and jaw digitally, as the approach to evaluate the repair effects and the basis of the following repair at return visit.

   Due to the considerable aging changes of hard and soft tissues and anatomic structure of young edentulous patients' oral system and the appearance of denture is basically a constant except occlusal surface abrasion, we specially design a custom gothic arch positioning plate with coordinate system and scale on the denture (Fig. 6.279), which can be used to determine the change of jaw position at return visit and also can establish an intraoral coordinate system to record the change of the jaw in different development stages throughout the whole life. The following is the approach we used:

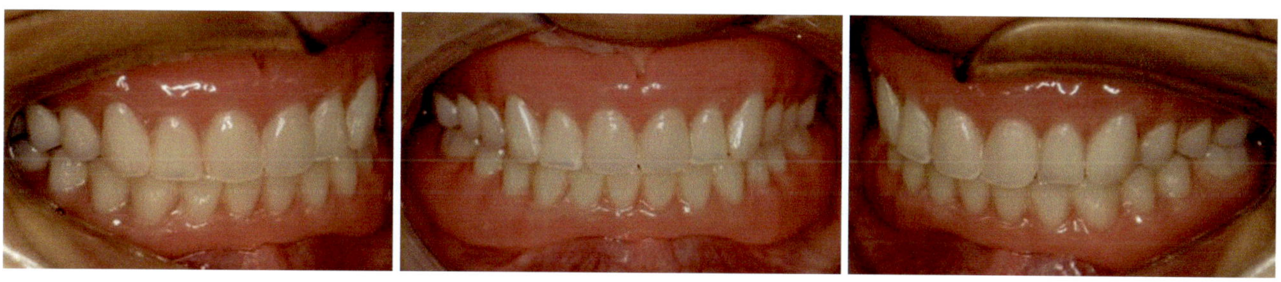

Fig. 6.278 Trying on

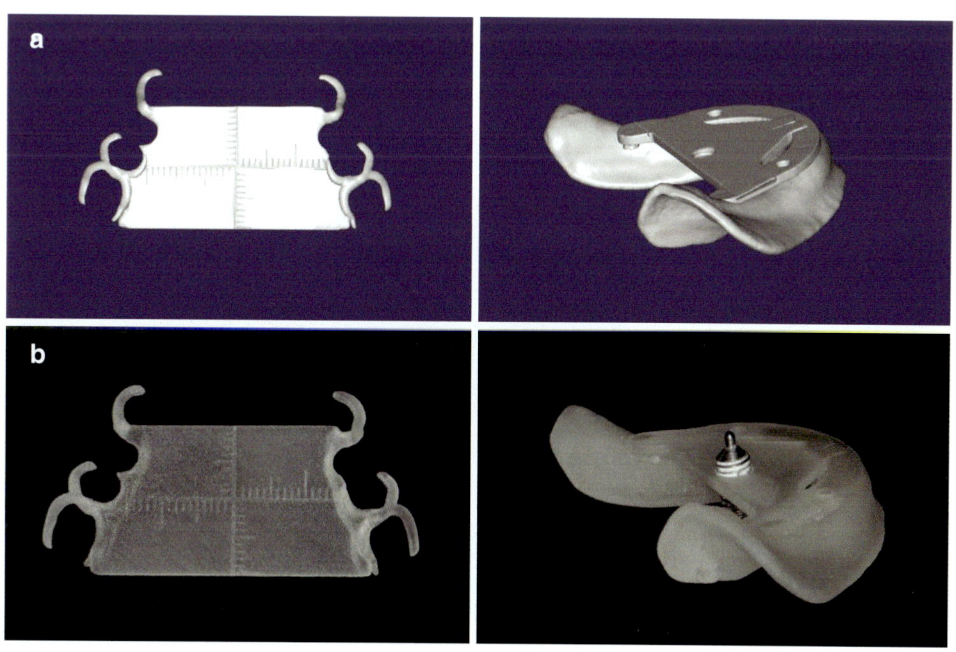

Fig. 6.279 Maxillary and mandibular custom gothic arch positioning plate. (**a**) Design data. (**b**) Print

After the first treatment, we made four blocking points on the maxillary positioning plate (Fig. 6.280) and then made CBCT images with the plate seated on the complete denture to obtain the relative position relationship between the jaw and positioning plate (Fig. 6.281). Next, we placed the maxillary guide on the maxillary denture and mandibular guide with tracing screw product on the mandibular ridges. Relining with bite silicone rubber is necessary if the tissue surface of the denture or the mandibular guide was not fit with alveolar ridge. Until the maxillary and mandibular guides were seated stably, we can describe the horizontal jaw position curve on the maxillary guide; due to that, there were no artificial teeth. After adjusting the height of tracing screw, we asked the patient to bite at CR position and do protrusive and lateral movements and recorded the coordinates of the CR position (Fig. 6.282).

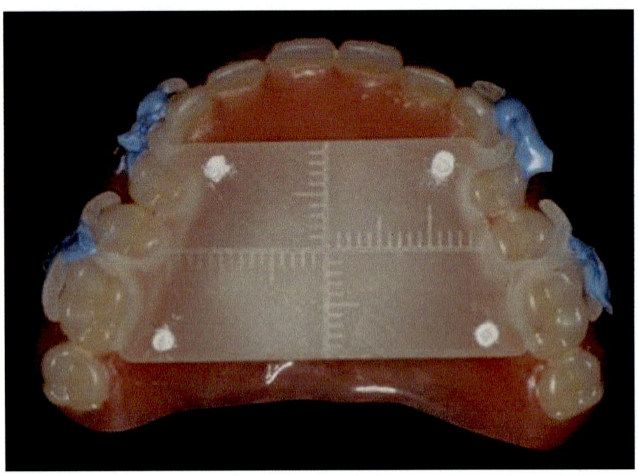

Fig. 6.280 Blocking points

Record the horizontal jaw position in the same way every 3 months in the first year (7–8 years old). When the coordinate deviation between two visits is large, complete denture should be fabricated again. The data recorded is two-dimensional.

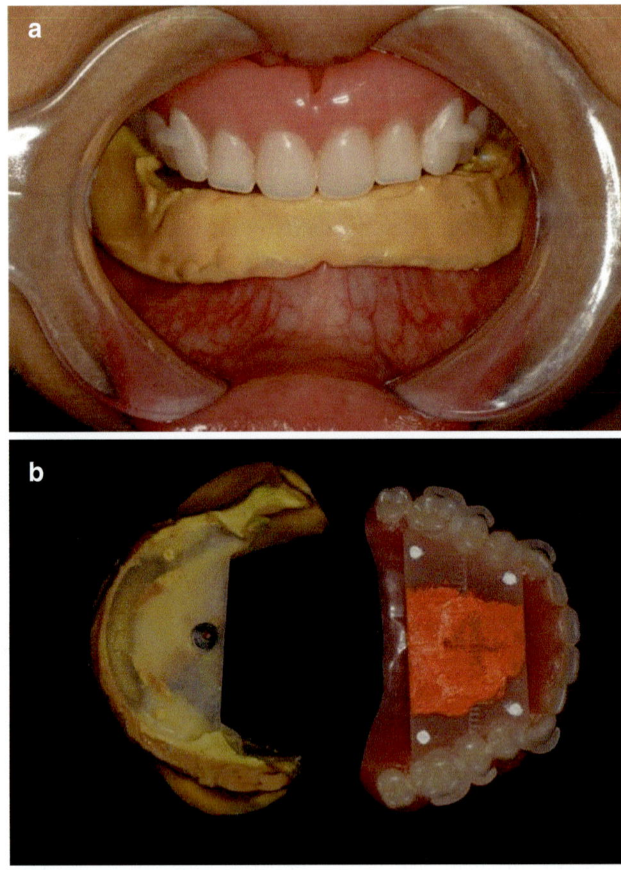

Fig. 6.282 Obtaining the relationship between horizontal jaw position. (**a**) Placed the custom gothic arch positioning plate. (**b**) The recorded relationship between horizontal jaw position

Fig. 6.281 Relative position relationship between the jaw and the positioning plate

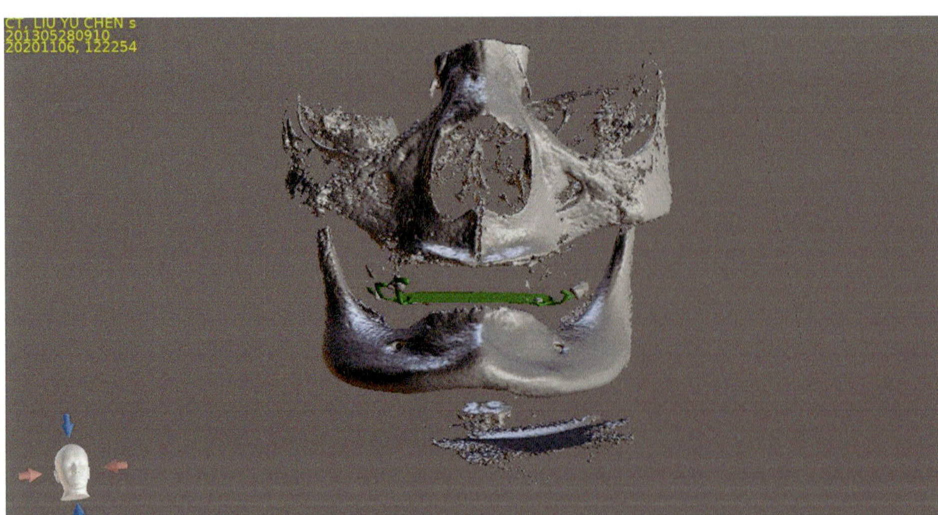

We make CBCT images with complete denture and maxillary positioning plate at return visit every year. Fit observation point data of the jaw were recorded every return visit through positioning plate to determine the change of the jaw. The data of the jaw and jaw position recorded is three-dimensional.

(b) Stage II: The first permanent prosthesis will be carried out with implant and removable treatment. According to the change trend of core indicators of observation points, implant will be placed at maxillary 13–14 and 23–24 teeth and mandibular 33–34 and 43–44 teeth in plan. Return visit every 3 months, and observe the data changes of observation points, and replace the denture periodically in accordance with specific conditions.

As mentioned at the beginning of this chapter, the remaining periodontal condition of patients with dentition defect in China is generally not good, the consciousness of patients' self-care is not strong, and the correct brushing and cleaning are difficult to be implemented in place. The basic treatment of dental pulp and periodontal is not in place, and other problems are common, which need to be looked at and solved urgently. Perfect basic treatment and scientific maintenance of health after restoration are the major premise of any successful restoration.

Dentists should remember that although RPD is suitable for almost all patients with dentition defects, the limitation of its curative effect is objective after all. According to the patients' complaints and the actual situation of the patients, the purpose of our repair is to improve the esthetics of the denture as much as possible on the basis of following the reasonable design, rather than pursuing the ultimate metal-free exposure for every case of clasp. And based on the three words of patient safety, "long-term, stable, and effective" are the pursuit of medical technology that we can never abandon.

References

1. Cochran DL. The scientific basis for and clinical experiences with Straumann implants including the ITI® Dental Implant System: a consensus report. J Clin Oral Implants Res. 2000;11(sl):33–58.
2. Stude S. A retrospective study of combined fixed-removable reconstructions with their analysis of failures. J Oral Rehab. 1998;25(7):513–26.
3. Vallittu PK, Kokkonen M. Deflection fatigue of a cobalt-chromium, titanium and gold alloy cast denture clasp. J Prosthet Dent. 1995;74(4):412–9.

Communication and Cooperation Between Clinicians and Technicians

7

Both clinician and technician play the most important roles in the whole treatment process of restoration, and their common goal is to provide prosthesis with beautiful appearance as well as functions to the patient.

To reach this goal, they are supposed to promote their cooperation except finishing their own tasks and responsibilities. Only when both of them realize that each other is a key partner in the treatment and it is significant to trust each other and maintain communication can the cases acquire satisfying treatment result.

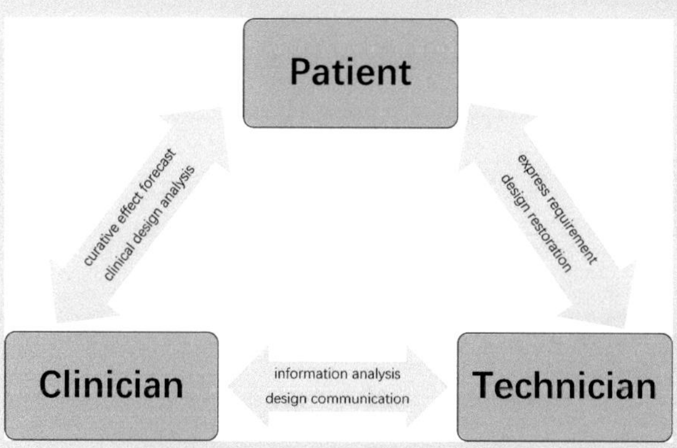

7.1 General Process of Clinician-Patient-Technician Communication

There are mainly three ways to increase the information capacity during communication: filling work authorization form, exchanging digital image data, and direct communication.

7.1.1 Fill Work Authorization Form

For there are a number of e-clasps, it's easy to get confused when filling the form, and sometimes it might cause misunderstanding. Undoubtedly, it would be easier if there is electronic form with pull-down options. However, design drawing sometimes is irreplaceable. The diagram below is work authorization form for e-clasp offered exclusively in this book. The front of it there is basic information of patient, smile exposed area, and framework design (Fig. 7.1).

On the back of the form, there is a diagram of 15 e-clasps introduced in this book (Fig. 7.2). It is simple and clear, easy to identify, and unique. Work authorization form is an important channel to increase the information capacity during communication between clinician and technician.

Example
Suppose a patient who missed A5, A6, B5, and B6, with A3 II°loose and B2 I°loose. Fill the form after analysis and design.

H. Yu, *Digital Removable Partial Denture Technology*, https://doi.org/10.1007/978-981-19-7923-1_7

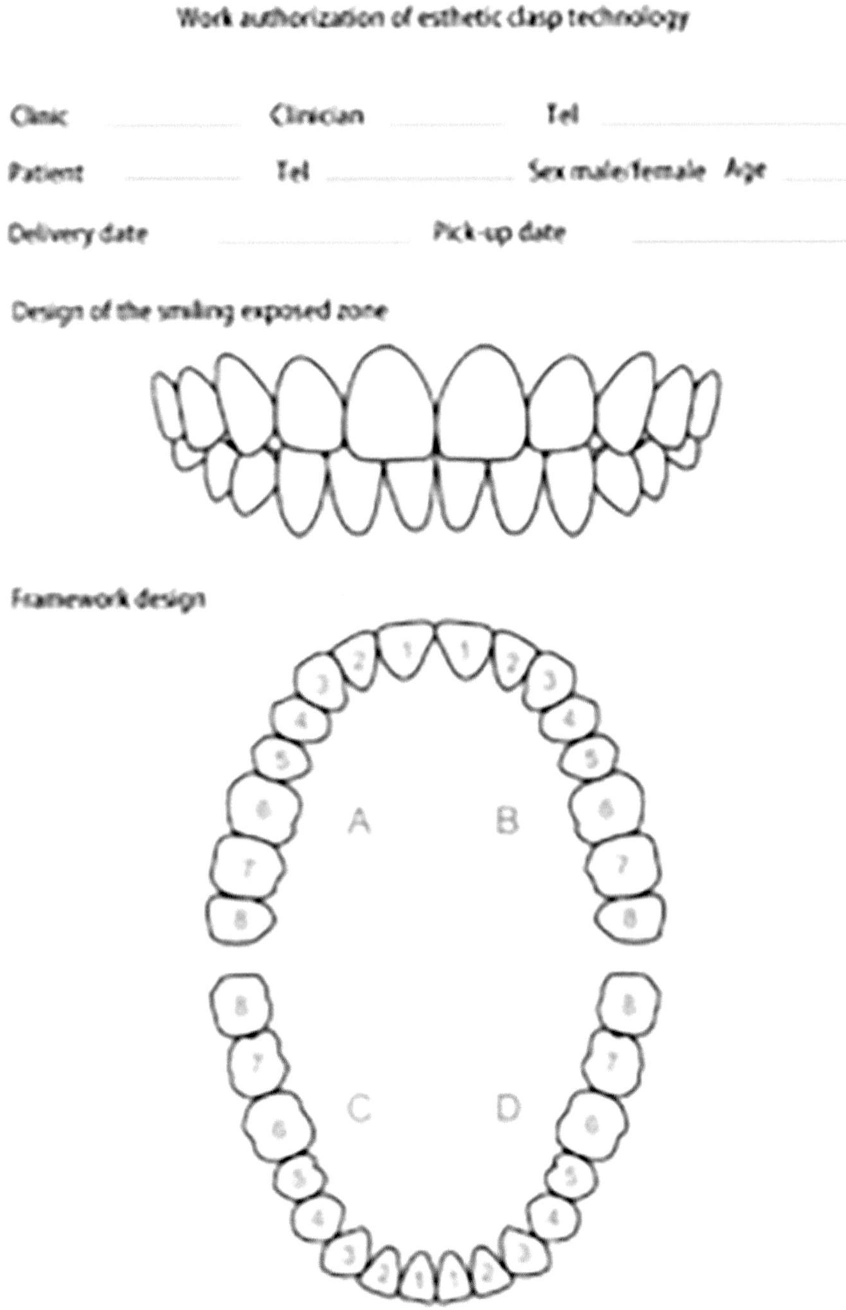
Work authorization of esthetic clasp technology

Clinic ________ Clinician ________ Tel ________

Patient ________ Tel ________ Sex male/female Age ________

Delivery date ________ Pick-up date ________

Design of the smiling exposed zone

Framework design

Fig. 7.1 Work authorization form for e-clasp (front)

Fig. 7.2 Work authorization form for e-clasp (back)

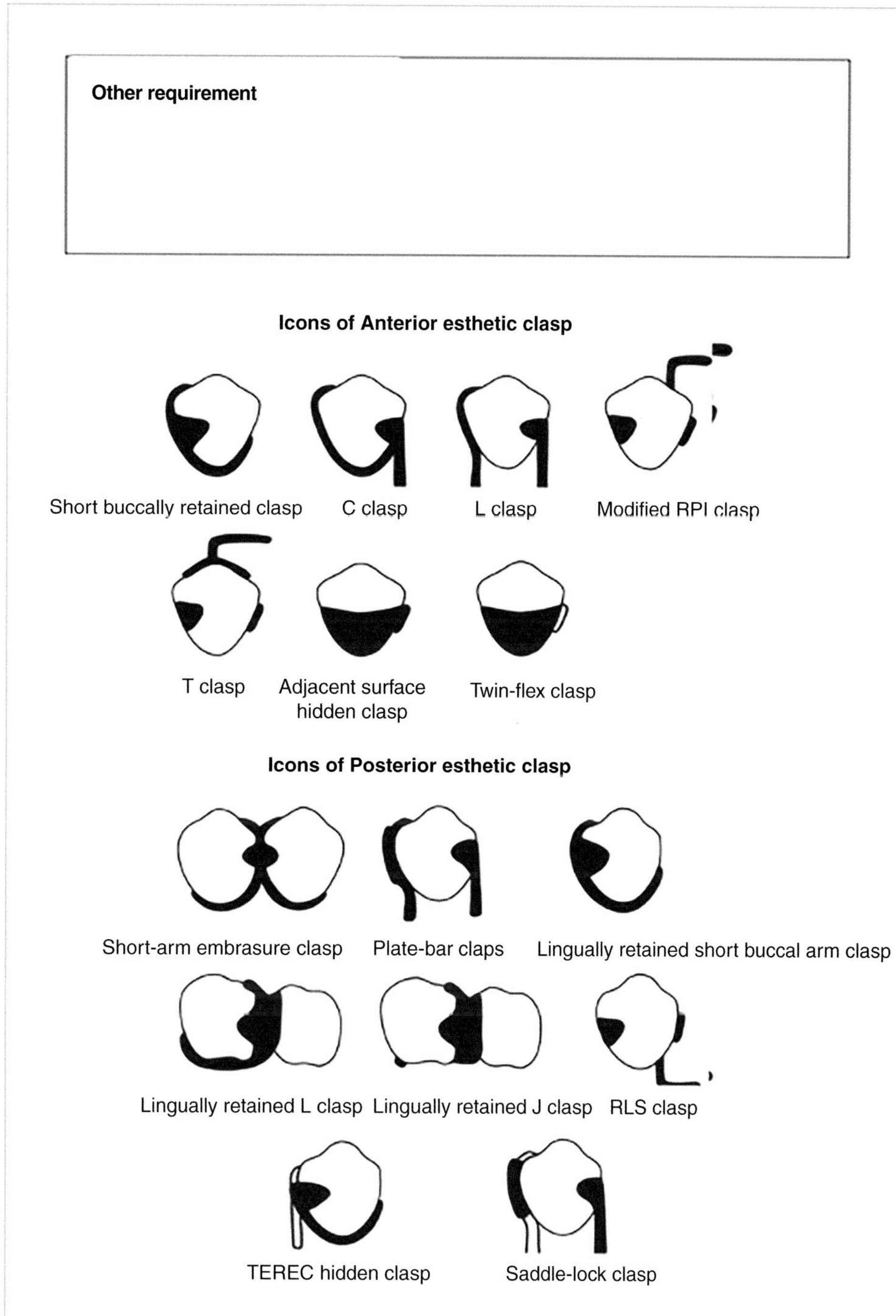

1. *Record the missing teeth* (Figs. 7.3 and 7.4).
2. *Record the agomphiasis* (Fig. 7.5).
3. *Describe the smiling exposed zone*. Through natural communications with patients, for example, asking about and recording their essential information, such as name and age, we can observe the exposed zone of the mouth when engaged in verbal activities, or we can observe the exposed zone in smile by letting the patient say “cheese” (Fig. 7.6).
4. *Design of smiling exposed zone*. According to the esthetic teeth showed by the smiling exposed zone, via comparing to the missing teeth, we decide the esthetic abutment. Then comparing the real oral exposure again, we decide the esthetic clasps and describe and simply label its name (Fig. 7.7).
5. *Design of non-esthetic area*. We don’t have to choose e-clasps here. We decide the abutment and describe and

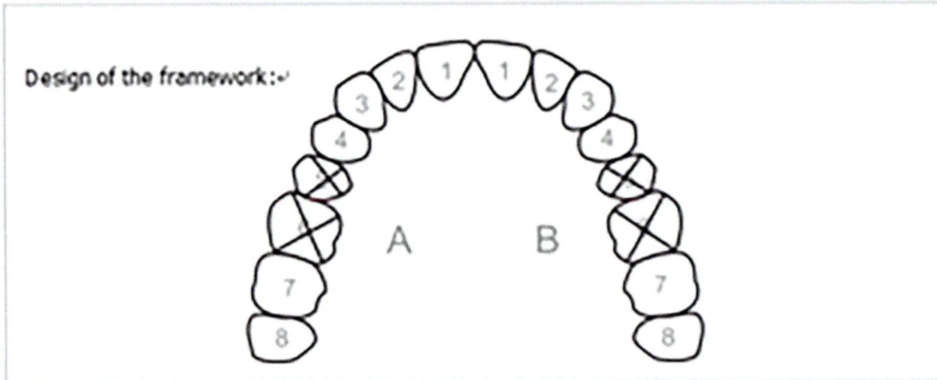

Fig. 7.3 Mark the missing teeth on the chart "Design of the framework"

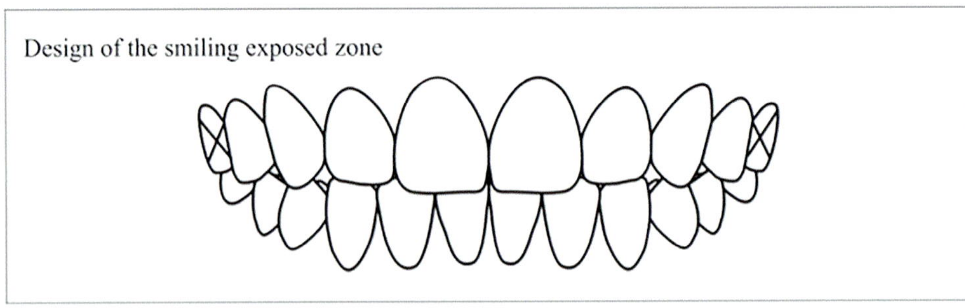

Fig. 7.4 Mark the missing teeth on the chart "Design of the exposed area in smile"

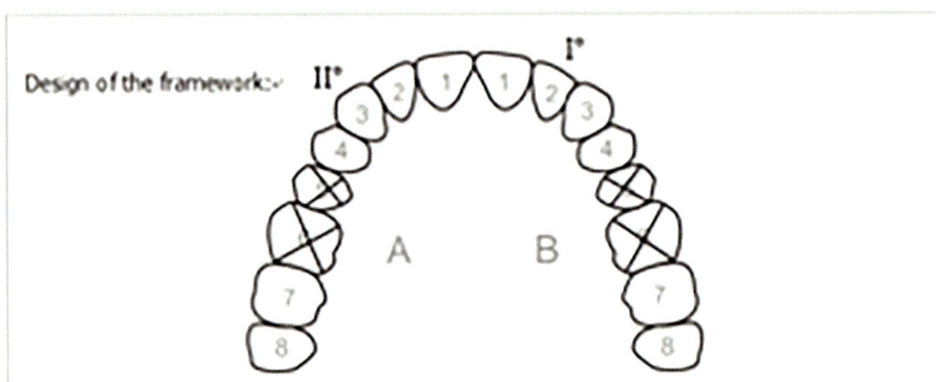

Fig. 7.5 Mark the agomphiasis and its mobility

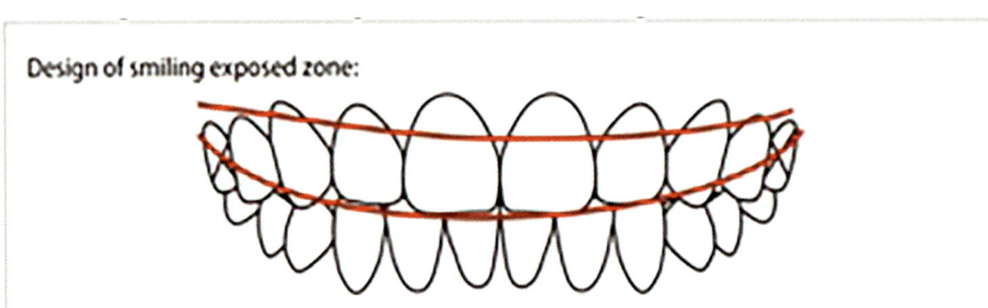

Fig. 7.6 Mark the exposed area in smile

simply label the name of clasps. Then we draw out other parts of the framework (Fig. 7.8).

6. *Other information*. If the patient would like to make an icing on the cake and laboratory conditions permit, we can authorize the technician to dye the artificial tooth. Specifically, the clinician does colorimetry in consulting room and recording the colorimetric message on the exposed area in smile (Fig. 7.9). The technician uses pho-

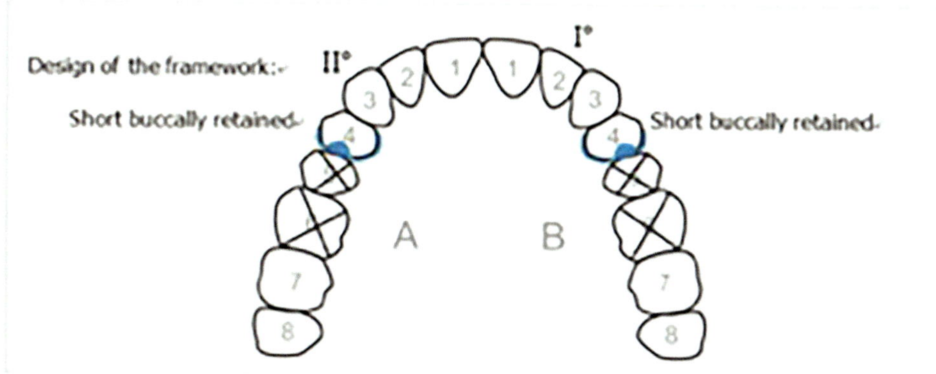

Fig. 7.7 Describe the esthetic clasps and simply label their name

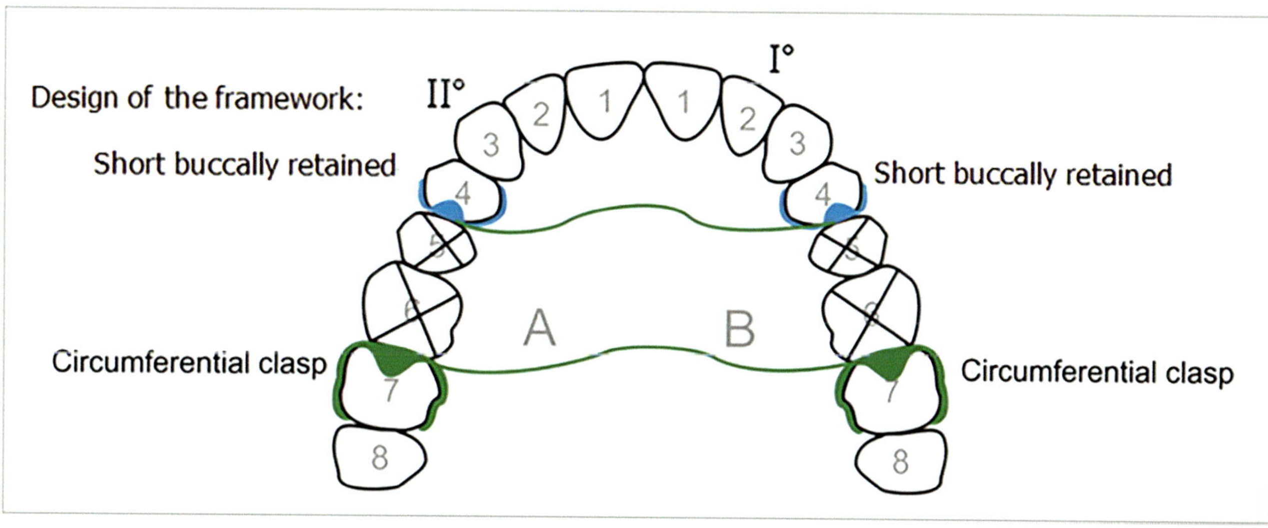

Fig. 7.8 Describe the traditional clasps and simply label their name

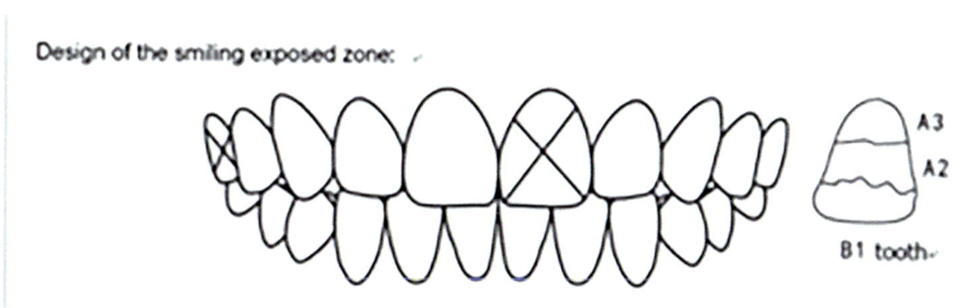

Fig. 7.9 Record the colorimetric message

tocurable resin to do personalized dyeing, according to the mark on the work authorization. Clinicians can record the colorimetric message on the blank of the chart "Design of smiling exposed zone."

7. *Accomplishing*. At this point, our work authorization is accomplished, in which the design of the exposed zone in smile is essential and is the important position reference for the wax pattern production of clasp (Fig. 7.10).

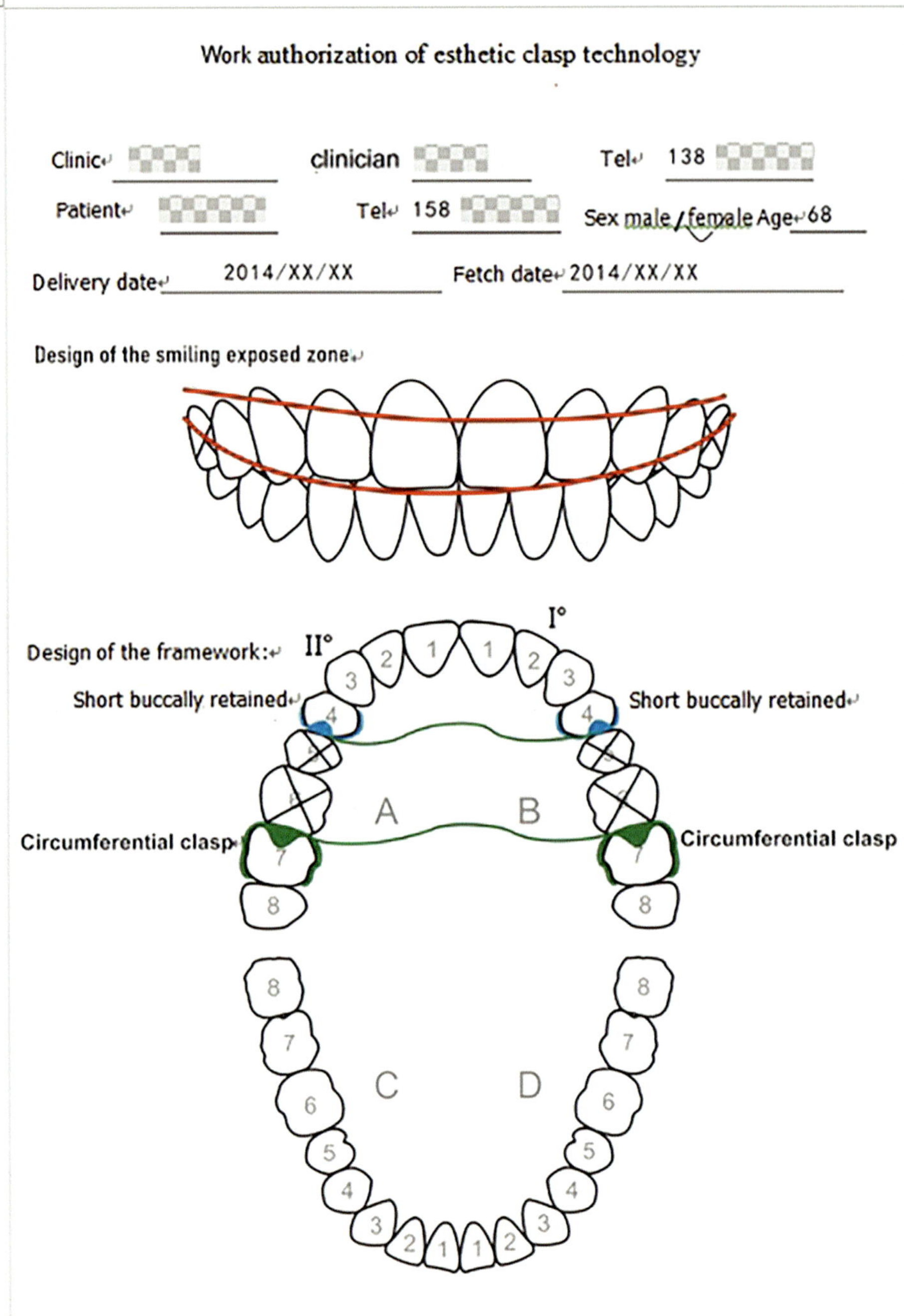
Work authorization of esthetic clasp technology

Clinic clinician Tel 138

Patient Tel 158 Sex male / female Age 68

Delivery date 2014/XX/XX Fetch date 2014/XX/XX

Design of the smiling exposed zone

Design of the framework: II° I°

Short buccally retained Short buccally retained

A B

Circumferential clasp Circumferential clasp

C D

Fig. 7.10 Accomplish the work authorization

7.1.2 Transfer Digital Image Data

After recording patient's image date by digital cameras in the consulting room (Fig. 7.11), clinicians can quickly transfer that to the technicians through the network to enrich communication information.

7.1.3 Communicate Directly

When technicians got the above information, clinicians and technicians can also communicate through telephone, interview face to face, and other ways to keep efficient communication. Clinicians and technicians are the most important two

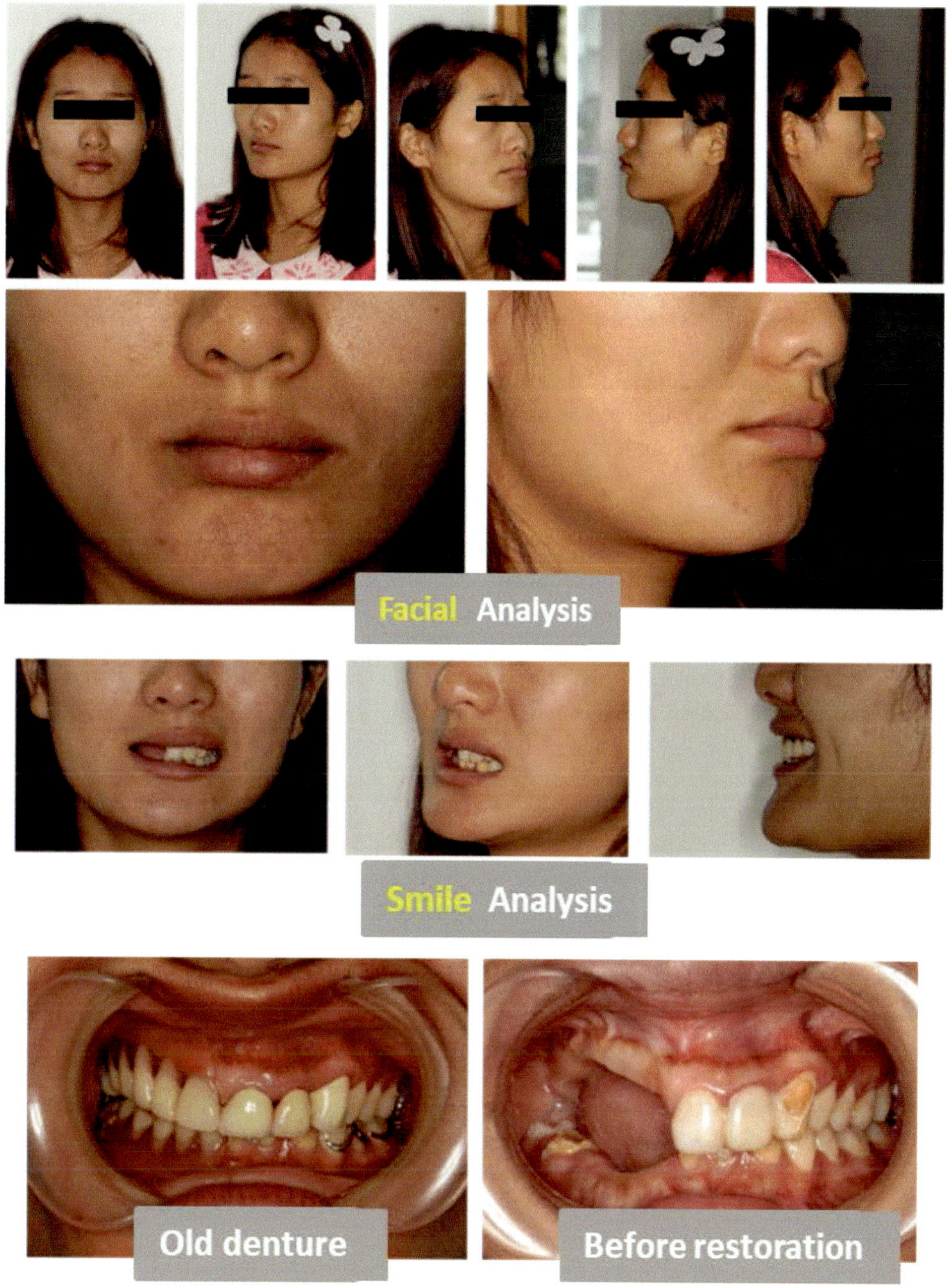

Fig. 7.11 Patient's image data

roles in the restoration of esthetic clasp. Only communicating effectively and trusting each other can they achieve the ultimate goal of satisfactory effect.

7.2 The Necessity of Digitalization in Clinician-Patient-Technician Communication and Cooperation

With the establishment of new medical model and clinician-patient relationship, clinicians are required to have good communication skills, learn to listen to patients' chief complaints, and pay attention to the way of language communication. Through good communication with patients, clinicians should respect their rights, gain their trust, help them establish the final achievable goals, and correct some unrealistic expectations in the meantime.

Along with the progress of society and science and technology, digital diagnosis and treatment and processing technology are becoming increasingly important in the field of stomatology. On one hand, digital technology shows its characteristics and superiorities in oral scanning, design, and production. On the other hand, it highlights a series of advantages such as convenience, accuracy, efficient, and unambiguous transmission of digital technology in clinician-patient-technician communication and cooperation.

7.2.1 The Basic Meaning of Digital Clinician-Patient-Technician Communication and Cooperation

The so-called digital clinician-patient-technician communication and cooperation mainly refers to using a series of digital technology and equipment (involving photography technology, scanning technology, multimedia technology, electronic colorimeter, oral and facial scanning system, digital analysis and design, digital production, and so on) to transform patient-related oral and maxillofacial information into digital information form for preservation, analysis, design, transmission, production, processing, etc. It ensures the accuracy and completeness of relevant information and is conducive to save storage space and materials, quickly search and trace information, facilitate clinician-patient-technician communication and discussion, and establish a database to facilitate the big data analysis and promote medical progress. Due to the complex form of dentition defect and the different health status of alveolar ridge and oral remaining teeth, the design and manufacture of denture is very complicated, which requires good and effective communication and exchange among clinicians, patients, and technicians, and makes use of digital technology and equipment for close cooperation to attain good final prosthetic effect.

7.2.2 The Necessity of Digitalization in Clinician-Patient-Technician Communication and Cooperation

1. *Meeting the needs of the development trend of digital oral diagnosis and treatment and manufacturing technology*

   With the rapid development of digital diagnosis and treatment technology and manufacturing and processing technology, as well as the promotion of national policies, the popularization of digital technology is bound to be the future development trend of the medical field. Using digital technology can support, improve, and promote the quality and efficiency of the entire medical system, facilitate patients to seek medical treatment, and improve patients' satisfaction.

   The traditional paper medical records is replaced by electronic ones, which benefits to the classification, preservation, and query of information. Digital impressions and models are also convenient to store and transmit. Digital colorimetry makes colorimetric results more accurate and intuitional. Digital design and analysis improve clinician-patient-technician communication, so that patients have the right to choose and know in advance.
2. *The need for the development of efficient and accurate medical care*

   With the popularization and application of digital technology, hospitals, clinics, and denture factories all over the world are able to communicate anytime and anywhere. Patients' requirements for the treatment process and prosthetic effect are getting higher and higher, which not only promotes the development and application of digital technology but also meets the needs of patients. The chairside dental technician can assist clinicians in data and information collection, digital analysis, computer-aided design, and computer-aided production.

   Efficient and accurate medical treatment requires both clinicians and technicians to supervise and manage the processes of denture analysis and design, tooth preparation, mold taking, occlusal and jaw position relationship recording, etc. Moreover, feedback problems to clinicians and patients in time put forward suggestions on the revision of production. For patients who require individuation or have special requirements, it's imperative to fully understand their gender, age, skin color, occupation, etc., conduct personalized colorimetry and tooth arrangement, and digitally obtain the patient's oral and maxillofacial information. In particular, the concept of esthetic restoration requires that dentures not only have masticatory function but also have to be beautiful and comfortable to meet the needs of patients. Therefore, we need the digital design and production to make the restoration system more accurate and more in line with clinical requirements while to save time and procedures; avoid communication obstacles among clinicians, patients, and technicians; and improve the accuracy of restoration and the efficiency of diagnosis and treatment.
3. *The need for clinician-patient-technician communication*

   There are common problems in the traditional production process, such as incomplete filling of processing design forms, poor quality of models or impressions, etc., resulting in technicians not well understanding the design intention of clinicians and the needs of patients. Digital technology can provide a good platform for communication and exchange between clinicians and technicians, which is able to completely deliver the patients' information and needs to technicians and clearly express the clinicians' design requirements. With the progress of society, patients' demand for restoration is getting higher and higher, and more personalized needs are highlighted, which also requires clinicians and technicians to carry out personalized analysis and design of patients; good communication and cooperation are needed among the three sides to achieve the final satisfactory results.

During the clinicians' operation, it is difficult to express clearly and simply to patients in words. Therefore, digital or multimedia technology can be a better choice to vividly show the steps and process of treatment, so that patients can be more at ease with treatment. This form of digital and multimedia technology has more advantages for low-level education or elderly patients. For the digital information and the process of digital analysis and design could be presented to patients, patients can fully understand the prosthetic effect and timely put forward suggestions for modification for full communication and exchange, in order to achieve satisfactory prosthetic effect.

Moreover, the mode of digital telemedicine can also provide diagnosis and treatment for patients who are inconvenient to come to the hospital, achieve good communication results, and improve the medical level in remote areas and townships. With the progress and development of dental technology, patients have proposed higher requirements for the quality and effect of oral restoration, from the traditional simple treatment of diseases to now paying attention to esthetic and esthetic effects. There are higher requirements for the shape, arrangement, and color of teeth, which urges a more clear and accurate communication between clinicians and patients in turn. Digital technology can not only well reappear patient information, analyze the designed restoration, and provide patients with prediction of prosthetic effect but also assist clinician-patient communication, transmit medical knowledge and information, deepen patient understanding, and improve patient satisfaction.

The three sides are able to communicate through network digital means such as telephone, video, e-mail, and so on, for example, using colorimeter in clinic to get colorimetric data which can be sent directly to the technician to create a lifelike restoration, using the intraoral scanner to obtain the oral information of the patient without making an impression, and using computer-aided design and computer-aided manufacturing technology to make model. Then, the technician can produce a restoration on the model without model transmission, avoiding deformation and damage of the model. Since good communication is an essential condition to ensure the quality and effect of restoration, clinicians, patients, and technicians should fully communicate with each other and find and solve problems with a scientific attitude, so as to improve the satisfaction of patients and the effect of restoration.

7.3 The Application of Digitalization in Clinician-Patient-Technician Communication and Cooperation

Digitalization has gradually penetrated into all aspects of the medical process, from electronic medical records at the initial stage of medical treatment to digital analysis and to the final production and design of digital models. The digital technology runs through the whole process and is conducive to good communication and cooperation among clinicians, patients, and technicians. The following digital technologies all benefit to that in the treatment process, improve the satisfaction of medical treatment, and avoid the rework rate and clinician-patient disputes.

1. *Multimedia technology* (Fig. 7.12): Multimedia video animation or photos can be used to show the treatment process to patients and communicate well with patients to avoid disputes and contradictions in the treatment process.

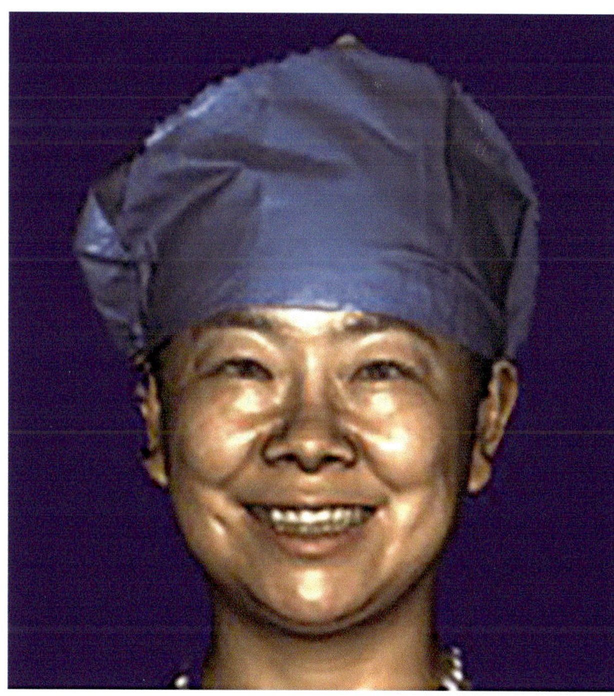

Fig. 7.12 Facial scanning

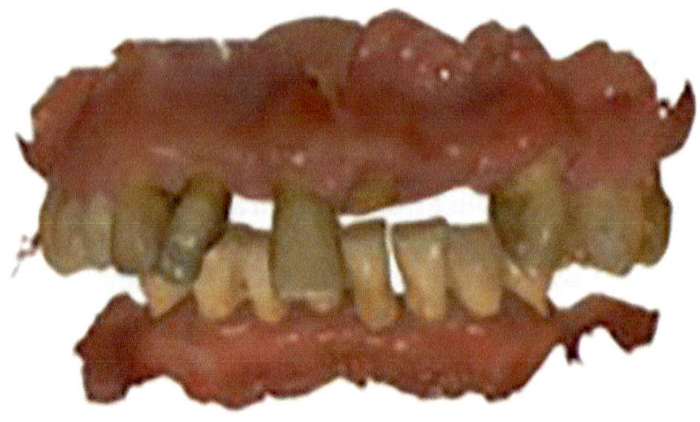

Fig. 7.13 Digital impression

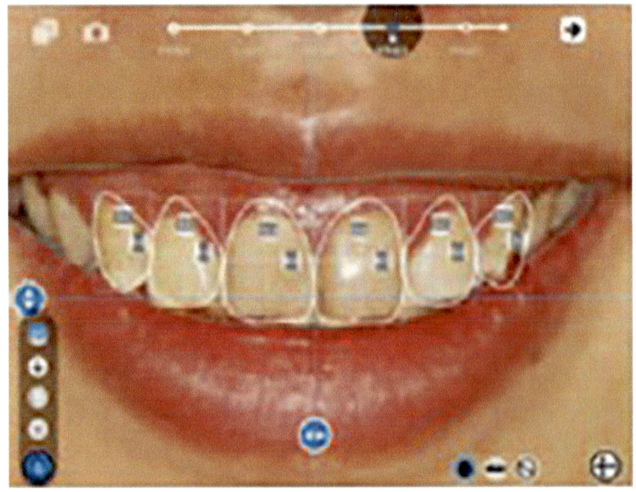

Fig. 7.14 Operating interface of Beauty Tooth Assistant

2. *Electronic medical records*: It can completely reflect all the diagnosis and treatment information of patients, so that clinicians can make a reasonable diagnosis and treatment plan according to their health status.
3. *Digital impression* (Fig. 7.13): It can clearly reappear the oral and maxillofacial conditions of the patients, so that the patients have a clearer understanding of their oral conditions. Then the clinicians need to explain the oral conditions to the patients in order to make them conceive a reasonable expectation for the prosthetic effect.
4. *Digital colorimetry*: Use the digital colorimeter to directly conduct colorimetry of natural teeth, on the precondition that eliminating the interference of objective and subjective factors in order to improve the accuracy of colorimetry. Meanwhile, show the expected restoration color to patients.
5. *Digital analysis and design*: Using digital analysis and prediction software to provide patients with visual foresight of postoperative effects, which can also provide clinicians with more treatment choice. By loading the oral and maxillofacial photos of the patients and referring to the anatomical characteristics, carry out the digital line surface analysis and design, which is convenient for the communication between clinicians and patients. The three sides can discuss and communicate the design effect, determine the final satisfactory repair effect and the best treatment plan, and improve the satisfaction of prosthetic effect. The commonly used digital line surface analysis and design software are Beauty Tooth Assistant (Fig. 7.14), Smile Designer Pro, Digital Smile System, Photoshop, Keynote, PowerPoint, etc.

   Preview steps for esthetic design analysis using digital techniques and methods (Fig. 7.15).
6. *Digital image data*: It is convenient for clinicians to conduct research and analysis; facilitate the communication between clinicians, patients, and technicians; complete transmission of esthetic information; improve the repair effect; and avoid clinician-patient disputes to a certain extent.
7. *Digital occlusal analyzer*: It detects the occlusal distribution, the occlusal balance, the distribution of bite force, etc., comprehensively and systematically analyzes the patient's occlusal status, and accurately guides clinicians and technicians to design and process the prosthesis.

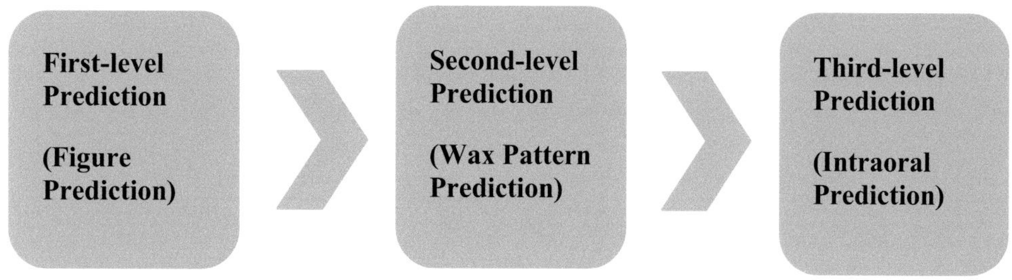

Fig. 7.15 Esthetic repair prediction process

7.4 The Prospect of Digitalization in Clinician-Patient-Technician Communication and Cooperation

To sum up, good communication among clinicians, patients, and technicians is the basis of our clinical work. In clinical operation, clinicians should think of the patients and take their safety as the purpose and as far as possible to reduce the damage to them. Clinicians and technicians should respect and cooperate with each other and maintain timely communication. Additionally, proactive perspective-taking creates a harmonious relationship between the three sides to provide better medical services for patients, finally successfully realizes the desire of patients' chief complaint, and reduces the occurrence of clinician-patient disputes and clinician-technician disputes.

Digital technology combines a series of high and new technologies, such as electronic information technology, material manufacturing technology, and multimedia technology, which has brought great changes to the development of stomatology. Different digital technologies are applied in all fields and stages of stomatology, which improves the production accuracy, saves resources and time, facilitates the preservation and transmission of information, and effectively avoids the disputes between clinicians, patients, and technicians.

Undeniably, digitization will bring greater revolution and development in the future. Using virtual reality technology including VR and AR can be helpful to achieve the further clinician-patient-technician communication and cooperation. VR (virtual reality) uses computer simulation to create a virtual world in three-dimensional space, providing users with sensory simulations such as vision, hearing, and touch, as if they were in the real world. AR (augmented reality) increases the perception of the real world through the information provided by the computer system and overlays the virtual objects, scenes, or system prompts generated by the computer into the real scene, showing the scene that can't be realized in the real world, so as to achieve the "enhancement" of reality and achieve a sensory experience beyond reality. From the above, this technology can be used in the future to predict the prosthesis and prostheses effect before the actual operation, to simulate the patient's face shape and smile after wearing a denture, and so on.

With the development and deepening of digital technology, networking, effect analysis prediction, four-dimensional technology, VR/AR technology, and chairside system will be popularized to facilitate more intuitive communication and exchange among clinician, patient, and technician. It will also lead to a new model for clinician-patient-technician communication and cooperation and further improve medical quality and patient satisfaction. Nowadays, digital technology has brought a new development direction for dental clinical and restoration production, and it will soon enter the all-digital era of high-efficiency and low-energy consumption in the near future!

Conclusion

Throughout the history of dentition defect restoration, removable partial denture (RPD) restoration technology has always been one of the important means of dentition defect restoration. More than 90 years ago, normalized RPD appeared in the modern sense, and the casting method was used to make RPD framework. Implant-supported RPD-combined restoration was adopted 40 years ago; 35 years ago, the design expert system of RPD was established. Framework was made with resin wax produced by 3D printing technology and casting technology 16 years ago; 14 years ago, selective laser melting made direct printing of metal supports possible. With the rapid development of digital technology, the application of various high and new digital technologies, like computer-aided design and computer-aided manufacture, has directly changed the subject basis of prosthodontics and of course brought new theoretical thinking.

In the face of dentition defect RPDS design, today, we can use almost all of the latest technology to restoration the known, such as implant-supported RPD, fixed-removable prostheses, the digitized segmented RPD, integration of PEEK or PEKK RPD, or implant surgery guide and tooth preparation guide for dentition defect, the principle of retention and stability support is derived from the design principle of RPD, fragmented digital restoration cannot effectively support the integration ability and demand of digital restoration, while the digital RPD is the best entry point for integrated or comprehensive restoration technology. On the one hand, it is because the effectiveness of traditional RPD is in urgent need of improvement, and although "hanging without dying," it has been ignored for a long time. Secondly, digitalization provides an integrated platform and historical opportunity for various new restoration technologies, which can effectively improve or solve various problems of RPD, making it an integrated restoration solution more acceptable to Chinese patients. At present, all kinds of classical restoration technologies have both advantages and disadvantages. Digital restoration technology provides new solutions, possibilities, and innovations for integrated restoration, so that all kinds of classical restoration technologies can give full play to their strengths and achieve the ultimate goal of "long-term, stable, and effective." From the perspective of clinical practice, guided prosthodontics is the embodiment of digital prosthodontics.

The underlying work we need to do now is the "revolution" of the discipline foundation for the future digital restoration. In view of the advantages of digital RPD, it is not comprehensive to say that RPD is "widely applicable." More accurately, it is theoretically suitable for all dental defects. "Cheap" is no longer the label for digital RPD. "Easy to get and wear" is clearly a weakness or a "feature," but it can never be an "advantage." Therefore, the biggest advantage of digital RPD should be "minimally invasive and reversible" and the "integration" of various high and new restoration technologies. On the other hand, the application of new digital composite materials, esthetic clasp and simulation base technology, etc. can greatly improve the esthetics of RPD, so the biggest disadvantages of RPD at present are insufficient functional recovery and poor comfort. It is worth noting that under the general background of integrated prosthodontics, high and new prosthodontics such as implant and esthetics are inseparable from the clinical design principles contained in classic restorative methods such as removable restoration and overdenture restoration.

The integrated application of digital technology in the field of RPD has given a new life of RPD. From taking impression to the design and precision machining production of restoration, constantly optimize the digital operation, reduce the cost of digital, from experience to digital, from artificial to intelligence, from man-made slow work to automatic production, from personal operation to network AI expert system to assist decision-making, known or unknown future of all kinds of advanced digital technology will continue to bring new content for digital RPD, constantly enrich and integrated type new scheme of prosthodontics.

Therefore, the digital RPD technology interpreted in this book combines various digital technologies, adopts innovative clasp design and digital new material application, and

H. Yu, *Digital Removable Partial Denture Technology*, https://doi.org/10.1007/978-981-19-7923-1

shows the new connotation of integrated prosthodontics, take "long-term, stable and efficient" as the goal, realized the low burden of disease and curative effect of high quality to two or more things, balance esthetics and function. It is a minimally invasive repair technology to improve the quality, efficacy, and efficiency of RPD. Also, it is the cognitive basis for further learning esthetic restoration and implant restoration, solid understanding of its related basic principles and clinical diagnosis and treatment scheme design, and standardizing clinical operation.

MIX
Papier aus verantwortungsvollen Quellen
Paper from responsible sources
FSC® C105338

If you have any concerns about our products,
you can contact us on
ProductSafety@springernature.com

In case Publisher is established outside the EU,
the EU authorized representative is:
Springer Nature Customer Service Center GmbH
Europaplatz 3, 69115 Heidelberg, Germany

Printed by Libri Plureos GmbH
in Hamburg, Germany